pReface

What sort of book is available to the surgeon early in his career that will extend his basic knowledge of anatomy and aid him as he is about to undertake a particular procedure? Works on surgical technique are much to the purpose, but generally more than one technique is available. Availability of several techniques, and opportunity to choose among them, is undoubtedly helpful to the experienced surgeon but may be confusing to the beginner. More basic than technical expertise, however, is the necessity of knowing precisely what physical change is to be accomplished, what structures are available for the procedure, what anomalies may be encountered, and what and where the structures are that must be identified or avoided. If the surgeon knows all this he is not only enabled to do a proper job, but is in a position to modify his technique to the situation, and even to develop original procedures of his own. This was the philosophy underlying our undertaking of a work on operative anatomy. This volume continues the effort begun with the presentation of Operative Anatomy of Thorax.

In order to present the anatomy pertinent to operations it is necessary in some instances to state briefly the aims of a procedure and the divergent methods used to achieve the desired results. The mode of presentation is to a great extent pictorial, through illustrations of anatomical dissections or by drawings of surgical procedures. Of necessity this involves some consideration of technique, but our primary concern is not with the maneuvers but with the structures involved. We have not attempted to portray pathologic conditions, except for some congenital anomalies, nor to present the range of the most current or preferred operations in each region. Rather we have attempted to choose procedures which best display the anatomy of each part or cast new light on areas perhaps inadequately considered elsewhere.

The depiction of a procedure does not necessarily mean its advocacy.

Again we are deeply grateful to authors and publishers who have allowed the use of published illustrations of evident precision and elegance.

We thank our colleagues of all ages for their stimulation and suggestions. Dr. George Musser, now of Denver, when a student made several of the preparations for the section on the liver. Dr. Paul H. Sugarbaker supplied the description of colonoscopy and the photographs obtained by that technique.

Several, both in Boston and elsewhere, have reviewed parts of the manuscript. We are particularly indebted to Dr. John E. Healy, Jr., of Houston, and Dr. William R. Waddell, of Denver, for their reviews of the section on the liver and the portal and biliary systems. We are indebted to Dr. Donald Goldstein, of the Peter Bent Brigham Hospital, for his help with the section on the female pelvis and perineum, and to Drs. J. Hartwell Harrison and Alan H. Bennett for their suggestions on the suprarenal glands and the urinary and male genital organs. Dr. Russell T. Woodburne, of Ann Arbor, responded to our queries with helpful and encouraging correspondence on matters regarding the bladder, as did Dr. William H. Boyce, of Winston-Salem, on matters concerning the kidney. Dr. Richard A. Norton, of Boston, generously discussed the variations of the pancreatic ducts, demonstrating the results of his endoscopic studies.

We continue to be grateful to Dr. Don W. Fawcett for continuing to place the facilities of the Department of Anatomy at our disposal, and to Dr. Francis D. Moore of the Department of Surgery, for his help and encouragement.

EDWARD A. EDWARDS
PAUL D. MALONE
JOHN D. MACARTHUR

Boston, Massachusetts

operative anatomy
of
abdomen and pelvis

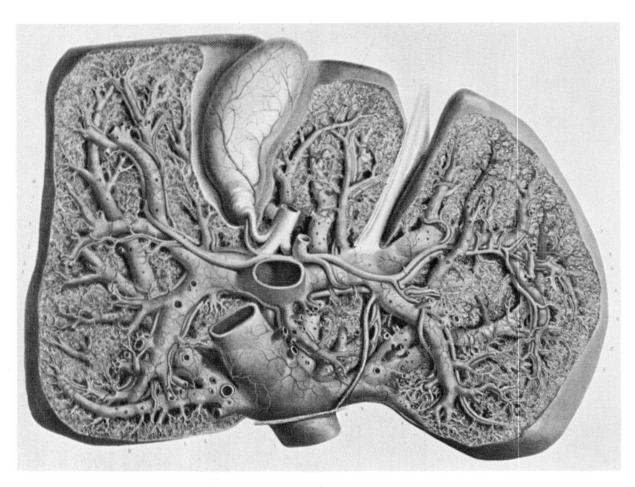

Hepatic distribution of blood vessels and ducts. (From Bourgery, J. M., and Jacob, N. H.: Traité complet de l'anatomie de l'homme, vol. 5. Paris, Librairie Anatomique, 1839.)

Edward A. Edwards, M.D.

Surgeon Emeritus, Peter Bent Brigham Hospital. Clinical Professor of Anatomy Emeritus, Harvard Medical School.

Paul D. Malone, A.B.

Director of Medical Illustration, Lahey Clinic Foundation. Member, Association of Medical Illustrators.

John D. MacArthur, M.D.

Surgeon in Chief, Cardinal Cushing Hospital, Brockton, Massachusetts. Assistant Clinical Professor of Surgery, Harvard Medical School, Lecturer in Surgery, Tufts University Medical School.

OPERATIVE ANATOMY
of
abdomen and pelvis

Lea & Febiger • Philadelphia
1975

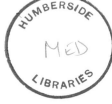
Library of Congress Cataloging in Publication Data

Edwards, Edward Allen, 1906–
     Operative anatomy of abdomen and pelvis.

     1. Abdomen—Surgery. 2. Pelvis—Surgery. 3. Anatomy, Surgical and topo-
graphical. I. Malone, Paul D., joint author. II. MacArthur, John D., joint author.
III. Title. [DNLM: 1. Abdomen—Anatomy and histology. 2. Abdomen—Surgery.
3. Pelvis—Anatomy and histology. 4. Pelvis—Surgery. WI900 E26o]
RD540.E35 1975   617'.55   74-23199
ISBN 0-8121-0491-9

Published in Great Britain by Henry Kimpton Publishers, London

Printed in the United States of America

CONTENTS

SECTION 1
THE Abdominal Wall and Peritoneum

SECTION 2

Major Vessels, Lymphatics, and Autonomic Nerves

SECTION 3

Stomach, Duodenum, Pancreas, Spleen

SECTION 4

The Liver; Biliary and Portal Systems

SECTION 5

The Bowel

SECTION 6

SUPRARENAl GlANds; URiNARY ANd MALE GENiTAL ORGANS

SECTION 7

FEMALE PELVIS AND PERINEUM

illustrations

SECTION 1
The Abdominal Wall and Peritoneum

SECTION 2

MAJOR VESSELS, LYMPHATICS, AND AUTONOMIC NERVES

SECTION 3

STOMACH, DUODENUM, PANCREAS, SPLEEN

SECTION 4

The Liver; Biliary and Portal Systems

SECTION 5
The Bowel

SECTION 6

Suprarenal Glands; Urinary and Male Genital Organs

SECTION 7

FEMALE PELVIS AND PERINEUM

SECTION 1
The Abdominal Wall and Peritoneum

1

THE AbdomiNAL WALL; SURGICAL APPROACHES

MUSCLES AND FASCIAS

The structure of this part of the body wall is of special interest (Fig. 1) because its incision affords entrance to the abdomen and access to the abdominal organs.

A continuous sac of the endoabdominal or transversalis fascia lines the osseous and muscular confines of the abdominal cavity. As traced in longitudinal and cross sections (Fig. 2), the fascia may be subdivided according to location into transversalis fascia beneath the anterolateral wall; the inferior capsule of the respiratory diaphragm above; the psoas, or prevertebral, fascia over the psoas muscle and the anterior lamella of the lumbodorsal fascia over the quadratus lumborum muscle posteriorly; and the parietal pelvic fascia on the pelvic diaphragm below.

The peritoneal sac lies within the endoabdominal fascia in close contact with the fascia anteriorly, but separated from the fascia posteriorly by the retroperitoneal fat and organs. In Figure 3 the renal fascia (fascia of Gerota) is seen as a separate sac lying within the retroperitoneum, enclosing the kidney, ureter, and gonadal vessels, closed above but having some continuity with the vesical fascia below. The retroperi-

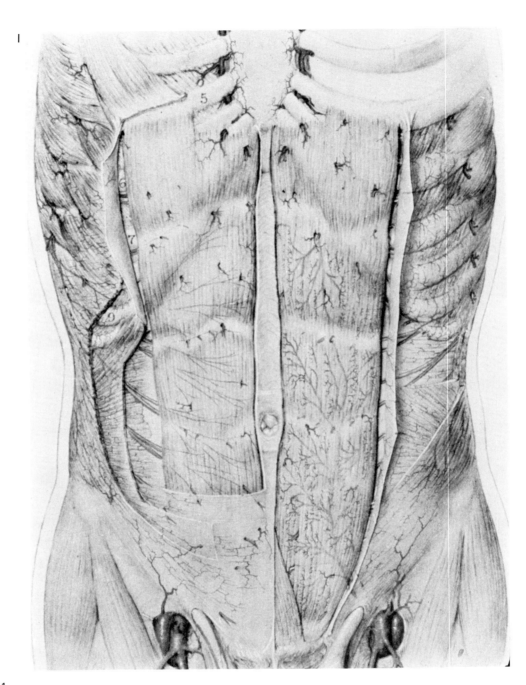

FIG. 1

The anterolateral abdominal musculature, nerves, and vessels.

I. Displayed from without. Note the rectus abdominis muscles with four tendinous intersections where the anterior sheath must be separated by sharp dissection. The left pyramidalis muscle is exposed. The transverse and oblique muscles are shown, all three aponeuroses joining to form the anterior rectus sheath in the lower abdomen. The nerves and vessels pass between the internal oblique and transversus abdominis muscles to reach the rectus muscles and overlying skin. The 10th intercostal nerve reaches the umbilicus.

II

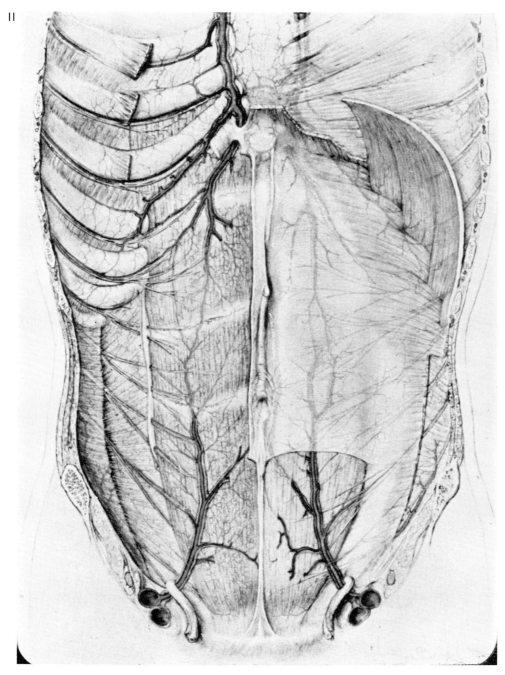

FIG. 1

The anterolateral abdominal musculature, nerves, and vessels (continued).

II. Displayed from within. The transversalis fascia has been removed. The ligamentum teres extends from the umbilicus upward; the median umbilical, or urachal, ligament extends downward. The posterior rectus sheath is intact on the right, its deepest stratum extending from the transversus abdominis, which is shown interdigitating with the costal origins of the diaphragm. The posterior sheath ends abruptly at the linea semicircularis. Below this line the rectus muscle is bare, and the inferior epigastric vessels lie upon it. At their origin these vessels lie medial to the turning of the spermatic cord at the internal abdominal ring. The inferior epigastric vessels are shown communicating with the superior epigastric and the intercostal. The superior epigastric artery is generally smaller than the inferior and is usually embedded within the substance of the rectus muscle. The course of the nerves through the rectus sheath and muscle is well shown on the left. (From Lesions of the rectus abdominis muscle simulating an acute intra-abdominal condition, Cullen, T. S., and Brödel, M., Bulletin of the Johns Hopkins Hospital, Vol. 61, pp. 295–316, 1937. ⓒ The Johns Hopkins University Press.)

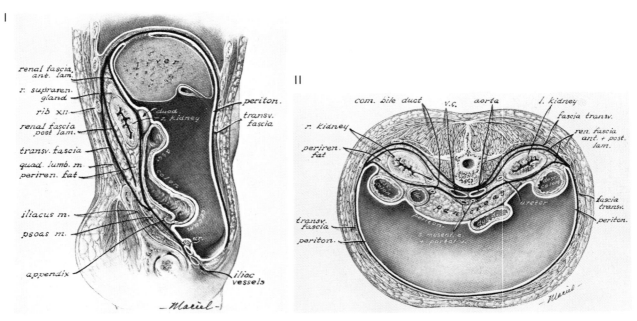

FIG. 2
Fascial and peritoneal relationships in the abdominal cavity. I. In right parasagittal section. II. In cross section. (From Altemeier and Alexander, Arch. Surg. 83:512–524, 1961. Copyright 1961, American Medical Association.)

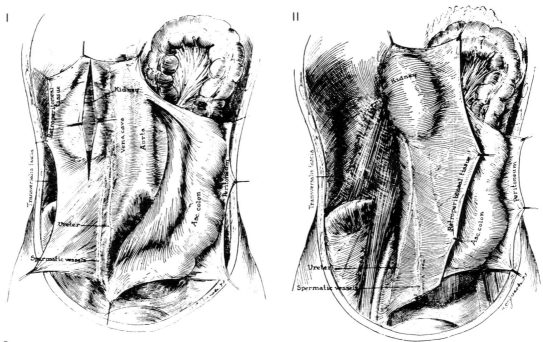

FIG. 3
The renal fascia: Its relationship (I) to the mesenteries, and (II) to the endoabdominal (transversalis) fascia. (From Tobin, 1944.)

toneal fat behind the renal fascia is the pararenal fat; that within the renal fascia is the perirenal fat. At its closed end above the kidney, the renal fascia has a somewhat tenuous connection with the connective tissue about the suprarenal gland. When the embryonic ascent of the kidney is arrested, as in iliac kidney, the suprarenal gland lies at its usual level and the renal fascia has no connection with it. The spaces within the renal fascia of each side are often continuous across the aorta, accounting for instances of crossed prolapse.

EXTRAPERITONEAL ABSCESSES

Abscesses lying outside of the peritoneal cavity may be classified according to location as anterior extraperitoneal; posterior retroperitoneal, or perinephric; retrofascial, or psoas; and pelvic extraperitoneal.

Anterior extraperitoneal abscesses point anteriorly between the peritoneum and the transversalis fascia. Their origin is overwhelmingly from the colon, appendix, or pancreas, occasionally from some other gastrointestinal source (Altemeier and Alexander, 1961; Stevenson and Ozeran, 1969). Rarely, they may originate from the pelvic organs.

Posterior retroperitoneal, or *perinephric, abscesses* lie between the peritoneum and the posterior endoabdominal fascia. The majority originate in the kidney and initially may be confined within the renal fascia. Others extend from the retroperitoneal surfaces of the gastrointestinal tract, or constitute metastatic infection.

In *retrofascial,* or *psoas, abscesses* the infection lies posterior to and outside the endoabdominal fascia, originating almost invariably from osteomyelitis of the spine. The retrofascial space extends into the thorax behind the fascia, here termed prevertebral, and downward within the psoas fascia. The abscess most often points in the groin, but it may extend to other parts of the thigh and leg or to the buttock or pelvis. By breaking into the renal fascia it may rarely spread to the opposite side (Ganguli, 1963).

Pelvic extraperitoneal abscesses may be subdivided into prevesical, rectovesical (in the male) or parametrial (in the female), pelvirectal, and retrorectal (presacral).

Drainage

Drainage of an *anterior extraperitoneal abscess* is usually accomplished by a short stab wound, with the finger and drain following the abscess toward its origin. A *perinephric abscess* is drained from behind through an incision resembling the upper end of a posterior kidney approach (see page 306). *Psoas abscesses* are today most commonly caused by pyogenic vertebral osteomyelitis (Oh and Banks, 1973). When a lumbar vertebra is involved, drainage may be achieved by a posterior exposure along the transverse processes at the desired level. Detachment of some of the fibers of origin of the quadratus lumborum muscle allows entrance to the psoas muscle, where the abscess leads to the vertebral body (see Fig. 2).

A *prevesical abscess* is readily drained by a suprapubic incision. A *rectovesical infection* in the male is most often an extension of a prostatic abscess. It is drained by a perineal exposure as for a radical prostatectomy (see page 343). In the female, a *parametrial infection* may rarely point anterolaterally (Cullen, 1917). Even when the infection is still within the broad ligament, Cullen suggested that it should be drained by an anterolateral muscle-splitting incision (Fig. 4), since vaginal drainage involved the danger of damaging the

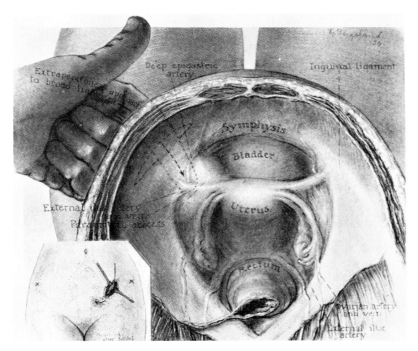

FIG. 4
Drainage of broad ligament abscess by suprainguinal approach. The external oblique aponeurosis is opened and the finger is pushed into the extraperitoneal space between the falx inguinalis and the inguinal ligament, at first lateral to the inferior epigastric and external iliac vessels, then over the brim of the pelvis. (From Douglass and Sheldon, 1931. By permission of Surgery, Gynecology & Obstetrics.)

ureter or uterine artery, or of entering the peritoneum. The drainage of *pelvirectal* and *retrorectal abscess* is described on page 251.

ANTEROLATERAL INCISIONS

The most frequently used approaches to the abdominal organs are those passing through the anterolateral wall. A *vertical incision* is the most versatile. A *paramedian incision* has the advantage over one made in the midline in that it avoids the confusion of entering the middle umbilical and falciform ligaments, which may be thick in the obese patient; and, more important, closure is stronger in the paramedian incision because above the linea semicircularis there exist both a posterior and an anterior aponeurotic sheath; this allows two lines of suture, strengthened also by the inter-position of the rectus muscle. The transversalis fascia and peritoneum are generally sutured as one layer if the perito-neum has been entered.

In the making of a paramedian incision, the rectus mus-cle is usually retracted laterally. If one splits the rectus mus-cle, the branches or trunks of the epigastric vessels will be divided. The intercostal and iliohypogastric nerves enter the rectus muscle at its lateral edge. For this reason a vertical incision lateral to the rectus muscle that divides two or more nerves is likely to result in atrophy of a segment of the rectus muscle and incisional hernia. A medial strip split from the main muscle is probably re-innervated from the intramus-cular branches of the divided nerves.

Transverse incisions (Fig. 5) are particularly useful for work in the mid-abdomen, especially in subjects of wide build. Incisional hernia rarely occurs after transverse inci-sions, especially if at least one or two of the three transverse and oblique muscles are split in the direction of their fibers rather than cut precisely in a transverse direction (Gurd, 1945; Keill *et al.,* 1973). The rectus muscle on one side may be divided, the other divided or retracted. The divided rectus does not retract widely, because of its attachment to the anterior sheath by the tendinous intersections.

Gurd emphasizes the necessity of placing the transverse incision a little above the umbilicus so that it can be ex-

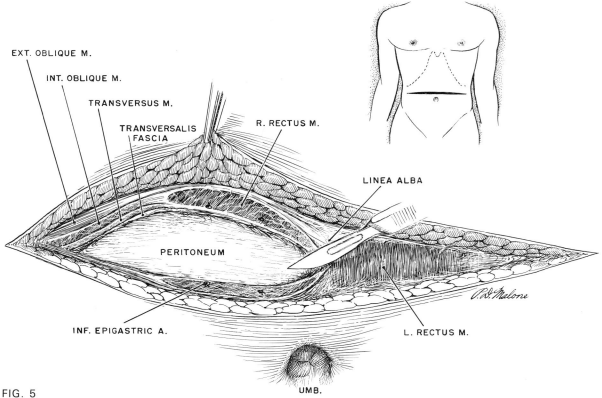

EXT. OBLIQUE M.

INT. OBLIQUE M.

TRANSVERSUS M.

TRANSVERSALIS FASCIA

R. RECTUS M.

LINEA ALBA

PERITONEUM

INF. EPIGASTRIC A.

L. RECTUS M.

UMB.

FIG. 5
Transverse mid-abdominal incision.

tended laterally if required, between the ribs and the iliac crests. Also, at this level, the internal oblique and transversus aponeuroses are relatively horizontal, so that their division as one layer approximates the line of their fibers. The rectus muscle is approximated in closure by sutures in the anterior sheath. If the incision lies above the umbilicus it is also above the linea semicircularis, so that a well-defined posterior as well as an anterior sheath is available for suture. The 'grid-iron,' or McBurney, incision for appendectomy is one which again splits each muscle in the direction of its fibers.

Satisfactory exposure for subcostal structures such as the gallbladder or spleen may be gained by an incision that parallels the costal border or is angled upward with an arm that divides or splits the rectus muscle. Intercostal nerves seen in the lower part of such incisions should be saved. Two or more intercostal nerves high under the arch are probably divided in subcostal incisions, but an incisional hernia is quite uncommon here.

A *suprapubic horizontal incision* constitutes an alternative to a paramedian incision for pelvic surgery. In the *Pfannenstiel incision* the skin is incised transversely within the pubic hair line, the anterior rectus sheaths are cut transversely, and the linea alba and peritoneum are opened in the midline. A *low transverse incision* with detachment of the rectus muscles from the pubis (*Cherney incision*) (Fig. 6) significantly increases exposure in the pelvis. The anterior rectus sheath is cut transversely, the division extending laterally to split the aponeuroses of the anterolateral muscles. The recti are divided at their exact fibrous origins from the pubes and retracted upward.

The inferior epigastric vessels lie at the lateral angles of the incision. The fascia and peritoneum are initially opened laterally to identify the location of the bladder. In closing the wound Cherney (1955) states that the rectus need not be directly sutured to the pubis; it is rather approximated to the deep surface of the lowermost part of the anterior rectus sheath. The pyramidalis muscles are allowed to fall onto the peritoneum and fascia without suture. According to Cherney, incisional hernia is rare.

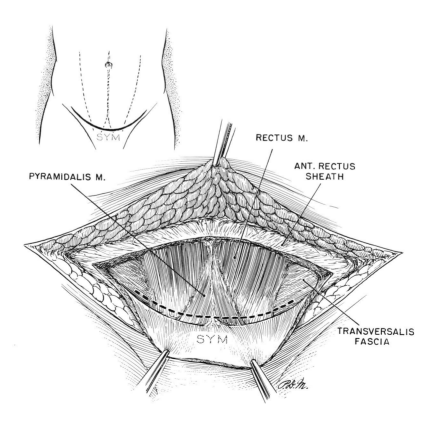

FIG. 6
Transverse low abdominal incision with rectus muscle detachment (Cherney incision).

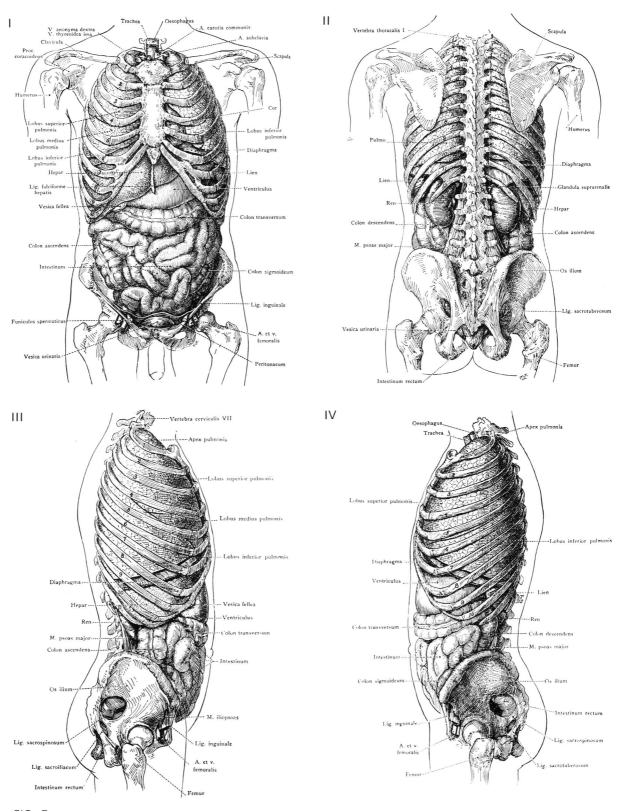

FIG. 7
Thoracoabdominal relationships. (From Medical Dept., U.S. Army, 1918.)

PROCEDURES TO INCREASE UPPER
ABDOMINAL EXPOSURE

Figure 7 shows the degree to which the intra- and extra-peritoneal organs of the upper abdomen are thoracoabdominal in position. Thoracoabdominal approaches will therefore give the most ample exposure for these organs. The varieties of such exposures are presented in our volume Operative Anatomy of Thorax (Edwards *et al.,* 1972).

Several procedures, short of making a thoracoabdominal incision, are available to increase upper abdominal exposure. Mobilization and retraction of the left lobe of the liver (Fig. 8) by division of the left portion of the coronary ligament ('triangular ligament') is often used to improve exposure of the structures beneath the left diaphragm once the abdomen has been opened. The *subcostal incision* with rectus muscle detachment (Fig. 9) gives excellent exposure of the entire upper abdomen. It is particularly useful for exposure of the suprarenal glands, the pedicles of the kidneys, and the major vessels of the upper abdomen.

Anterior abdominal incisions have been extended across the lower sternum or the ribs and their cartilages in a number of ways, all tending to increase exposure. These include removal of the xiphoid (Saint and Braslow, 1953); the splitting of the lower sternum with extension into the left 4th intercostal space (Wangensteen); the division of the left 6th and 7th cartilages (Clute and Albright); the creation of a retractable left costochondral flap by medial and lateral division of three or four ribs and cartilages (Baudet-Navarro); and the incision of the lower cartilaginous costal border (the Marwedel operation, modified by Gambee and Ingala, 1948) (Fig. 10).

These maneuvers are described by Clute and Albright (1938) and by Shackelford (1955). Pertinent to such incisions is the possibility of an unusually low position of the pleural reflection at the costophrenic sinus. On the average, the pleura reaches the 6th intercostal space at the side of the sternum, the 8th costochondral junction in the mid-clavicular line, and the 10th rib in the mid-axillary line. The pleura may lie one cartilage or space higher on either side. Variations in its lower limit never carry the left pleura below the costal border, but the right pleura cuts across the angle

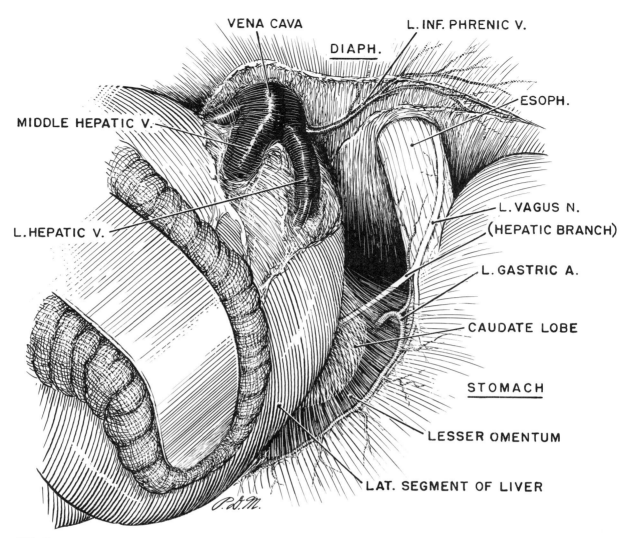

FIG. 8
Mobilization and retraction of the left lobe of the liver. The veins shown, or an aberrant biliary duct, are subject to injury in this maneuver (see pages 156 and 158).

between the xiphoid and the costal arch in about one third of individuals (Melnikoff, 1923).

APPROACHES TO THE RETROPERITONEUM

Approaches to the retroperitoneum may be transperitoneal, primarily retroperitoneal, or thoracoabdominal. *Transperitoneal approaches* vary according to the location and type of laparotomy incision used. The posterior peritoneum may be incised directly, as over the lower vena cava or aorta,

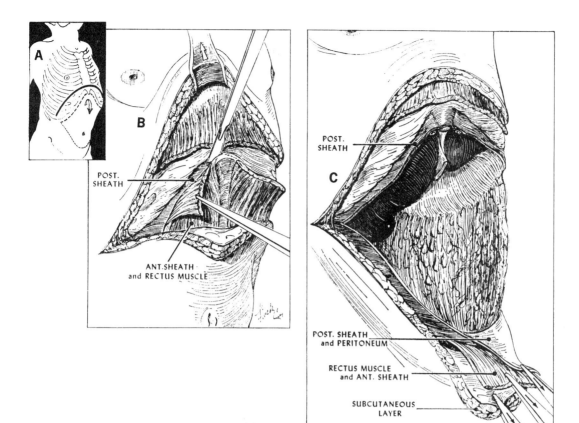

FIG. 9
Subcostal incision with rectus muscle detachment. A. The incision extends through the anterior rectus sheath above the edges of the costal arch. B. The rectus muscles and their posterior sheaths are divided below the costal arch. C. Exposure on opening the peritoneum. (From Vasko, 1966. By permission of Surgery, Gynecology & Obstetrics.)

or in the region of the suprarenal glands after one has passed through the omental bursa.

Such incisions in the lower abdomen are limited by the presence of the vessels of the small and large intestines. The widest exposures are obtained by opening the peritoneum lateral to portions of the gastrointestinal organs to open up the plane of embryonic post-rotational fusion; blunt dissection then can free these organs to their midline attachment, where their arterial supply lies. Common examples of this procedure are the *Kocher maneuver* (see Fig. 73), and *paracolic incisions* to mobilize the colon for exposure of the kidneys, vena cava, aorta, or sympathetic trunks (see Fig. 42).

An incision through the spleno-renal ligament allows a retroperitoneal exposure of the spleen, pancreas, and upper

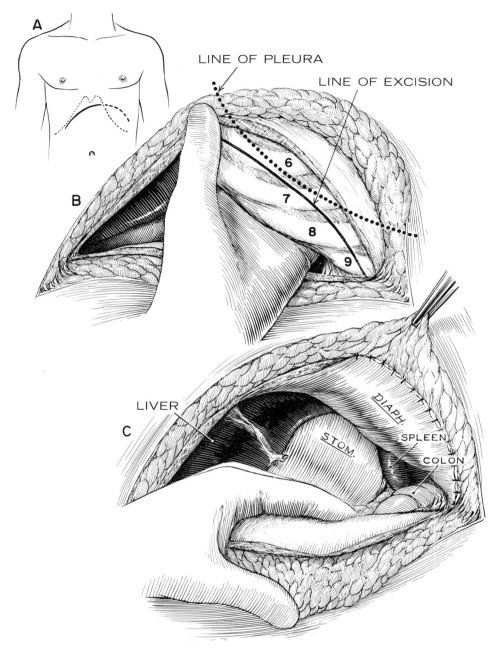

FIG. 10

Costal arch resection for left subdiaphragmatic approach. A. The initial curved incision (solid line) divides the right rectus muscle and, after initial exploration, is extended across the left rectus and the anterior surface of the left costal arch (broken line). B. The costal border has been cleared. Identifiable intercostal nerves should be pushed aside and saved. The fingers are stripping the transversus muscle, transversalis fascia, and peritoneum from under the costal border. The attachment of the diaphragm is palpated along the line which will indicate the limit of excision of the costal cartilages. C. The peritoneum and transversus muscle are sutured to the anterior line of resection of muscle and fascia. During closure, the left lower edge of muscle and fascia will be sutured to this initial line of suture. (After Gambee and Ingala, 1948.)

aorta. Downward extension of this incision elevating the colon gives exposure of the entire abdominal aorta (see Fig. 37). An incision to the left of the mesentery, continued around the right colon, exposes the entire infrarenal retroperitoneum (see Fig. 36).

Primary retroperitoneal incisions range from the front of the abdomen to the back. A *low anterior incision,* vertical or transverse, constitutes a standard approach to the bladder, the prostate (either suprapubic or retropubic), or the uterus for extraperitoneal cesarean section (see page 398). It is helpful to start with a distended bladder to elevate the peritoneum. In the upper abdomen, *extraperitoneal incisions* may be used to open anterior subphrenic abscesses, or, by going through the diaphragm to the left of the xiphoid, to drain the pericardium. A *mid-abdominal extraperitoneal paramedian incision* is of limited usefulness because of the frequent lack of sufficient extraperitoneal fat in this location to facilitate displacement of the peritoneum without tearing and because of the distance from the midline around to the retroperitoneal structures.

Anterolateral oblique or *transverse incisions* are adequate for exposure of structures below the kidney, such as the ureter, infrarenal cava, sympathetic trunks, and the iliac vessels and nodes. The oblique and transverse muscles are split in the direction of their fibers, but may be divided if exposure is difficult. The incision is initially deepened through the transversalis fascia in the most posterior part of the wound, for here one comes upon the constant bolster of retroperitoneal fat. Once the fatty interval is entered posteriorly the plane between fascia and peritoneum becomes more obvious anteriorly.

Additional relaxation can be obtained by extending the incision medially through the edge of the rectus sheath. The intercostal vessels and nerves are encountered between the internal oblique and transversus muscles, entering the lateral edge of the rectus muscle. For further relaxation the rectus muscle may be divided. One should note that the upper ureter generally adheres to the medially displaced peritoneum. The lateral end of the incision can be extended into the flank for further exposure of the ureter and kidney. A *long oblique incision* with rectus muscle division can be used for exposure of the aorta and iliac vessels (see page 58).

The posterior route is the most direct for uncovering the kidneys and suprarenal glands. Since these structures lie partly above the 12th rib it is pertinent to examine the lower limit of the pleura here. The pleura frequently lies below the 12th rib, particularly in the costovertebral angle, oftener on the right than on the left (Melnikoff, 1923). Thus the pleura should be looked for below the 12th rib in a posterolateral kidney exposure, especially if one is dividing the posterior lumbocostal ligament (Fig. 11).

I

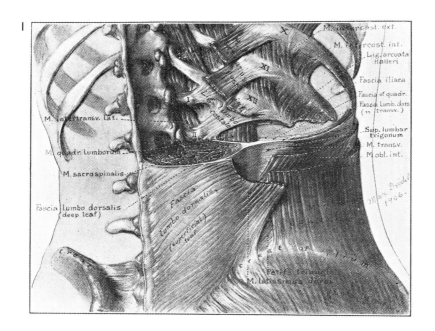

II

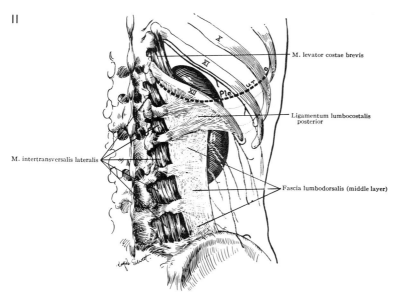

FIG. 11
Relationships pertinent to posterior approaches to the retroperitoneum. I. Muscles and fascias of the lumbar region. (From Kelly and Burnam, 1914.) II. Posterior topography of the kidney and pleura. (From Anson and McVay, 1971, after Kelly and Burnam, 1914.)

If the 12th rib is rudimentary, or absent, and does not reach the lateral border of the erector spinae muscle, the pleura is sure to be entered if the incision is carried into the angle between this muscle and the 11th rib. As Ochsner and Graves (1933) emphasized, the pleura will always escape injury if the dissection can be carried out below a horizontal line crossing the spinous process of the 1st lumbar vertebra (Fig. 12).

Exposure of the upper pole of the kidney, especially on the left side, or of the suprarenal gland is improved by removing a long 12th rib or the 11th rib, subperiosteally, with upward retraction of the pleura and division of the posterior costal origin of the diaphragm (see Figs. 154 and 155).

The infradiaphragmatic splanchnic nerves and celiac ganglion, as well as the sympathetic trunk, can be reached by a *posterior incision* through the lumbodorsal and transversalis fascias and medial retraction of the erector spinae and quadratus lumborum muscles. When it was performed for hypertension, this operation was often combined with a supradiaphragmatic retropleural removal of these nerves (see Fig. 54).

Nagamatsu (1963) introduced a *dorso-abdominal incision* allowing bilateral aorto-iliac lymph node dissection as

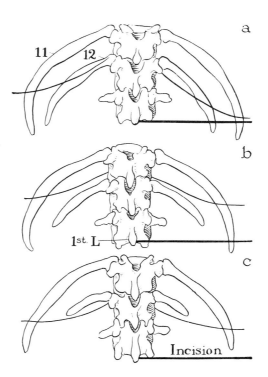

FIG. 12
Variations in the posterior lower limit of the pleura. A horizontal incision at the level of L I will always lie below the pleura. (From Ochsner and Graves, 1933.)

for cancer of the testis (Fig. 13). This is a right-sided incision removing portions of the 11th and 12th ribs, and dividing the posterior lumbocostal ligament below the pleura. This allows upward retraction of the diaphragm and pleura. The incision continues obliquely downward and forward and ends by dividing both rectus muscles as in a Cherney incision (see Fig. 6). The peritoneum and its contents are rolled to the left, a division of the inferior mesenteric artery allowing the structures to clear the entire aorto-iliac field to a level just above the renal vessels, where the course of the superior mesenteric artery bars higher exposure.

Thoracoabdominal exposures of the retroperitoneum vary from a relatively short posterior diaphragmatic incision, giving limited access to the retroperitoneum, as for a transthoracic sympathectomy and biopsy of the suprarenal gland and the kidney, to wider incisions which enter the upper peritoneal cavity as for the removal of large tumors of the suprarenal gland or kidney (see Edwards *et al.,* 1972, and Fig. 170). In the thoracoabdominal incision for aorto-iliac lymph node dissection of Cooper and his colleagues (1950) the diaphragm and retroperitoneum are opened widely, exposing the higher as well as the lower nodes, but this is satisfactory for work on one side only.

The hazards in retroperitoneal exposures are summarized by Young (1969). The commonest complication is injury to the ureter. Adhesions about the right kidney increase the danger of injury to the duodenum and pancreas; adhesions

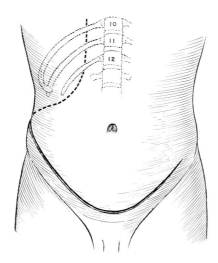

FIG. 13
Incision for dorsolumbar flap exposure for bilateral aortic lymph node dissection (Nagamatsu).

about the left kidney, the danger of injury to the jejunum and tail of the pancreas. Lumbar veins are easily torn. Anomalous venae cavae in unexpected positions should be anticipated (see Chapter 5). Any of the branches of the aorta may be injured in removing large tumors or scarred masses of lymph nodes.

PERINEAL APPROACHES TO THE PELVIS

In the male, radical prostatectomy constitutes the only common occasion for perineal entry (see page 343). Procedures involving perineal approaches to the genital organs in the female are more common and various. They include the operations of vaginal hysterectomy (see Chapter 25). A wider exposure is available through the paravaginal Shuchard incision utilized in cancer of the cervix (Schauta, 1908). This exposure allows the removal of parametrial tissue and visualization of the ureter.

The removal of the anorectum for carcinoma is regularly accomplished through the perineum, at times aided by removal of the coccyx. This is easier in the female since the pelvic outlet is usually roomier, and the peritoneal reflection is closer to the anus, the distance averaging 5.5 cm. in the female vs. 7.5 cm. in the male.

The term 'Kraske operation,' as used today, denotes the sacral approach to the anorectum, with removal of the coccyx and varying portions of the sacrum and the origin of the sacrotuberous and sacrospinous ligaments. The presence of the sacral, sciatic, and pudendal nerves (Fig. 14) limits the extent of removal of the sacrum. Injury to the 3rd sacral nerves risks the danger of bladder and rectal incontinence. MacCarty and his co-workers (1952) state that neither incontinence nor perineal anesthesia follows bilateral removal of the 4th and 5th sacral nerves. The added loss of the 3rd sacral nerve on one side will give unilateral perineal anesthesia, but bladder and rectal function will be normal or near normal. If the 3rd, 4th, and 5th sacral nerves on both sides or both pudendal nerves are sacrificed, vesical and rectal dysfunction and bilateral perineal sensory loss will ensue.

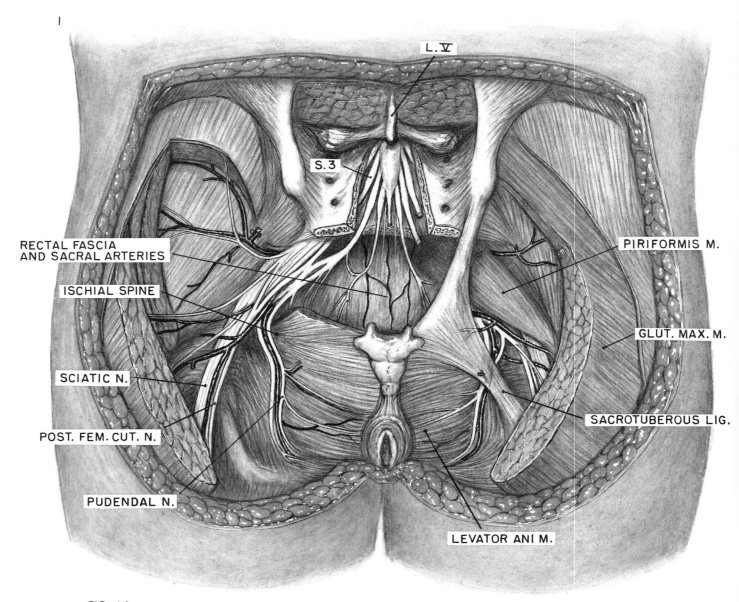

L. Ⅴ

S. 3

RECTAL FASCIA
AND SACRAL ARTERIES

PIRIFORMIS M.

ISCHIAL SPINE

SCIATIC N.

GLUT. MAX. M.

POST. FEM. CUT. N.

SACROTUBEROUS LIG.

PUDENDAL N.

LEVATOR ANI M.

FIG. 14
Relationships limiting sacral approaches to the pelvis.
I. Nerves and blood vessels related to the sacrum, buttocks, and perineum. The fourth and fifth segments of the sacrum have been removed, with adjacent parts of ligaments and muscles on the left side. The sacral plexus is shown formed from the anterior rami of the sacral nerves. The rectum and its blood vessels and lymphatics remain covered by the rectal fascia.

REFERENCES

Altemeier, W. A., and Alexander, J. W.: Retroperitoneal abscess.
    Arch. Surg. 83:512–524, 1961.
Anson, B. J., and McVay, C. B.: Surgical Anatomy, 5th ed. Phila-
    delphia, W. B. Saunders, 1971.

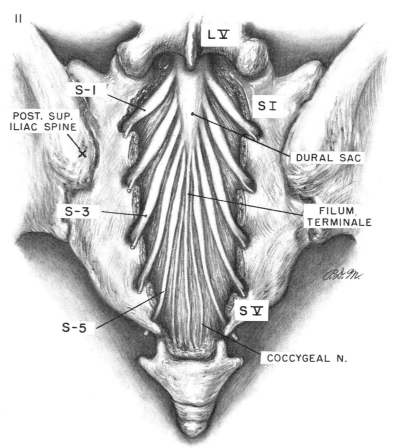

FIG. 14

Relationships limiting sacral approaches to the pelvis (continued).

II. Neural structures in the sacral canal. The dural-subarachnoid sac extends lower than the level of the second sacral vertebra in 46 per cent, sometimes 2 cm. or less from the sacral hiatus. (Trotter, 1947.)

The third sacral foramen lies 3 or 4 cm. below the posterior superior iliac spine. The iliac spine can be palpated at a skin dimple 4 or 5 cm. lateral to the spine and body of the second sacral vertebra. The possibility of partial or (rarely) total lack of the bony roof to the sacral canal, or the presence of six or of four sacral vertebrae, suggests the advisability of consulting a roentgenogram of the sacrum prior to planning any excision of this bone. (I, after Waldeyer, 1899, II, from personal dissection.)

Cherney, L. S.: Transverse low abdominal incision with detachment of the recti from the pubis. Follow-up study of eight hundred cases. J.A.M.A. 157:23–26, 1955.

Clute, H. M., and Albright, H. L.: Cutting the costal arch for upper abdominal exposure. Surg. Gynec. Obstet. 67:804–809, 1938.

Cooper, J. F., Leadbetter, W. F., and Chute, R.: The thoracoabdominal approach for retroperitoneal gland dissection. Its application to testis tumors. Surg. Gynec. Obstet. 90:486–496, 1950.

Cullen, T. S.: The surgical methods of dealing with pelvic infections. Surg. Gynec. Obstet. 25:134–146, 1917.

Cullen, T. S., and Brödel, M.: Lesions of the rectus abdominis muscle simulating an acute intra-abdominal condition. Bull. Johns Hopkins Hosp. 61:295–316, 1937.

Douglass, M., and Sheldon, D.: The treatment of pelvic cellulitis. Surgical drainage of parametric exudates. Surg. Gynec. Obstet. 52:1121–1128, 1931.

Edwards, E. A., Malone, P. D., and Collins, J. J., Jr.: Operative Anatomy of Thorax. Philadelphia, Lea & Febiger, 1972.

Gambee, L. P., and Ingala, A.: The costal arch resection—A substitute for the transthoracic approach to upper abdominal pathology. West. J. Surg. Obst. Gynec. 56:605–610, 1948.

Ganguli, P. K.: Radiology of Bone and Joint Tuberculosis with Special Reference to Tropical Countries. Bombay, Asia Publishing House, 1963.

Gurd, F. B.: Anatomical principles involved in abdominal incisions. Surg. Clin. N. Amer. 25:271–284, 1945.

Keill, R. H., Keitzer, W. F., Nichols, W. K., Henzel, J., and DeWeese, M. S.: Abdominal wound dehiscence. Arch. Surg. 106:573–577, 1973.

Kelly, H. A., and Burnam, C. F.: Diseases of the Kidneys, Ureters and Bladder, with Special Reference to the Diseases in Women. New York, Appleton, 1914.

MacCarty, C. S., Waugh, J. M., Mayo, C. W., and Coventry, M. B.: The surgical treatment of presacral tumors. A combined problem. Proc. Staff Meet. Mayo Clin. 27:73–84, 1952.

Medical Department, United States Army: Manual of Surgical Anatomy, 1918. (No author or publisher named.)

Melnikoff, A.: Die chirurgische Anatomie des Sinus costodiaphragmaticus. Arch. klin. Chir. 123:133–196, 1923.

Nagamatsu, G. R.: A new extraperitoneal approach for bilateral retroperitoneal lymph node dissection in testis tumor. J. Urol. 90:588–590, 1963.

Ochsner, A., and Graves, A. M.: Subphrenic abscess. An analysis of 3,372 collected and personal cases. Ann. Surg. 98:961–990, 1933.

Oh, W., and Banks, H.: Osteomyelitis of the spine. Presented at a meeting of the New England Surgical Society, April, 1973.

Saint, J. H., and Braslow, L. E.: Removal of the xyphoid process as an aid in operations on the upper abdomen. Surgery 33:361–366, 1953.

Schauta, F.: Die erweiterte vaginale Totalexstirpation des Uterus bei Kollumkarzinom. Wien, Šafář, 1908.

Shackelford, R. T.: Bickham-Callander Surgery of the Alimentary Tract. Vol. III. Philadelphia, W. B. Saunders, 1955.

Stevenson, E. O. S., and Ozeran, R. S.: Retroperitoneal space abscesses. Surg. Gynec. Obstet. 128:1202–1208, 1969.

Tobin, C. E.: The renal fascia and its relation to the transversalis fascia. Anat. Rec. 89:295–311, 1944.

Trotter, M.: Variations of the sacral canal: Their significance in the administration of caudal analgesia. Curr. Res. Anesth. Analg. 26:192–202, 1947.

Vasko, J. S.: Valuable approach to upper abdominal cavity. Surg. Gynec. Obstet. 122:844–845, 1966.

Waldeyer, W.: Das Becken. Chirurgie und Gynäkologie. Bonn, F. Cohen, 1899.

Young, J. D., Jr.: Surgery of Retroperitoneal Diseases. Chapter 16 in Urologic Surgery, Glenn, J. F., and Boyce, W. H., Eds. New York, Hoeber Medical Division, Harper & Row, 1969.

2

special aspects of visceral and peritoneal topography

THE ABDOMEN IN THE NEONATE

The abdomen of the newborn differs from that of the adult in the presence of patent umbilical vessels and other structures which undergo involution. There are differences also in the shape of the abdominal cavity, in the disposition of the viscera, and in their form and relative size.

The umbilical arteries and vein become occluded after birth, by contraction and later tissue ingrowth, but the arteries can be cannulated during the first day or two of postnatal life; the vein can usually be opened even in the adult (see page 206). The ductus venosus (see Fig. 121) closes at birth and has not been proved dilatable in the adult (see page 208). Within the abdomen, the two arteries and the vein are at this time more prominent than the ligaments they will become (Fig. 15). The upper end of the true urachus has descended with the bladder to a level below the umbilicus.

The urachus is normally closed by birth and is represented by the median umbilical ligament. The upper part of the ligament is made up of heavy fibrous strands which extend to the umbilical arteries, tending to pull them medially (see also page 315). A small umbilical hernia is often

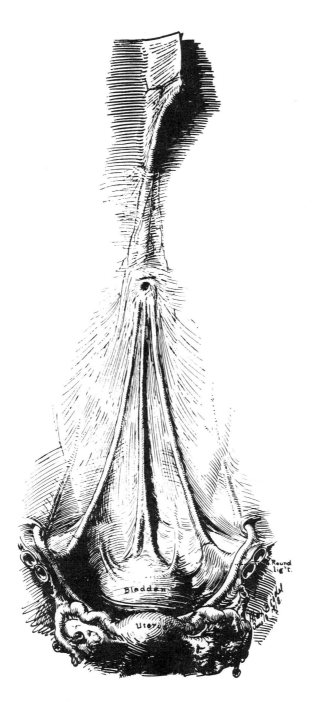

FIG. 15
Vestigial structures of the anterior abdominal wall, viewed from within. Above, the round ligament is lost in the abdominal wall about 8 cm. above the umbilicus. The obliterated hypogastric arteries extend from the internal iliac arteries, not defined in the illustration. The median umbilical ligament extending upward from the bladder apex is unusually prominent in this subject. The line of each inferior epigastric artery can be seen medial to the round ligament of the uterus then behind the rectus muscle. (From Cullen, 1916.)

present, more frequently in black than in white infants, and twice as often in girls (Gray and Skandalakis, 1972). Most small umbilical hernias close spontaneously within the first year of life, and Gross (1953) says some may close in several years. The testes lie high in the scrotum. The processus vaginalis closes shortly before or after birth. Spontaneous closure with cure of a congenital inguinal hernia is not to be expected.

The abdomen at birth is relatively wide and protuberant. The pelvic cavity is narrow and the intestine, exclusive of the rectum, lies almost wholly outside of the pelvis. The abdominal visceral mass (Fig. 16 A) presents an oval anterior surface, with its long axis transverse. With the assumption of the upright posture, the small and large intestines begin to enter the pelvis. By adult life, the visceral mass (Fig. 16 B) is again ovoid, but with its long axis vertical.

The liver is large, its lower edge close to the umbilicus. The spleen is small and not visible from the front. Its size

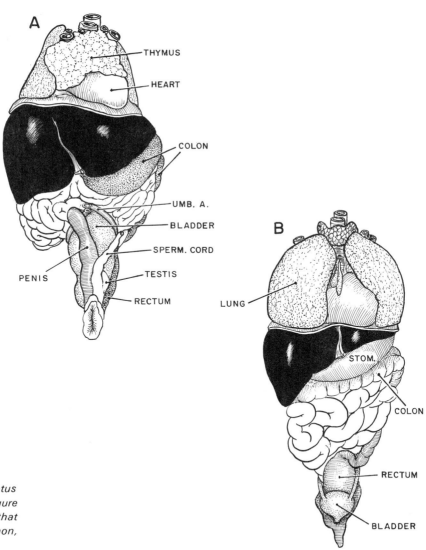

FIG. 16
Visceral mass (A) of a full-term fetus and (B) of an adult. In B the figure is reduced to the same length as that of the fetus in A. (After Scammon, 1953.)

is relatively the same in the child and in the adult (Scammon, 1923). The stomach is small and hidden by the liver. The intestine is short (see page 232). The small cecum lies within the iliac fossa, but appears high because of the low-lying liver (Scammon, 1923). The ascending colon is short, the hepatic flexure poorly marked. The transverse colon is long and wide, and may be thrown into folds. The sigmoid lies above the pelvis. The rectum is capacious. The cecum tapers into the wide appendix without a distinct boundary.

Scammon noted that most commonly the lower cecum and the appendix are bent upward, anteriorly or posteriorly, at an acute angle with the upper cecum. Less often, the cecum forms a cone, with the apex downward. The diameter of the appendix at birth is about one-fourth that of the cecum, as against one-eighth that of the cecum in the adult (Kelly, 1909). Teniae and haustra are poorly defined, reaching full development at the fourth year (Scammon, 1923).

Much of the urinary bladder at birth lies above the pelvis in both sexes. Whether it is empty or distended, its anterior surface is in close contact with the abdominal wall for about two-thirds of the distance from the symphysis pubis to the umbilicus. The internal urethral orifice lies behind the symphysis pubis (Symington, 1887) (see Fig. 171). By four or five years the bladder has descended enough so that a pouch of peritoneum separates the abdominal wall and the symphysis pubis from the empty bladder. Both the kidneys and the suprarenal glands are large at birth, and the kidneys show surface markings of lobulation (see Fig. 151). The para-aortic bodies (of Zuckerkandl) may be quite prominent. Data on the weights of the viscera of the newborn, compared with those of the adult, are presented by Scammon (1953).

THE VISCERA IN SITUS INVERSUS

Reversal in position from right to left of all the thoracic and abdominal viscera and blood vessels, the structures presenting in mirror image of the usual, is known as *situs inversus totalis.* The incidence among one and a half million patients seen at the Mayo Clinic was reported by Mayo and Rice (1949) as 1 in 20,408. Most of such individuals are normal, but in about 20 per cent bronchiectasis and malformations of the nasal sinuses are also present, to form the triad known as Kartagener's syndrome.

Partial, or *thoracic, situs inversus* is more common, dextrocardia being seen about once in 8500 screening roentgenograms (Gray and Skandalakis, 1972). The incidence at birth of this anomaly is undoubtedly greater, since partial situs inversus is often associated with other congenital anomalies, especially of the heart, which are severe enough to be incompatible with life.

Splenic anomalies have a particular association with thoracic situs inversus (Gray and Skandalakis). This may take the form of agenesia of the spleen (asplenia). Cardiac defects and spina bifida may be present. In polysplenia, the second splenic anomaly to accompany the situs inversus, the organ is replaced by multiple distinct splenic masses. These differ from accessory spleens, which exist along with a spleen of usual form (see Chapter 9).

INTRAPERITONEAL SPACES AND THEIR DRAINAGE

The localization of fluids within the peritoneum is determined partly by the subdivision of the peritoneal cavity by anatomic barriers, modified by forces of gravity and respiratory movement, and varying somewhat according to the source of the fluid. Two transverse barriers divide the cavity into three horizontal regions (Fig. 17). The upper of these barriers is constituted by the transverse colon and mesocolon, the lower by the pelvic brim, bolstered by the psoas muscles and the iliac vessels. The resultant *supracolic* and *infracolic regions* are irregularly divided into right and left halves by the bodies of the vertebrae, the aorta, and the inferior vena cava, plus the mesentery of the small intestine in the infracolic region. The *right subhepatic space* (see Boyd, 1966) includes the depression often called the hepatorenal pouch (of Morison); the *left subhepatic space* is mainly the omental bursa. The *pelvis* is partly divided by the pelvic colon and its mesentery. The spaces into which these regions are subdivided are shown in Figure 17.

Of 194 intraperitoneal abscesses studied by Altemeier and his colleagues (1973), almost half were located in the

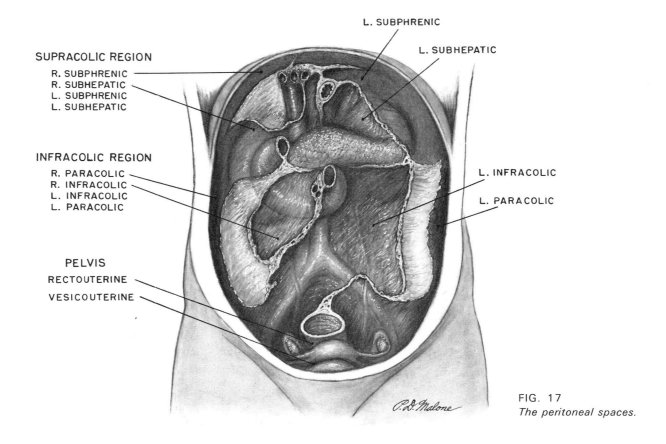

SUPRACOLIC REGION
  R. SUBPHRENIC
  R. SUBHEPATIC
  L. SUBPHRENIC
  L. SUBHEPATIC

INFRACOLIC REGION
  R. PARACOLIC
  R. INFRACOLIC
  L. INFRACOLIC
  L. PARACOLIC

PELVIS
  RECTOUTERINE
  VESICOUTERINE

L. SUBPHRENIC
L. SUBHEPATIC

L. INFRACOLIC
L. PARACOLIC

FIG. 17
The peritoneal spaces.

right lower quadrant, or at the junction of the right infracolic and paracolic spaces; the remainder were distributed over other locations (Table 1). Localization was determined to a great extent by the initiating process. When an intraperitoneal abscess was the residual of diffuse peritonitis, the abscess was most often found in the hepatorenal (right subhepatic) and rectovesical (or rectouterine) pouches, the paracolic, and the subphrenic spaces. When the infection was more localized, the resultant abscess was often found in contiguity with the initiating infection (Table 2).

The significance of contiguity has also been emphasized by the etiological study of left subphrenic abscess by Neuhof and Schlossmann (1942). They found lesions of the stomach, duodenum, and spleen most often responsible for infection in this space. In a review of 3,372 cases of subphrenic abscess (using the term to include subhepatic abscesses as well), Ochsner and Graves (1933) found that diseases of the appendix, stomach, and duodenum were responsible for 60 per cent of all the cases; other causes included diseases of

TABLE 1

*Location and Type of 540 Intra-abdominal Abscesses.**

Location and Type	Number of Cases	Per Cent
Intraperitoneal		
Right lower quadrant	86	16
Left lower quadrant	28	5
Pelvic	27	5
Subphrenic	27	5
Morison's pouch, or subhepatic	10	2
Interloop	8	1
Giant horseshoe	6	1
Lesser sac	2	0.3
Subtotal	194	36
Retroperitoneal		
Anterior retroperitoneal	92	17
Posterior retroperitoneal	79	15
Retrofascial	32	6
Subtotal	203	38
Visceral		
Hepatic	69	13
Pancreatic	34	6
Tubo-ovarian	26	5
Gallbladder and biliary tract	13	2
Kidney	1	0.2
Subtotal	143	26
Total	540	100

*From Altemeier *et al.,* 1973.

the liver and biliary system. This correlates with the fact that the number of abscesses found on the right was double that on the left.

The two spaces that are most dependent in the supine position are the right subhepatic (*hepatorenal*) and the *rectovesical pouches* (Fig. 18). Yet subhepatic abscess may result from a diffuse peritonitis even though the patient is placed in a semi-erect (Fowler's) position, and subphrenic abscess may not infrequently follow pelvic infection.

The upward movement of peritoneal fluid appears to depend partly on capillary action (in the interserous spaces) and the subphrenic suction which Overholt (1930) demon-

TABLE 2
*Relationship of Locations of Intra-abdominal
Abscesses to Primary Diseases.**

Primary Disease	Location of Abscess	Number
Appendicitis	Right lower quadrant	76
	Pelvic	16
	Anterior retroperitoneal	19
	Subphrenic	8
	Interloop	3
Diverticulitis of colon	Left lower quadrant	20
	Pelvic	9
	Right lower quadrant	5
	Anterior retroperitoneal	2
	Interloop	2
	Subphrenic	1
	Subhepatic	1
Pancreatitis and pancreatic tumor	Retroperitoneal	19
	Lesser sac	16
	Intraperitoneal	4
Peptic ulcer	Right subphrenic	5
	Left lower quadrant	5
	Right upper quadrant	2
	Left subphrenic	5
	Subhepatic	2
	Pelvic	1
	Interloop	1

*From Altemeier *et al.,* 1973.

strated during inspiration. Even the presence of pneumo-peritoneum fails to halt an upward progression of fluid (Overholt, 1930; Autio, 1964).

The spread of fluid loosed in the peritoneal cavity was studied by Mitchell (1940) through the use of radiopaque material injected into human fetuses. Mitchell's findings have been well confirmed by general observations on the accidental introduction of barium suspensions in patients, and a postoperative study of the spread of oily contrast medium by Autio (1964). Mitchell used 48 fetuses, injecting the barium mixture in various places to mimic the escape of fluid from various organs. His findings on the spread of fluid from a ruptured duodenal ulcer are shown in Figure

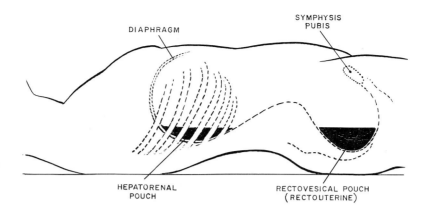

FIG. 18
Peritoneal spaces dependent in the supine position. (After Basmajian, 1971.)

DIAPHRAGM

SYMPHYSIS PUBIS

HEPATORENAL POUCH

RECTOVESICAL POUCH (RECTOUTERINE)

19. Contrary to former belief the fluid ran downward over the colic barrier, thence to the pelvis and the right paracolic gutter. Once in the paracolic gutter the fluid did pass upward to the right subhepatic and subphrenic spaces. The phrenicocolic ligament precluded flow along the left paracolic gutter to the left subhepatic and subphrenic spaces. Instead, fluid passed from the infracolic space or the pelvis upward over the colon to the left subphrenic space. Some communication was shown between the two subhepatic spaces.

Intraperitoneal abscesses other than subphrenic and subhepatic or pelvic are usually drained by an anterior laparotomy incision. *Pelvic abscesses* may be drained through the anterior wall of the rectum in the male, and through the posterior vault of the vagina in the female if the abscess is

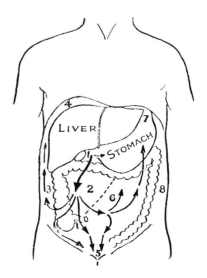

FIG. 19
Sequence of spread of effusion from the gastroduodenal area. (From Mitchell, 1940.)

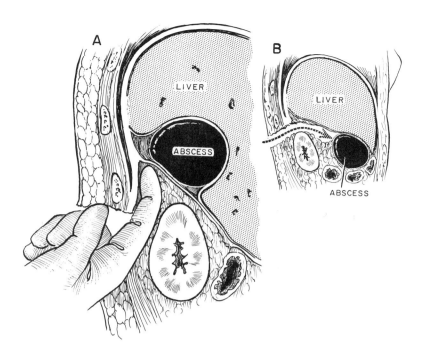

FIG. 20
Posterior extraperitoneal approach to right subhepatic abscesses. B shows approach to an anteriorly placed abscess through the same incision. (After Ochsner and Graves, 1933.)

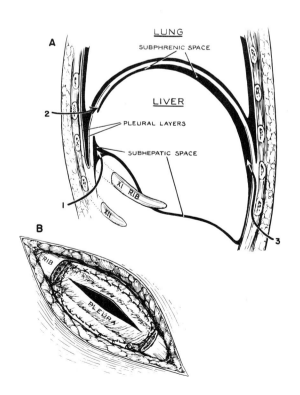

FIG. 21
Approaches to the subphrenic and subhepatic spaces. A. Direction of approaches. B. Incision through rib bed (approach 2) after suture-closure of the costodiaphragmatic recess. (From Boyd, 1958.)

located in the recto-uterine pouch. *Subphrenic* or *subhepatic abscesses* may be approached extraperitoneally. For a right subphrenic abscess (Fig. 20) the incision is made subcostally and the abscess entered bluntly. This may also be possible for left subphrenic abscesses. Posterior or subhepatic abscesses can be approached by a posterior incision. The 12th rib is removed subperiosteally (Fig. 20), and a horizontal incision is made through the bed of the rib at the level of the spine of the 1st lumbar vertebra. At this level the incision will miss the pleura, even if the latter is exceptionally low (see Fig. 12). The incision is deepened by incising the diaphragm or displacing it upward, entering the abscess.

A transpleural and transdiaphragmatic approach may be used for subhepatic or hepatic abscess (Fig. 21). Some surgeons favor an anterior transperitoneal approach for all subphrenic and subhepatic abscesses because it affords opportunity to explore the abdomen in the face of an often uncertain diagnosis. The drainage of extraperitoneal abscess is discussed in Chapter 1.

REFERENCES

Altemeier, W. A., Culbertson, W. R., Fullen, W. D., and Shook, C. D.: Intra-abdominal abscesses. Amer. J. Surg. 125:70–79, 1973.

Autio, V.: The spread of intraperitoneal infection. Studies with roentgen contrast medium. Acta Chir. Scand., Suppl. 321, 1964.

Basmajian, J. V.: Grant's Method of Anatomy, 8th ed. Baltimore, Williams & Wilkins, 1971.

Boyd, D. P.: The anatomy and pathology of the subphrenic spaces. Surg. Clin. N. Amer. 38:619–626, 1958.

Boyd, D. P.: The subphrenic spaces and the emperor's new robes. New Eng. J. Med. 275:911–917, 1966.

Cullen, T. S.: Embryology, Anatomy, and Diseases of the Umbilicus. Together with Diseases of the Urachus. Philadelphia, W. B. Saunders, 1916.

Gray, S. W., and Skandalakis, J. E.: Embryology for Surgeons. The Embryological Basis for the Treatment of Congenital Defects. Philadelphia, W. B. Saunders, 1972.

Gross, R. E.: The Surgery of Infancy and Childhood. Its Principles and Techniques. Philadelphia, W. B. Saunders, 1953.

Kelly, H. A.: Appendicitis and Other Diseases of the Vermiform Appendix. Philadelphia, J. B. Lippincott, 1909.

Mayo, C. W., and Rice, R. G.: Situs inversus totalis. A statistical review of data on 76 cases with special reference to disease of the biliary tract. Arch. Surg. 58:724–730, 1949.

Mitchell, G. A. G.: The spread of acute intraperitoneal effusions. Brit. J. Surg. 28:291–313, 1940.

Neuhof, H., and Schlossmann, N. C.: Left subphrenic abscess. Surg. Gynec. Obstet. 75:751–758, 1942.

Ochsner, A., and Graves, A. M.: Subphrenic abscess. An analysis of 3,372 collected and personal cases. Ann. Surg. 98:961–990, 1933.

Overholt, R. H.: Air in the peritoneal cavity. Its effect on the position and activity of the diaphragm. Arch. Surg. 21:1282–1290, 1930.

Scammon, R. E.: A Summary of the Anatomy of the Infant and Child. Chapter III *in* Pediatrics, Abt, I.A., Ed. Vol. 1. Philadelphia, W. B. Saunders, 1923.

Scammon, R. E.: Developmental Anatomy. Section I in Schaeffer, J. P., *et al.,* Eds.: Morris' Human Anatomy, 11th ed. New York. Blakiston, 1953.

Symington, J.: The Topographical Anatomy of the Child. Edinburgh, Livingstone, 1887.

iNGuiNAL ANd fEMORAL HERNiA

THE PATH OF INGUINAL AND OF FEMORAL HERNIAS

Figure 22 shows the inguinal ligament and related structures viewed from within. The medial end of the ligament on the pubic tubercle is hidden by the rectus abdominis muscle. Its posterior expansion—the lacunar ligament—is seen attaching to the pecten—the ridge behind the tubercle—and continuing as the pectineal ligament (of Cooper). The pectineal (Cooper's) ligament clothes the iliopectineal line of the pelvis.

Femoral hernia occurs through the femoral ring—the entrance to the femoral canal. In a much-dissected anatomical specimen, the boundaries of the ring are the lacunar ligament medially, the femoral vein laterally, and the inguinal and pectineal ligaments anteriorly and posteriorly. However, McVay and Savage (1961) have shown that, when the ring is intact, the falx inguinalis and adherent transversalis fascia form the medial boundary, the falx normally extending 1 or 2 cm. lateral to the lacunar ligament. The pectineus fascia continues the posterior relationship of a femoral hernia below the pectineal ligament. A femoral hernia makes its appearance in the subcutaneous fat of the upper thigh, medial to the saphenous hiatus (see Fig. 28 A).

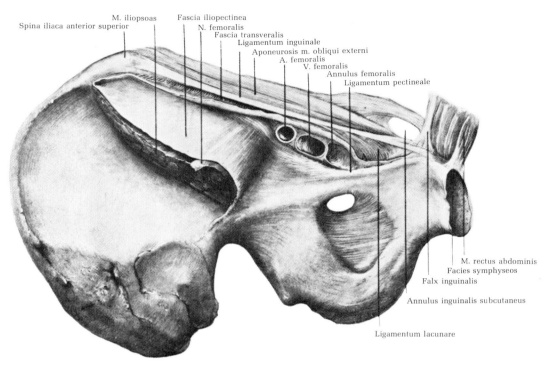

Spina iliaca anterior superior — M. iliopsoas — Fascia iliopectinea — N. femoralis — Fascia transveralis — Ligamentum inguinale — Aponeurosis m. obliqui externi — A. femoralis — V. femoralis — Annulus femoralis — Ligamentum pectineale — M. rectus abdominis — Facies symphyseos — Falx inguinalis — Annulus inguinalis subcutaneus — Ligamentum lacunare

FIG. 22
Structures behind the inguinal ligament. (From Anson and McVay, 1971.)

Femoral hernia is commoner in women than in men, consistent with the presence in women of a wider pelvis and femoral canal; yet even in women inguinal hernia is more frequently encountered than femoral.

In its passage through the abdominal wall the processus vaginalis and the testis push before them thin extensions of each layer. The extension of the internal oblique muscle constitutes a substantial sheath—the cremaster muscle. The processus normally closes shortly before or at birth, only that part about the testis remaining as a mesothelial-lined sheath—the tunica vaginalis. Even when the processus closes, the path of descent of the testis leaves the tract of weakness in the abdominal wall traversed by an indirect hernia. When the entire length of the processus remains open, it constitutes an open tunnel for the passage of the so-called congenital inguinal hernia. Because an indirect hernia of any type follows the pathway of the processus, its sac (Fig. 23) will be found anterior to the pedicle of the testis, that is, the spermatic cord.

In the female a processus vaginalis also develops, but,

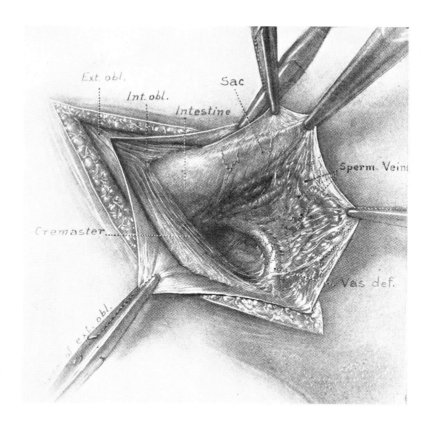

FIG. 23
Relationships of the sac of an indirect inguinal hernia. (From Martin, 1908.)

although the processus extends through the abdominal wall, the ovary is diverted to the pelvis, the gubernaculum developing into the round ligament. The obliterated processus and the round ligament course through the subcutaneous inguinal ring to blend with the fibrous tissue of the labium majus. Rarely, the processus vaginalis in the female persists to allow the formation of a congenital inguinal hernia.

From within the abdomen (Fig. 24), the internal ring is seen to lie lateral to the inferior epigastric vessels in the lateral inguinal fovea. Medial to these vessels lies the inguinal triangle (Hesselbach's triangle), through which direct inguinal hernia occurs. The pulsation of the inferior epigastric artery may occasionally be felt through a greatly enlarged subcutaneous inguinal ring. Usually determination of its location, establishing whether a direct or indirect hernia is present, must await opening of the inguinal canal.

The bladder when empty lies close to the medial inguinal fovea, and when distended overlies the fovea. Thus the bladder is invariably medial to a femoral hernia, is frequently medial to a direct hernia, and may actually herniate beside

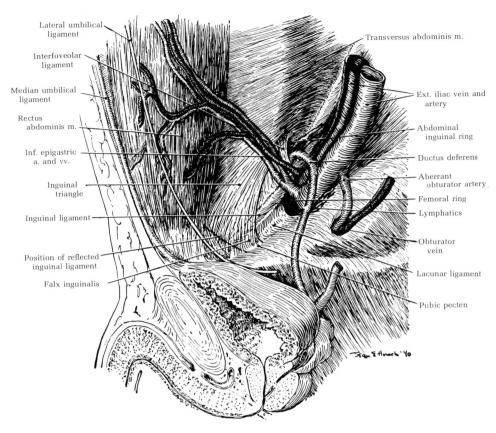

Lateral umbilical ligament

Interfoveolar ligament

Median umbilical ligament

Rectus abdominis m.

Inf. epigastric a. and vv.

Inguinal triangle

Inguinal ligament

Position of reflected inguinal ligament

Falx inguinalis

Transversus abdominis m.

Ext. iliac vein and artery

Abdominal inguinal ring

Ductus deferens

Aberrant obturator artery

Femoral ring

Lymphatics

Obturator vein

Lacunar ligament

Pubic pecten

FIG. 24

Internal view of anterior abdominal wall. The lacunar ligament is drawn too wide, and the falx inguinalis too narrow. The falx should lie at the medial edge of the femoral ring. (From Anson, B. J.: Morris' Human Anatomy, 12th ed. Copyright, 1966, McGraw-Hill Book Company, New York. Used with permission of McGraw-Hill Book Company.)

either sac (Fig. 25). Bladder injury thus constitutes a regular hazard during repair of femoral and direct inguinal hernia. Since the portion of bladder involved is extraperitoneal, it will not be seen within the sac but may be a part of its wall. The proximity of the bladder during dissection is signaled by the coarsely lobulated pale yellow fat which overlies it, and by the prominent elongated blood vessels which lie upon its wall (see Fig. 172). Infrequently, the bladder may present within the sac of a femoral or an indirect inguinal hernia, or as a part of a sliding hernia.

In sliding hernia (Fig. 26) the wall of the protrusion is at least partly constituted by large bowel or, less commonly, by the bladder presenting its retroperitoneal surface. Most often the hernia is indirect inguinal in type, with cecum

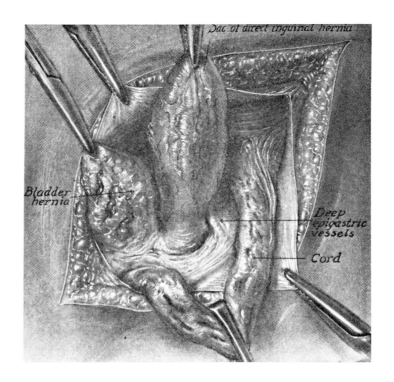

FIG. 25
Bladder hernia accompanying direct inguinal hernia. (From Watson, 1938.)

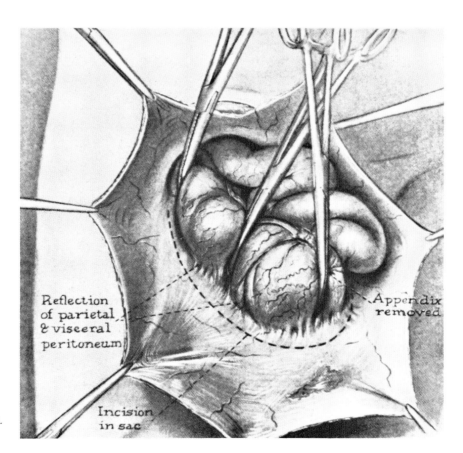

FIG. 26
Inguinal view of sliding hernia. (From Bevan, 1935.)

involved on the right, and sigmoid colon on the left. A sliding hernia of bladder more often occurs in a direct inguinal or femoral position. The relationship of the bowel to the peritoneum when a sac is present is shown in Figure 26. Rarely there may be no peritoneal sac, the herniating organ having rotated so as to present its bare area only.

EXPOSURE THROUGH THE INGUINAL CANAL; INGUINAL LIGAMENT REPAIR; RESECTION OF THE SPERMATIC CORD

Both inguinal and femoral hernias may be approached by opening the inguinal canal (Fig. 27), their contents may

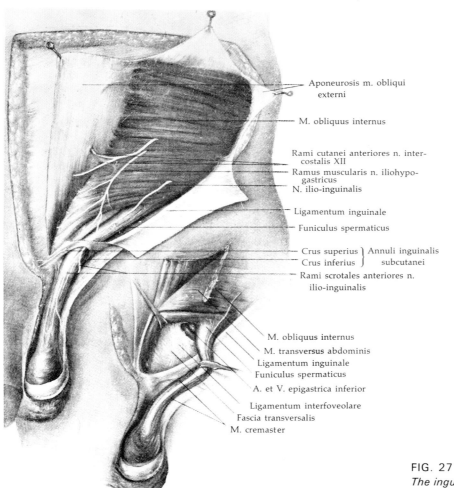

Aponeurosis m. obliqui externi

M. obliquus internus

Rami cutanei anteriores n. intercostalis XII
Ramus muscularis n. iliohypogastricus
N. ilio-inguinalis

Ligamentum inguinale
Funiculus spermaticus

Crus superius ⎫ Annuli inguinalis
Crus inferius ⎰ subcutanei
Rami scrotales anteriores n. ilio-inguinalis

M. obliquus internus
M. transversus abdominis
Ligamentum inguinale
Funiculus spermaticus
A. et V. epigastrica inferior
Ligamentum interfoveolare
Fascia transversalis
M. cremaster

FIG. 27
The inguinal canal. (From Anson and McVay, 1971.)

be reduced, and the defect in the abdominal wall repaired. The canal is entered by a supra-inguinal incision through the external oblique aponeurosis. The spermatic cord and an indirect sac will be surrounded by the cremaster muscle, which must be incised to delineate these structures. A direct inguinal hernia or a femoral hernia is not covered by cremaster muscle or fascia. Exposure of the sac of either of these types will require displacement of the spermatic cord. The transversalis fascia will be encountered in its juxtaperitoneal position as part of the sac of an indirect or a direct inguinal hernia. In the case of a femoral hernia, the neck of the sac will be exposed (see Fig. 31 I).

Indirect hernia in infancy is often treated by simple removal of the sac. In most cases of inguinal or femoral hernia, however, the surgeon attempts to strengthen the abdominal wall by a repair to overcome the presumed underlying weakness. The many techniques available may be classified as inguinal ligament or pectineal (Cooper's) ligament repairs, on the basis of which of the two structures some more flexible part of the abdominal wall is sutured to.

Inguinal ligament repairs are much used in instances of inguinal hernia, and the structure sutured to the ligament is usually the falx inguinalis. It has been remarked that 'conjoined tendon,' the older term for the falx, is erroneous, since the lower borders of the internal oblique and transversus muscles are neither conjoined nor tendinous. The two muscles are indeed usually separable in the middle of their arching, but the transversus is aponeurotic here (Fig. 27). Medially, the two aponeuroses are joined in the falx. One can therefore utilize the transversus aponeurosis for suture to the inguinal ligament in the lateral part of the canal, continuing the line of suture in the falx medially. In the Bassini operation the suturing is done behind the cord. The falx inguinalis often arches too high over the canal to allow its suture to the inguinal ligament without excessive tension. It can be relaxed by a short incision in the lower part of the anterior rectus sheath (see Fig. 31 II). The defect in the sheath needs no repair, the rectus muscle preventing herniation.

As sutures are passed through the inguinal ligament, one must avoid injury to the external iliac and inferior epigastric vessels, and the femoral nerve.

The spermatic cord is sometimes sectioned as an aid in the repair of large or recurrent hernias. This step is taken when the cord is bulky in hernias of long standing. Although this does not necessarily cause necrosis of the testis because of the existence of collateral blood supply (see Fig. 181), it is apparent from reports of great numbers of such procedures that damage to the testis may result (Harrison, 1971). Burdick and Higinbotham (1935), in a review of 200 patients in whom the cord was sectioned during hernia repair, reported four cases of postoperative necrosis of the testis. In patients followed for a long time, atrophy occurred in 27 per cent.

Heifetz (1971), reporting on 109 such operations, found fever and testicular swelling in 72 patients, testicular necrosis in 1, late atrophy in 39, and the development of hydrocele in 4. Heifetz believes these complications will be fewer if the scrotal part of the hernial sac is left intact, and the testis is not displaced from its scrotal lodgment. It would seem that, if the vas and the artery and veins immediately surrounding it were left intact, this would not seriously hamper a solid repair, and it might prevent ischemic damage, especially since, in older men, the testicular artery is often already occluded by arteriosclerosis (Edwards and LeMay, 1955).

FEMORAL HERNIA; PECTINEAL LIGAMENT REPAIRS OF FEMORAL AND INGUINAL HERNIAS

It is simple to approach a femoral hernia over the subinguinal prominence it produces (Fig. 28). Once the contents are replaced and the sac removed, repair is effected by suturing the inguinal ligament to the pectineal fascia or, if the tissues are lax enough, to the pectineal ligament which lies at the superior limit of the fascia. Such a repair is satisfactory for an easily reducible hernia, and in the case where the hernia is discovered in the course of some other procedure in the groin.

An inguinal approach to a femoral hernia is more generally desirable for two reasons. The first is the possible coexistence of an inguinal hernia. The second is that section

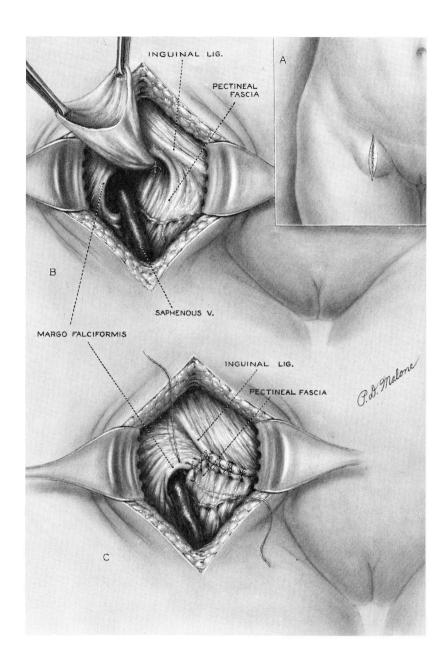

INGUINAL LIG.

PECTINEAL FASCIA

A

B

SAPHENOUS V.

MARGO FALCIFORMIS

INGUINAL LIG.

PECTINEAL FASCIA

P. D. Malone

C

FIG. 28
*Subinguinal repair of femoral
hernia.*

of the inguinal ligament from below, in order to reduce an
obstructed femoral hernia, entails the danger of hemorrhage
from the blind division of an aberrant obturator artery. The
incidence of the anomaly is 33 per cent on any one side
(see page 65). No figures are available on the frequency with
which the aberrant artery courses anterior to the femoral
ring, where it is vulnerable when the ligament is divided,
or posterior, where it is not (Fig. 29). A vein connecting the
inferior epigastric and obturator veins is fairly constant along

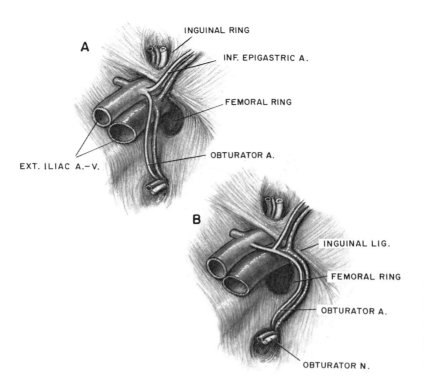

A

INGUINAL RING

INF. EPIGASTRIC A.

FEMORAL RING

OBTURATOR A.

EXT. ILIAC A.–V.

B

INGUINAL LIG.

FEMORAL RING

OBTURATOR A.

OBTURATOR N.

FIG. 29
Relations of the aberrant obturator artery to the femoral ring. In A, the artery would escape injury if the inguinal ligament and the neck of a femoral hernia were divided from below; in B, it would be vulnerable.

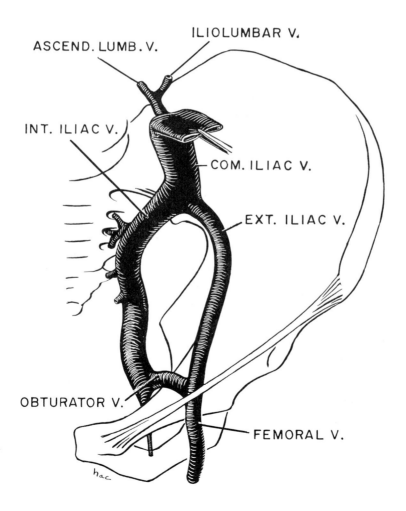

ASCEND. LUMB. V.

ILIOLUMBAR V.

INT. ILIAC V.

COM. ILIAC V.

EXT. ILIAC V.

OBTURATOR V.

FEMORAL V.

hac

FIG. 30
Anomalously large obturator vein. The communication from the external iliac crossed the femoral ring.

the same location and thus is in relationship to the inguinal ligament. This vein can be huge, as in the case shown in Figure 30.

In the earliest pectineal ligament repairs the inguinal ligament was the relatively mobile structure approximated to the pectineal ligament (Seelig and Tuholske, 1914; Koontz, 1963). This was shortly followed by suture of the falx inguinalis to the pectineal ligament. This operation is carefully described by McVay and Anson (1949). McVay (1954) recommended this repair for femoral, direct inguinal, and large indirect inguinal hernias. The steps in these procedures are shown in Figure 31. Note that McVay uses an incision in the rectus sheath to relax the falx in the repair of inguinal hernia, but usually finds it unnecessary in the repair of femoral hernia.

HERNIA REPAIR FROM WITHIN; PREPERITONEAL REPAIR

Occasionally, during laparotomy, the surgeon is unexpectedly confronted by a femoral or inguinal hernia. In such cases, the contents may be withdrawn and the neck of the peritoneal sac closed from within. This is a particularly useful maneuver when the hernia represents the previously unrecognized cause of an intestinal obstruction. While the obstruction is thus resolved, the hernia recurs frequently, if not consistently, after this simple repair. A secure repair can be obtained by incising the peritoneum around the neck of the sac and suturing the fascia, as in a planned preperitoneal approach.

Hernia repair by suture of the defect in the transversalis fascia is the aim of the so-called preperitoneal repair. As Nyhus (1971) says, the cure of all groin hernias must restore the integrity of the fascia, and he finds this step alone sufficient. An extraperitoneal view of groin hernias clearly shows the aperture in the fascia through which the peritoneum protrudes. Such views are inadvertently obtained in the course of exposures of the bladder, pelvic ureters, and the prostate, and the occasion has been grasped by many surgeons to repair the hernias thus exposed (Nyhus and Harkins, 1964).

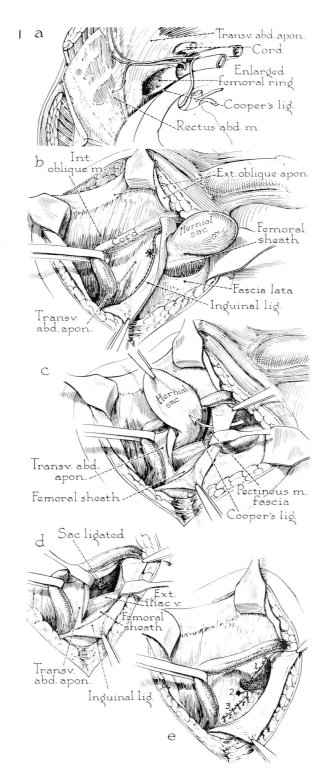

FIG. 31

Pectineal (Cooper's) ligament repair of hernia. (From McVay, C. B.: Hernia, 1954. Courtesy of Charles C Thomas, Publisher, Springfield, Illinois.)

I. Repair of a right femoral hernia. a. Abdominal wall viewed from within after removal of peritoneum and preperitoneal tissue. An anomalous obturator artery is shown, but located lateral and posterior to the femoral ring. b. Operative view: The external oblique aponeurosis is opened. The hernial sac is shown as though exposed in its infrainguinal position. The asterisk and dotted line mark the incision into the transversalis fascia to expose the neck of the sac. c. The sac has been pulled up into the inguinal exposure. d. The sac has been removed after replacement of its contents. The pectineal (Cooper's) ligament is indicated by the broad black line. e. The repair by suture of the transversus aponeurosis (medially the falx) (1) to the pectineal (Cooper's) ligament, (2) to pectineal fascia and femoral sheath, and (3) to the femoral sheath alone. No relaxing incision was necessary.

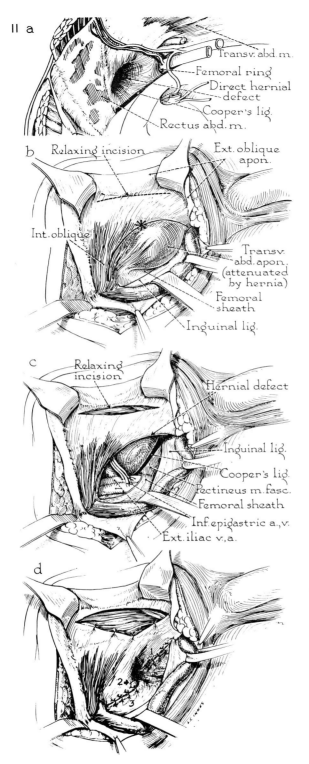

ll a

Transv. abd. m.

Femoral ring

Direct hernial defect

Cooper's lig.

Rectus abd. m.

b Relaxing incision

Ext. oblique apon.

Int. oblique

Transv. abd. apon. (attenuated by hernia)

Femoral sheath

Inguinal lig.

c Relaxing incision

Hernial defect

Inguinal lig.

Cooper's lig.

Pectineus m. fasc.

Femoral sheath

Inf. epigastric a., v.

Ext. iliac v., a.

d

2
3

FIG. 31

Pectineal ligament repair of hernia (continued).

II. Repair for a right direct inguinal hernia. a. Abdominal wall viewed from within. b. Operative view: The inguinal canal is opened, the bulge of the hernia is seen. The asterisk marks the line of incision through aponeurosis and fascia, to expose the sac and delineate a strong edge of falx inguinalis. The line of the proposed relaxing incision is indicated. c. The attenuated aponeurosis and fascia have been excised to expose the sac and the structures to be used in repair. As is often the case with direct hernia, the sac is a wide bulge, and it is not opened or removed. d. Suture of the falx to the lower structures along the line 1, 2, 3, as in I.

Nyhus (1971) practiced deliberate preperitoneal approach and repair of femoral and inguinal hernias in over 1200 cases. He makes the exposure through a transverse incision above the level of the inguinal canal and the internal spermatic ring. The incision passes through the three anterolateral muscles and enough of the rectus sheath to allow medial retraction of the rectus muscle. Division of the transversalis fascia gives entrance to the preperitoneal space in which the hernial sac is seen. The sac is drawn upward, its contents are reduced, and the sac is then removed. When there is a long inguinal sac Nyhus sections it, leaving its distal part intact. Hydrocele is an infrequent complication following this procedure.

Repair involves a firm closure of the fascia of the hernial ring. Nyhus agrees with older writers on the existence of a special thickening of the transversalis fascia, the iliopubic tract, lying internal to the inguinal ligament, and extending from the iliac fascia to the superior border of the pubis (Fig. 32). He admits that in some instances it consists of only a few fibers. In such cases the needle must engage a good width of fascia to compensate for the thinness of the tract. His technique in the three types of groin hernia is shown

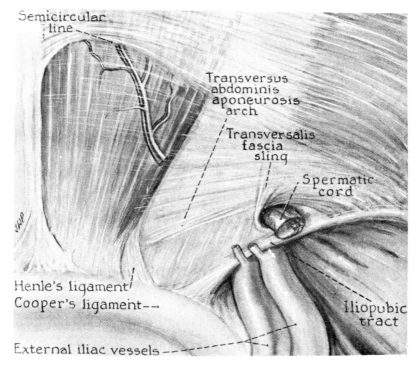

FIG. 32

Preperitoneal view of anterior abdominal wall, emphasizing the iliopubic tract, a thickening of the transversalis fascia, lying internal to the inguinal ligament. The pectineal ligament is here labeled Cooper's ligament; Henle's ligament is an occasionally encountered extension of the rectus tendon. The transversalis fascia sling separating the internal ring from the inferior epigastric vessels is a tenuous structure, also called the interfoveolar ligament. (From Condon, 1964.)

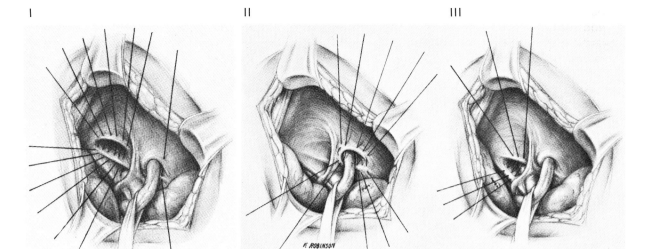

I   II   III

FIG. 33

Preperitoneal repair of hernia. The repair is shown after withdrawal or section of the hernial sac and closure of the peritoneal defect. I. Right direct inguinal hernia: The ring is closed by suture of the arch of the transversus abdominis and its fascial lining to the iliopubic tract. A single suture is placed lateral to the spermatic cord to correct a lax internal ring. II. Right indirect inguinal hernia: The superior crus of the internal ring is sutured to the inferior crus (iliopubic tract). III. Right femoral hernia: Sutures are placed between the iliopubic tract and the pectineal ligament. (From Nyhus, 1971.)

in Figure 33. For direct hernia (Fig. 33 I), the overlying falx inguinalis, as well as the fascia, is secured by the suture at the upper border of the defect; below, the pectineal ligament may be included with the iliopubic tract if the tract is attenuated. A relaxing incision in the rectus sheath (see Fig. 31 I) may be required. An indirect inguinal hernia (Fig. 33 II) is closed by fascial approximation alone; a femoral hernia (Fig. 33 III) is closed by suture of the displaced iliopubic tract to the pectineal ligament.

REFERENCES

Anson, B. J.: Morris' Human Anatomy, 12th ed. New York, Blakiston, 1966.

Anson, B. J., and McVay, C. B.: Surgical Anatomy, 5th ed. Philadelphia, W. B. Saunders, 1971.

Bevan, A. D.: in Discussion on Graham, R. R.: The operative repair of sliding hernia of the sigmoid. Ann. Surg. 102:784–792, 1935.

Burdick, C. G., and Higinbotham, N. L.: Division of the spermatic cord as an aid in operating on selected types of inguinal hernia. Ann. Surg. 102:863–874, 1935.

Condon, R. E.: The Anatomy of the Inguinal Region and Its Relationship to Groin Hernias. Chapter 2 *in* Hernia, Nyhus, L. M., and Harkins, H. N., Eds. Philadelphia, J. B. Lippincott, 1964.

Edwards, E. A., and LeMay, M.: Occlusion patterns and collaterals in arteriosclerosis of the lower aorta and iliac arteries. Surgery 38:950–963, 1955.

Harrison, J. H.: Resection of the spermatic cord in inguinal hernia repair (Editorial). Amer. J. Surg. 121:631–633, 1971.

Heifetz, C. J.: Resection of the spermatic cord in selected inguinal hernias. Twenty years of experience. Arch. Surg. 102:36–39, 1971.

Koontz, A. R.: Historical analysis of femoral hernia. Surgery 53:551–555, 1963.

McVay, C. B.: Hernia. The Pathologic Anatomy of the More Common Hernias and Their Anatomic Repair. Springfield, Charles C Thomas, 1954.

McVay, C. B., and Anson, B. J.: Inguinal and femoral hernioplasty. Surg. Gynec. Obstet. 88:473–485, 1949.

McVay, C. B., and Savage, L. E.: Etiology of femoral hernia. Ann. Surg. 154(Suppl.): 25–32, 1961.

Martin, E.: Operations for Inguinal Hernia. Chapter 41 *in* Gynecology and Abdominal Surgery, Kelly, H. A., and Noble, C. P., Eds. Vol. II. Philadelphia, W. B. Saunders, 1908.

Nyhus, L. M.: The Preperitoneal Approach and the Iliopubic Tract Repair of Groin Hernias. Chapter 70 *in* The Craft of Surgery, Cooper, P., Ed., 2nd ed. Vol. II. Boston, Little, Brown, 1971.

Nyhus, L. M., and Harkins, H. N., Eds.: Hernia. Philadelphia, J. B. Lippincott, 1964.

Seelig, M. G., and Tuholske, L.: The inguinal route operation for femoral hernia; with a supplementary note on Cooper's ligament. Surg. Gynec. Obstet. 18:55–62, 1914.

Watson, L. F.: Hernia. Anatomy, Etiology, Symptoms, Diagnosis, Differential Diagnosis, Prognosis, and the Operative and Injection Treatment, 2nd ed. St. Louis, C. V. Mosby, 1938.

SECTION 2
Major Vessels, Lymphatics, and Autonomic Nerves

4

abdominal AORTA
and its branches

TOPOGRAPHY; DIAMETER

The major topographic landmarks for the abdominal aorta and its branches are shown in Figure 34. The abdominal aorta begins at the aortic hiatus, marked by the arcuate ligament of the diaphragm and the usual origin of the inferior phrenic arteries at the level of the 12th thoracic vertebra. Externally this level is 2 or 3 cm. below the tip of the xiphoid process (Feller and Woodburne, 1961). The aorta usually bifurcates over the body of the 4th lumbar vertebra, a level marked externally by the umbilicus and the line between the most lateral parts of the iliac crests. The level of this trans-cristal line ranges from the 3rd lumbar disc to the body of the 5th lumbar vertebra; it is likely to be at the lower range in women (Edwards, 1951). Location of the bifurcation of the aorta shows a similar range, with a tendency to downward displacement with age (Adachi, 1928).

The range of variation of vertebral level of origin of the major branches of the abdominal aorta is shown in Table 3, based on Adachi (1928), George (1935), Cauldwell and Anson (1943), and Feller and Woodburne (1961). One or both inferior phrenic arteries may arise from the celiac or

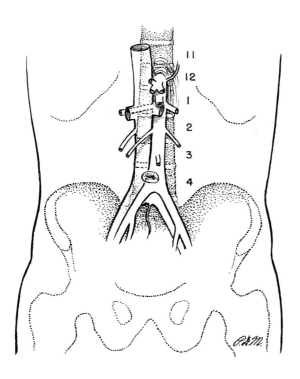

FIG. 34
Levels of branching of the abdominal aorta.

the superior mesenteric. The celiac and superior mesenteric arteries may rarely possess a common stem. Small supra-renal branches arise irregularly from the aorta at this same high level. Accessory renal arteries are most likely to be given off inferior to the major renal arteries. A gonadal artery may arise from a renal.

Four pairs of lumbar arteries originate at the levels of the first four lumbar vertebrae or the discs below, then course

TABLE 3
*Vertebral Level of Origin of Major Branches of the Abdominal Aorta.**

Artery	Most Frequent	Range
Inferior Phrenic	T XII disc	T XI to L I disc
Celiac	T XII disc or L I	T XI to L I disc
Superior Mesenteric	L I	T XII to L II
Renal	L I	T XII to L II disc
Gonadal	L II	L I to L III disc
Inferior Mesenteric	L III	L II to L III disc
Common Iliac (aortic bifurcation)	L IV	L III disc to L V

*Based on Adachi (1928), George (1935), Cauldwell and Anson (1943), and Feller and Woodburne (1961).

laterally over the bodies of the corresponding vertebrae. One or two 5th lumbar arteries may be present, usually coming off the median sacral artery close to that vessel's take-off from the back of the aortic bifurcation.

According to Roessle and Roulet (1932), the internal diameter of the abdominal aorta and of the common iliac arteries have the following values, averaged for the two sexes: At birth the aorta at the diaphragm is 2.1 cm. in diameter, in its lower part, 1.3 cm.; the common iliac, 1.1 cm. The vessels widen with age. At the seventh decade the corresponding measurements are given as: 5.5 cm., 4.8 cm., and 2.8 cm.

COLLATERALS FOR THE ABDOMINAL AORTA

Collaterals in obstruction of the infrarenal segment of the abdominal aorta were studied by aortography and dissection by Edwards and LeMay (1955). In these cases, the superior rectal artery was the single largest vessel reaching the iliac systems (Fig. 35). When the inferior mesenteric is occluded at its take-off, flow through the superior rectal comes from

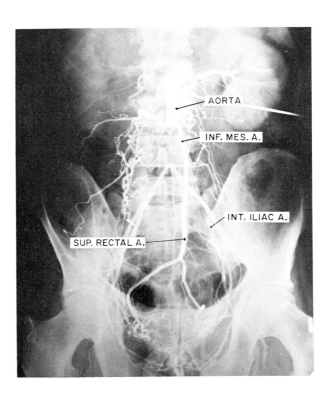

FIG. 35
Collaterals in localized obstruction of the lower aorta. The inferior mesenteric through the superior rectal artery is the major affluent of the anastomoses. The superior rectal artery characteristically bifurcates on the rectum; the middle and inferior rectal arteries conduct the flow to the iliac systems. (From Edwards, 1957.)

the much enlarged marginal artery of the colon, thus remotely from the superior mesenteric. Many smaller vessels send branches downward to the iliac arteries in instances of aortic or common iliac artery obstruction. These include the lower intercostal and lumbar arteries and the adipose capsular branches of the renals. The superior to inferior epigastric pathway, important in aortic coarctation, does not seem as significant in arteriosclerosis.

Observations on obstruction of the upper abdominal aorta are fragmentary. Presumably supradiaphragmatic arteries—the internal thoracic and intercostals—conduct blood to the upward-coursing branches of the internal iliac and the lumbar and inferior epigastric arteries, and thus to the aorta below the obstruction. Occlusion of either the celiac or superior mesenteric arteries can be overcome by flow through the pancreaticoduodenal arteries; that of the inferior mesenteric by flow from the superior mesenteric through the marginal artery of the large bowel; and that of the renal arteries by flow through collateral branches derived from parietal vessels, although hypertension may result from persistent partial renal ischemia. Instances have been recorded of survival after occlusion of several visceral arteries or of the upper abdominal aorta, the parietal arteries acting as a collateral source (see page 215).

EXPOSURES OF THE LOWER AORTA AND
THE RENAL ARTERIES

An exposure of the lower aorta which may require a view of the renal arteries, but no higher, is usually gained by a transperitoneal laparotomy. In thin individuals, the peritoneum is incised directly over the aorta and iliac vessels. In others a U-shaped incision is made in the posterior peritoneum from below the duodenojejunal junction downward and around the cecum and ascending colon (Fig. 36). The jejunum, ileum, and cecum and ascending colon, with their mesenteries, can now be reflected upward.

The frequently occluded inferior mesenteric artery must be divided; if patent it is freed from its surroundings. The testicular or ovarian arteries generally escape notice in the arteriosclerotic patient, since they are usually occluded

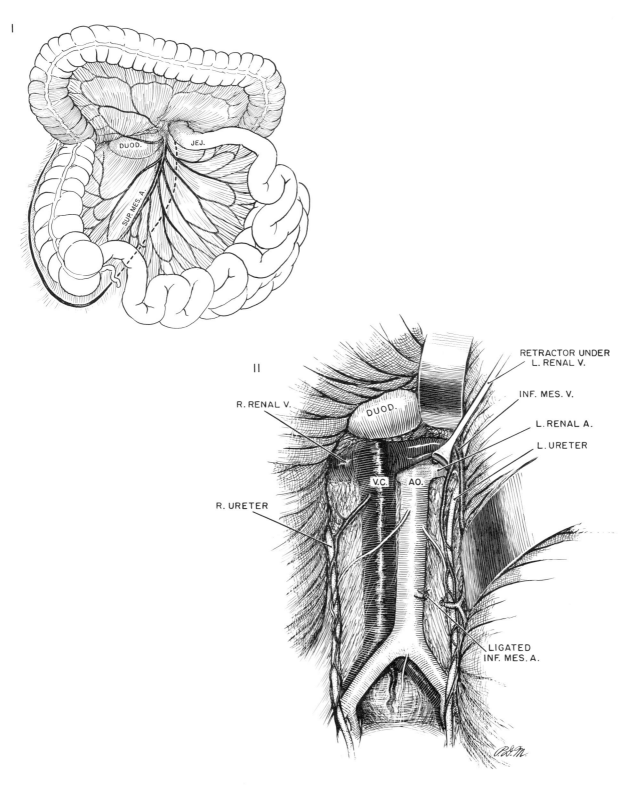

FIG. 36
Exposure of the lower aorta. I. Incision in the posterior peritoneum for elevation of the bowel. II. Extent of the exposure.

(Edwards and LeMay, 1955). On the left the left colic artery is seen ascending beneath the peritoneum, along with the inferior mesenteric vein. The vein turns medially behind the duodenojejunal junction. Division of the inferior mesenteric vein alone produces no recognizable changes, but it may play a part in bowel necrosis when added to division of the inferior mesenteric artery (Ottinger et al., 1972). Laterally, the ureter on each side descends 2 to 4 cm. from the aorta, to cross the brim of the pelvis over the bifurcation of the common iliac artery.

Above the origin of the inferior mesenteric artery three structures cross the aorta anteriorly: the transverse part of the duodenum, with the pancreas above it, and, on a deeper plane and somewhat higher, the left renal vein. The duodenum and pancreas, and the left renal vein, must be retracted to see the origin of the renal arteries. The left renal vein may have one component anterior and one posterior to the aorta ('renal collar'); rarely it may be entirely retro-aortic (see Fig. 40). Mobility for retraction of the renal vein may be gained by dividing the left suprarenal and the gonadal veins, and freeing the initial part of the superior mesenteric artery which overlies it above. It appears that the renal vein may be divided if necessary (Neal and Shearburn, 1967; DeLaurentis, 1970). It usually need not be reconstituted, since the left ascending lumbar and the hemiazygos vein offer an excellent collateral pathway peculiar to the left side (Edwards, 1958). A view of the origin of the right renal artery is often facilitated by dividing one or two lumbar veins here to allow retraction of the cava. Brener and his associates (1974) have reported on anomalies of the cava and the renal vein complicating abdominal aortic surgery.

More intimately, the aorta and iliac vessels are surrounded by a substantial sheath and by the heavy aortic and iliac nerve plexuses and the aortic lymph nodes. Three or four strands of the presacral nerves (superior hypogastric plexus) are seen in front of the aortic bifurcation (see Fig. 211). The bifurcation sits astride the termination of the left common iliac vein and the beginning of the inferior vena cava. The origins of the lumbar and the median sacral arteries and left lumbar veins are also related to the posterior surface of the aorta. Small retro-aortic veins are common, and large anomalous veins may also be present. These are persistent portions of the embryonic left inferior vena cava and intercaval anastomoses (see Fig. 40). Posterolaterally, on the right, the aorta is in contact with the infrahepatic vena cava; in its upper extent it is in contact with the cisterna chyli (see Fig. 45), and in some instances with the azygos vein, deep to the right crus of the diaphragm. Posterolaterally, on the left, lies the left lumbar sympathetic trunk, and, at a higher level, the hemiazygos vein (see Fig. 48).

A better view at the renal level is obtained, after the abdomen has been entered, by incising the peritoneum around the splenic flexure of the colon. This organ and the duodenojejunal flexure, plus the root of the mesentery, are now retracted to the right, after division of the usually thin material constituting the suspensory muscle of the duodenum, or ligament of Treitz. This differs from the approach for the entire abdominal aorta shown in Figure 37, in that there the organs retracted include the spleen. A similar approach for the right renal artery is effected by incising the peritoneum to the right of the hepatic flexure of the colon and the duodenum, retracting these structures and the head of the pancreas to the left (see Fig. 168). Trippel and O'Conor (1962) expose both renal arteries through a 'chevron,' or subcostal, incision (see Fig. 9), then mobilize the peritoneum and intraperitoneal organs from either side toward the midline.

The aortic bifurcation, iliac arteries, and the lower lumbar sympathetic trunks can be exposed extraperitoneally. The incision is made in the lower quadrant of the desired side, with or without division of the rectus muscle just below the umbilicus. If required, the incision may be carried across the opposite side, creating a low transverse incision. Rob (1963), to expose the infrarenal aorta and the iliac arteries, has used a higher left extraperitoneal incision starting at the tip of the 12th rib, continuing across the left rectus muscle below the umbilicus.

Operations on the lower aorta and iliac arteries for aneurysm or obstruction carry a small incidence of ischemic damage to the colon and rectum, bladder, or spinal cord. Necrosis of the bowel has been explained by the division of a previously patent inferior mesenteric artery (Birnbaum *et al.,* 1964; Ottinger *et al.,* 1972), or of an anomalous vessel connecting the two mesenteric arteries (Gonzalez and Jaffe,

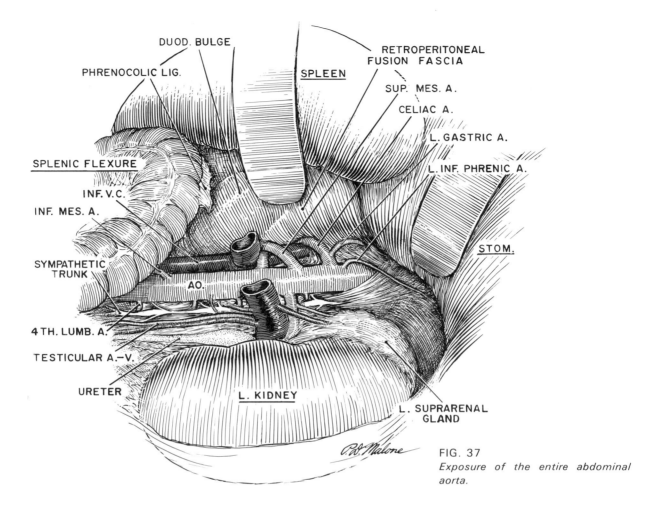

DUOD. BULGE

PHRENOCOLIC LIG.

SPLEEN

RETROPERITONEAL
FUSION FASCIA

SUP. MES. A.

CELIAC A.

L. GASTRIC A.

SPLENIC FLEXURE

L. INF. PHRENIC A.

INF. V.C.

INF. MES. A.

STOM.

SYMPATHETIC
TRUNK

AO.

4 TH. LUMB. A.

TESTICULAR A.–V.

URETER

L. KIDNEY

L. SUPRARENAL
GLAND

FIG. 37
*Exposure of the entire abdominal
aorta.*

1966); by concomitant injury of the inferior mesenteric vein (Ottinger *et al.*); or by the failure to reconstitute flow through at least one internal iliac artery (Smith and Szilagyi, 1960). Zimberg and Sullivan (1964) report a rare complication of midgut necrosis, based on prior occlusion of the superior mesenteric and celiac arteries. Internal iliac obstruction is presumed to be the cause of the extremely rare necrosis of the bladder (Campbell, 1960). Additional matter relating to complications of ligation of the internal iliac artery is presented below. Paraplegia has occurred after operations on the abdominal aorta, although it is much rarer than after procedures on the thoracic aorta. Skillman and his colleagues (1969) have collected several instances of this catastrophe after excision of an abdominal aortic aneurysm. It is presumably due to the division of a lumbar artery that had given rise to the arteria radicularis magna. The source of this significant vessel to the cord is most often a 2nd lumbar artery, but its origin ranges from the 8th thoracic to the 4th lumbar (Suh and Alexander, 1939; see also Edwards *et al.,* 1972).

EXPOSURES OF UPPER ABDOMINAL AORTA AND CELIAC AND SUPERIOR MESENTERIC ARTERIES

Exposure of the abdominal aorta at this high level is made by mobilizing the spleen, duodenojejunal flexure, pancreas, and left colon, and retracting them to the right (Fig. 37). Some mobility is gained by loosening the tissues about the proximal superior mesenteric artery. The initial incision may be abdominal (Bergan, 1967; Buscaglia *et al.,* 1969), or left thoracoabdominal, especially if it is required to secure the lower thoracic, in addition to the abdominal, aorta (DeBakey *et al.,* 1956; Starzl and Trippel, 1959). Any of these approaches are easily extended downward to make available the renal arteries or the entire course of the abdominal aorta. A limited view of the upper abdominal aorta, as for initial control in ruptured aneurysm, is available through the omental bursa.

A special impetus to surgical exposure about the origin of the celiac artery has been given by the recognition of the 'median arcuate ligament syndrome,' wherein the celiac and perhaps the superior mesenteric artery are compressed by the median arcuate ligament of the diaphragm and possibly by the celiac nerve plexus as well (Lindner and Kemprud, 1971). Opening the lesser omentum brings these structures into view behind the posterior wall of the omental bursa (see Fig. 152). Exposure of the first few centimeters of the superior mesenteric artery can be gained through the same approach, or by entering the bursa through the gastrocolic omentum (Jackson, 1963). The upper border of the pancreas must be displaced downward by dividing the pancreatic plexus of the nerves which course to the organ from the celiac and superior mesenteric plexuses (Yoshioka and Wakabayashi, 1958). Care must be taken to avoid injury to the superior mesenteric vein or veins, the inferior mesenteric vein, and the splenic vessels (see Fig. 72).

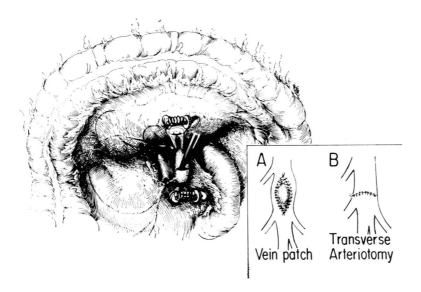

FIG. 38
Superior mesenteric artery embolectomy. The embolus is usually lodged proximal to the site of the arteriotomy shown. (From Bergan, 1967.)

The superior mesenteric artery can be exposed below the transverse mesocolon to the right of the duodenojejunal junction (Fig. 38). The artery is mobilized above the terminal duodenum after dividing the suspensory ligament and displacing the pancreas upward (Shaw and Maynard, 1958; Jackson, 1963) (see Fig. 76). The first large branch of the artery seen is the midcolic artery, and its origin is the usual site of lodgment of an embolus.

In operations for chronic occlusion of the origin of the celiac or superior mesenteric artery the vessel is frequently vascularized by a bypass graft taken from the infrarenal aorta. For the celiac artery, the path is through the transverse mesocolon, then retropancreatic or prepancreatic. For the superior mesenteric artery, the aorta is approached either through the common anterior infrarenal path (as above) or through a right retroperitoneal dissection (see Fig. 118). The posterior aspect of the superior mesenteric artery is available through either aortic approach, and the graft is placed between the two vessels.

VARIETIES OF BRANCHING OF THE
INTERNAL ILIAC ARTERIES

The internal iliac artery is subject to considerable variation in its branching (Adachi, 1928; Roberts and Krishingner, 1967). The artery commonly divides into a smaller posterior and a larger anterior division, as in Figure 39. In roughly half of all subjects the posterior division gives off the superior gluteal, iliolumbar, and lateral sacral arteries. In others the inferior gluteal and, uncommonly, the internal pudendal as well also stem from the posterior division.

The anterior division has both parietal and visceral branches. The parietal are the inferior gluteal and obturator arteries. With extreme rarity, the inferior gluteal may be the major artery of the lower limb, with the popliteal its direct continuation, as in the early embryo (Adachi, 1928). The obturator arises from the external iliac, usually in common with the inferior epigastric artery, in 48 per cent of individuals (Pick *et al.,* 1942). In only about one third of these individuals is the anomaly present on both sides; the incidence of anomalous origin for all obturator arteries is therefore about 30 per cent. The course of the aberrant obturator is significant in relation to femoral hernia (see page 45).

The internal pudendal, which may be considered the visceral branch to the external genitalia, comes off the anterior division alone, or shares a common stem with the inferior gluteal artery ('gluteopudendal trunk'). A separate dorsal artery of the penis ('accessory internal pudendal') may arise from the anterior division of the iliac, or the obturator artery ('normal,' or aberrant), to run on the superior aspect of the pelvic diaphragm and then beneath the pubic arch.

Other visceral branches of the internal iliac vary in both origin and number, but many originate close to or in common with the umbilical artery. The proximal umbilical artery maintains a lumen after birth; superior vesical arteries are constant branches. Additionally, in the male, the deferential artery is almost always a distinct vessel arising from the umbilical (Braithwaite, 1952). The inferior vesical artery, often arising from the pudendal, or from a combined gluteo-pudendal trunk, gives off five or six branches to the prostate (collectively called the prostatic artery) and to the base of the bladder (Flocks, 1937; Roberts and Krishingner, 1967). Clegg (1955) found that the prostatic artery occasionally arose from the middle or even the superior rectal artery at the side of the rectum. The uterine artery is most often a separate branch of the anterior division, next most often a branch of the umbilical (Roberts and Krishingner). The vaginal artery either replaces the inferior vesical or is com-

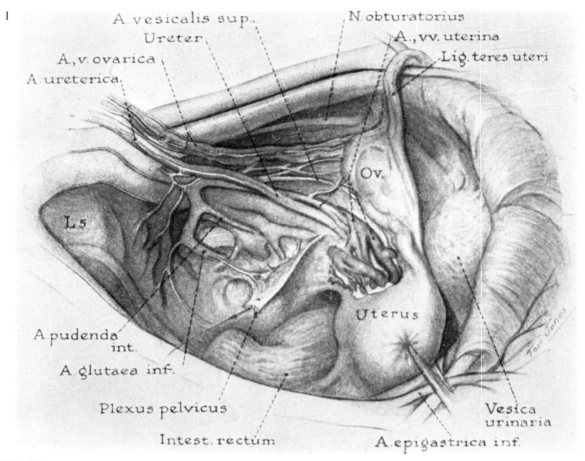

FIG. 39
Arteries, veins, and nerves on the side wall of the female pelvis.
  I. Arteries and veins beneath the peritoneum. The course of the ureter is clearly shown.

bined with it (see Fig. 215). Roberts and Krishingner could find a middle rectal artery in 66 per cent of specimens examined. When present it arose most often from the internal pudendal, or from a gluteopudendal trunk.

LIGATION OF THE INTERNAL ILIAC ARTERY

Unilateral or bilateral ligation of the internal iliac has often been performed to control hemorrhage, especially in gynecologic surgery or after obstetrical delivery (Siegel and Mengert, 1961; Reich and Nechtow, 1961) and in fracture of the pelvis; to limit bleeding in operations as for carcinoma of the cervix or abdominoperineal resection of the colon

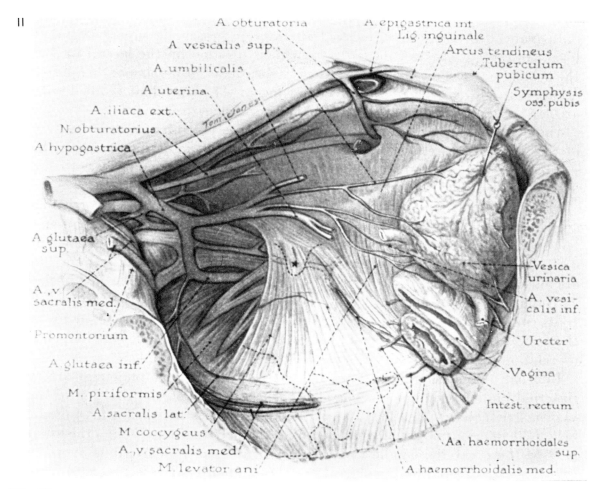

II

A. obturatoria
A. vesicalis sup.
A. umbilicalis
A. uterina
A. iliaca ext.
N. obturatorius
A. hypogastrica
A. glutaea sup.
A., v. sacralis med.
Promontorium
A. glutaea inf.
M. piriformis
A. sacralis lat.
M. coccygeus
A., v. sacralis med.
M. levator ani

A. epigastrica int.
Lig. inguinale
Arcus tendineus
Tuberculum pubicum
Symphysis oss. pubis
Vesica urinaria
A. vesicalis inf.
Ureter
Vagina
Intest. rectum
Aa. haemorrhoidales sup.
A. haemorrhoidalis med.

FIG. 39

Arteries, veins, and nerves on the side wall of the female pelvis (continued).

II. Arteries and nerves of deeper dissection. The ovarian artery has been removed, and the uterine artery divided. The obturator artery has an aberrant origin from the inferior epigastric. Its course lateral to the external iliac vein is unusual. Arteries to the bladder, vagina, and terminal rectum are shown. The middle rectal (hemorrhoidal) stems from the internal pudendal in this subject. The asterisk marks the position of the ischial spine. Posteriorly the major bulk of the sciatic nerve is being formed by the union of the lumbosacral trunk (L-4,5) with the anterior rami of S-1,2. The superior gluteal artery leaves between the lumbosacral trunk and S-1. Below the sciatic nerve lies the inferior gluteal artery above the anterior rami of S-3,4. (From Curtis et al., 1942. By permission of Surgery, Gynecology & Obstetrics.)

(McGregor, 1959), or hindquarter amputation; or in the treatment of aneurysm of the internal iliac artery.

Exposure of the internal iliac artery can be extraperitoneal, but bilateral ligation is usually done transperitoneally. In the latter instance, unless the cecum lies low and needs mobilization, the right artery is approached directly through the peritoneum. The left artery is approached by incising the posterior peritoneum lateral to the sigmoid, to enable the bowel and its vessels to be pushed medially with the peritoneum. On either side, the ureter is reflected from its position anterior to the iliac bifurcation. The internal iliac vein lies postero-medial to the artery and is crossed medially by the anterior division of the artery. The external iliac vein lies lateral to the internal iliac artery. The union of the two veins and the initial portion of the common iliac vein lie behind the most proximal part of the internal iliac artery.

The collaterals for the vessel include the inferior mesenteric, the lumbar and sacral, and the ovarian arteries, from above; and the medial and lateral femoral circumflex arteries, from below. Ligation of the internal iliac artery has failed to control hemorrhage from fracture of the pelvis (Peltier, 1965; Huittinen and Slätis, 1973), probably because of these collaterals. Rare instances are also reported of ischemic necrosis of the perineum, buttocks, or bladder following the arterial ligation (Finaly, 1925; Tajes, 1956). Failure to restore internal iliac flow in the course of operations on the aorta has also been implicated in the uncommon instances of ischemic damage to the viscera (see above).

REFERENCES

Adachi, B.: Das Arteriensystem der Japaner. Vol. II. Kyoto, Kenkyusha, 1928.

Bergan, J. J.: Recognition and treatment of intestinal ischemia. Surg. Clin. N. Amer. 47:109–126, 1967.

Birnbaum, W., Rudy, L., and Wylie, E. J.: Colonic and rectal ischemia following abdominal aneurysmectomy. Dis. Colon Rectum 7:293–302, 1964.

Braithwaite, J. L.: The arterial supply of the male urinary bladder. Brit. J. Urol. 24:64–71, 1952.

Brener, B. J., Darling, R. C., Frederick, P. L., and Linton, R. R.: Major venous anomalies complicating abdominal aortic surgery. Arch. Surg. 108:159–165, 1974.

Buscaglia, L. C., Blaisdell, F. W., and Lim, R. C., Jr.: Penetrating abdominal vascular injuries. Arch. Surg. 99:764–769, 1969.

Campbell, D. A.: in Discussion on Smith, R. F., and Szilagyi, D. E., Arch. Surg. 80:820–821, 1960.

Cauldwell, E. W., and Anson, B. J.: The visceral branches of the abdominal aorta: Topographical relationships. Amer. J. Anat. 73:27–57, 1943.

Clegg, E. J.: The arterial supply of the human prostate and seminal vesicles. J. Anat. 89:209–216, 1955.

Curtis, A. H., Anson, B. J., Ashley, F. L., and Jones, T.: The blood vessels of the female pelvis in relation to gynecological surgery. Surg. Gynec. Obstet. 75:421–423, 1942.

DeBakey, M. E., Creech, O., Jr., and Morris, G. C., Jr.: Aneurysm of thoracoabdominal aorta involving the celiac, superior mesenteric, and renal arteries: Report of four cases treated by resection and homograft replacement. Ann. Surg. 144:549–573, 1956.

DeLaurentis, D. A.: Renal vein ligation (Letter to the editor). J.A.M.A. 214:1889, 1970.

Edwards, E. A.: Operative anatomy of the lumbar sympathetic chain. Angiology 2:184–198, 1951.

Edwards, E. A.: Choice of therapy for peripheral arteriosclerosis. New Eng. J. Med. 256:875–880, 1957.

Edwards, E. A.: The anatomy of collateral circulation. Surg. Gynec. Obstet. 107:183–194, 1958.

Edwards, E. A., and LeMay, M.: Occlusion patterns and collaterals in arteriosclerosis of the lower aorta and iliac arteries. Surgery 38:950–963, 1955.

Edwards, E. A., Malone, P. D., and Collins, J. J., Jr.: Operative Anatomy of Thorax. Philadelphia, Lea & Febiger, 1972.

Feller, I., and Woodburne, R. T.: Surgical anatomy of the abdominal aorta. Ann. Surg. 154(Suppl.):239–252, 1961.

Finaly, R.: Over stoornissen ten gevolge van onderbinden der beide arteriae hypogastricae. Nederl. T. Geneesk. 69:1115–1119, 1925.

Flocks, R. H.: The arterial distribution within the prostate gland. Its role in transurethral prostatic resection. J. Urol. 37:524–548, 1937.

George, R.: Topography of the unpaired visceral branches of the abdominal aorta. J. Anat. 69:196–205, 1935.

Gonzalez, L. L., and Jaffe, M. S.: Mesenteric arterial insufficiency following abdominal aortic resection. Arch. Surg. 93:10–20, 1966.

Huittinen, V. M., and Slätis, P.: Postmortem angiography and dissection of the hypogastric artery in pelvic fractures. Surgery 73:454–462, 1973.

Jackson, B. B.: Occlusion of the Superior Mesenteric Artery. Springfield, Charles C Thomas, 1963.

Lindner, H. H., and Kemprud, E.: A clinicoanatomical study of the arcuate ligament of the diaphragm. Arch. Surg. 103:600–605, 1971.

McGregor, R. A.: Ligation of the hypogastric arteries in combined abdominoperineal surgery. Dis. Colon Rectum 2:166–168, 1959.

Neal, H. S., and Shearburn, E. W.: Division of the left renal vein as an adjunct to resection of abdominal aortic aneurysms. Amer. J. Surg. 113:763–765, 1967.

Ottinger, L. W., Darling, R. C., Nathan, M. J., and Linton, R. R.: Left colon ischemia complicating aorto-iliac reconstruction. Arch. Surg. 105:841–846, 1972.

Peltier, L. F.: Complications associated with fractures of the pelvis. J. Bone Joint Surg. 47-A:1060–1069, 1965.

Pick, J. W., Anson, B. J., and Ashley, F. L.: The origin of the obturator artery. A study of 640 body-halves. Amer. J. Anat. 70:317–343, 1942.

Reich, W. J., and Nechtow, M. J.: Ligation of the internal iliac (hypogastric) arteries: A life-saving procedure for uncontrollable gynecologic and obstetric hemorrhage. J. Int. Coll. Surg. 36:157–168, 1961.

Rob, C.: Extraperitoneal approach to the abdominal aorta. Surgery 53:87–89, 1963.

Roberts, W. H., and Krishingner, G. L.: Comparative study of human internal iliac artery based on Adachi classification. Anat. Rec. 158:191–196, 1967.

Roessle, R., and Roulet, F.: Mass und Zahl in der Pathologie. Berlin, Springer, 1932.

Shaw, R. S., and Maynard, E. P., III: Acute and chronic thrombosis of the mesenteric arteries associated with malabsorption. A report of two cases successfully treated by thromboendarterectomy. New Eng. J. Med. 258:874–878, 1958.

Siegel, P., and Mengert, W. F.: Internal iliac artery ligation in obstetrics and gynecology. J.A.M.A. 178:1059–1062, 1961.

Skillman, J. J., Zervas, N. T., Weintraub, R. M., and Mayman, C. I.: Paraplegia after resection of aneurysms of the abdominal aorta. New Eng. J. Med. 281:422–425, 1969.

Smith, R. F., and Szilagyi, D. E.: Ischemia of the colon as a complication in the surgery of the abdominal aorta. Arch. Surg. 80:806–821, 1960.

Starzl, T. E., and Trippel, O. H.: Reno-mesentero-aorto-iliac thromboendarterectomy in patient with malignant hypertension. Surgery 46:556–564, 1959.

Suh, T. H., and Alexander, L.: Vascular system of the human spinal cord. Arch. Neurol. Psych. 41:659–677, 1939.

Tajes, R. V.: Ligation of the hypogastric arteries and its complications in resection of cancer of the rectum. Amer. J. Gastroent. 26:612–618, 1956.

Trippel, O. H., and O'Conor, V. J., Jr.: Renovascular hypertension. Surg. Clin. N. Amer. 42:109–130, 1962.

Yoshioka, H., and Wakabayashi, T.: Therapeutic neurotomy on head of pancreas for relief of pain due to chronic pancreatitis. A new technical procedure and its results. Arch. Surg. 76:546–554, 1958.

Zimberg, Y. H., and Sullivan, J. M.: Midgut gangrene after resection of an infrarenal aortic aneurysm. Case report and discussion of the collateral flow potential of the abdominal viscera. Amer. J. Surg. 107:785–788, 1964.

ThE iNfERiOR VENA CAVA; MAJOR lyMphATiC pAThWAYS

TOPOGRAPHY OF THE INFERIOR VENA CAVA

The inferior vena cava may be divided into infrarenal, renal, and hepatic segments, the last-named including its terminal intrathoracic portion. The vena cava begins by the confluence of the common iliac veins on the 5th lumbar vertebra, a bit below the aortic bifurcation, and overlain on the left by this bifurcation (see Fig. 36). It ascends on the right anterior aspect of the lumbar vertebrae. The renal veins enter at the 2nd lumbar level. The cava lies behind the epiploic foramen for about 4 cm. (see Fig. 101), then enters the caval groove of the liver at the level of the 12th thoracic vertebra. It passes through the diaphragm at the level of the 8th thoracic vertebra. The intrathoracic cava is only about 1 cm. long, partly outside and partly within the pericardium.

ANOMALIES OF THE INFERIOR VENA CAVA

The numerous embryonic changes undergone by the great veins of the abdomen set the stage for the many anomalies of the inferior vena cava. These may be divided into those affecting the cava above or below the renal veins.

TABLE 4

*Classification of Anomalies
of the Inferior Vena Cava.*

Topographic Classification	Embryologic Equivalent
I. Major anomalies	
A. In the suprarenal segment	Prerenal cava
1. Azygos continuation (with right, left, or double infrarenal cava)	Persistent supracardinal system ('Absence of the vena cava')
2. Reception of the portal vein	
3. Reception of a right pulmonary vein	
B. In the infrarenal segment	Postrenal cava
1. Double infrarenal (post-ureteric) cava	Persistent left postrenal cava, or persistent supracardinal system. Persistent left supracardinal vein
2. Left infrarenal (post-ureteric) cava	
3. Lateral pre-ureteric cava ('Retrocaval ureter')	Persistent posterior cardinal vein or peri-ureteric ring
4. Medial pre-ureteric cava	Persistent subcardinal vein
5. Coexistent pre-ureteric and post-ureteric cavae	
6. Reception of a portal tributary	
II. Lesser variations	
1. Partial azygos continuation	
2. Infrarenal caval rudiments	
a. Abridged left or right cava	
b. Renal collar: intercaval anastomoses and caval diverticula	
3. Lateral pre-ureteric veins	Persistent posterior cardinal vein
4. Medial pre-ureteric and para-aortic veins	Persistent subcardinal vein

*From Edwards, 1951.

Edwards (1951) proposed a classification based on the gross anatomy of the cava, and correlated his topographic classification of the anomalies with the embryological terms often used in naming them (Table 4). Major anomalies (Fig. 40 I) occur with a frequency variously reported as from 1.5 to 4.4 per cent. As to the lesser variations identified by Edwards (Fig. 40 II), there is hardly an individual who does not harbor some such variation in the inferior vena cava or its major tributaries.

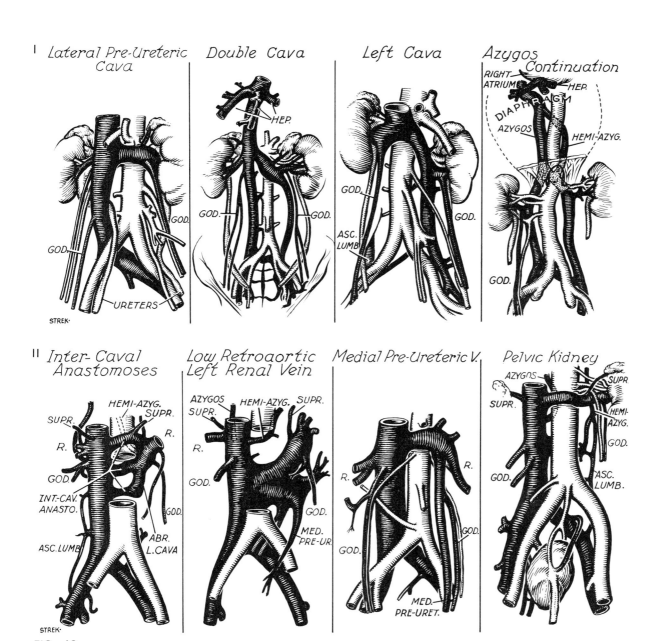

FIG. 40

Anomalies of the inferior vena cava. I. Major anomalies. II. Minor variations. Abr. L. Cava—abridged left vena cava; Int.-Cav-Anasto.—intercaval anastomosis; Asc. Lumb.—ascending lumbar, God.—gonadal, Hemi. Azygo.—hemiazygos, Hep.—hepatic, Med. Pre. Ur.—medial pre-ureteric, R.—renal, Supr.—suprarenal, veins. (From Edwards et al., 1961, adapted from Edwards, 1951.)

THE VERTEBRAL VENOUS SYSTEM

The extravertebral venous plexus (Fig. 41 I) and the intravertebral plexus (Fig. 41 II), together with connecting veins, constitute a chain of vessels which has been termed the 'vertebral venous system' (Batson, 1957). The plexuses ex-

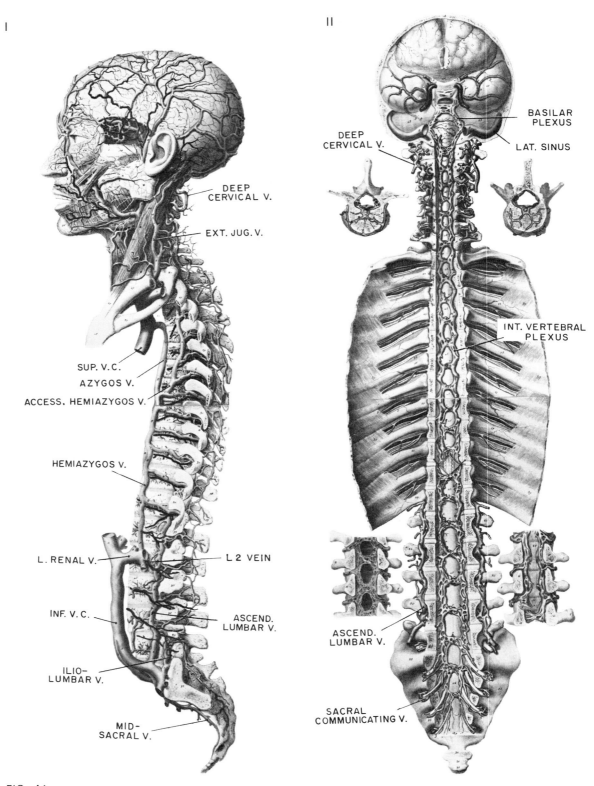

I

II

DEEP
CERVICAL V.

EXT. JUG. V.

SUP. V.C.

AZYGOS V.

ACCESS. HEMIAZYGOS V.

HEMIAZYGOS V.

L. RENAL V.

L 2 VEIN

INF. V.C.

ASCEND.
LUMBAR V.

ILIO-
LUMBAR V.

MID-
SACRAL V.

BASILAR
PLEXUS

DEEP
CERVICAL V.

LAT. SINUS

INT. VERTEBRAL
PLEXUS

ASCEND.
LUMBAR V.

SACRAL
COMMUNICATING V.

FIG. 41
The vertebral venous system and its communications. I, Extravertebral, and II, intravertebral components. (From Breschet, [1829–1830].)

tend from sacral veins below to the intracranial basilar venous sinus above. Connecting longitudinal channels include: in the neck—the deep cervical and the external, internal, and anterior jugular veins, and (not shown in the Figure) the posterior jugular and ascending cervical; in the thorax—the azygos and hemiazygos veins; in the abdomen—the inferior vena cava and iliac veins, and the azygos, hemiazygos, and ascending lumbar veins. The ascending lumbar veins lie in front of the vertebral transverse processes, behind the psoas major muscles, which have been removed in the figure. The large lower end of each ascending lumbar ends in the common iliac vein (see Fig. 52). The left ascending lumbar communicates with the left renal via the second lumbar vein, which also receives the lower end of the hemiazygos vein. On the right, comparable connections between the second lumbar and azygos veins and the renal segment of the inferior vena cava are inconstant.

The normal absence of valves in the vertebral venous system and many of its connecting veins facilitates venous flow between regions and is consistent with the presumed use of the system as a path for emboli of tumor or bacterial cells between the regions involved.

COLLATERALS FOR CAVAL OBSTRUCTION

Collaterals of the infrarenal vena cava in man were studied by Filler and Edwards (1962) with venography. The pathways comprise vessels starting below the obstruction and discharging blood into the cava and other veins at the renal level. Of these veins, the most prominent are the ascending lumbar and gonadal veins. The ovarian veins, when varicosed, are potential sources of recurrent embolism. Less important are the superficial abdominal, the deep circumflex iliac, and the iliolumbar veins. The blood from these vessels must go through anastomotic channels before being discharged to higher levels. The vessels receiving the blood from these channels include the renal vena cava and the left renal, azygos, hemiazygos, lumbar, intercostal, and vertebral veins (Fig. 41).

Major pathways after occlusion at the renal level include the portal system, the ascending lumbar vein, and vertebral veins. In these instances the ascending lumbar vein empties, not at the renal level, but higher into the hemiazygos and azygos veins. For collateral circulation in obstruction at the hepatic level, the ascending lumbar and vertebral veins alone are available (Filler and Edwards, 1962).

EXPOSURES OF THE INFERIOR VENA CAVA

The infrarenal segment of the vena cava is readily available through a right abdominal extraperitoneal exposure. This is usually accomplished by an oblique incision in the right flank similar to that used for lumbar sympathectomy (Fig. 42). Extension of the incision into the rectus sheath, with medial retraction of the muscle, improves the exposure, especially of veins entering the cava from the left. Moran and his colleagues (1969) advise an approach through the bed of the 12th rib, which brings the renal level of the vena cava into view. A simultaneous exposure of the cava and

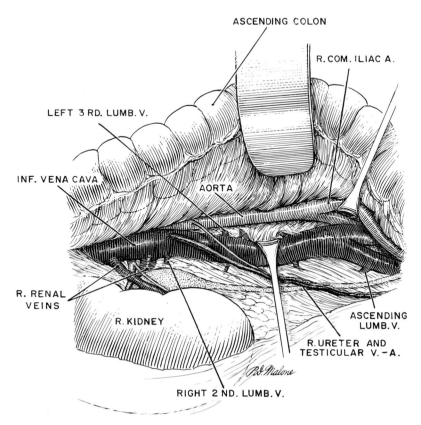

FIG. 42
Relationships of the inferior vena cava. This anatomic exposure is more extensive than that usually seen at operation, as for interruption below the renal veins. In the operative exposure, the ureter and gonadal vessels would be retracted with the peritoneum. (From Edwards, 1975.)

both ovarian veins can be made through laparotomy, mobilizing the duodenum and ascending colon to expose the cava and right ovarian vein, and the descending colon to expose the left ovarian vein.

The renal level of the cava is available by the incision of the 12th rib bed previously mentioned, or by the same methods used to expose this level of the aorta (pp. 58–61), or as part of anterior exposures of the kidney pedicles or suprarenal glands (see Figures 153 and 168).

Visualization of the hepatic segment of the cava, as for injury, is usually accomplished by transhepatic dissection (Chapter 12). The transthoracic portion is available through a right or mid-sternal thoracotomy; from the abdomen a limited view may be obtained by incising the diaphragm (see page 174). Membranous obstruction of the terminal inferior vena cava has been reported mainly from Japan (Yamamoto *et al.,* 1968; Hirooka and Kimura, 1970). The caval obstruction may be accompanied by occlusion of the orifices of the middle and left hepatic veins. Correction has been accomplished by rupturing or dilating the caval membrane by a finger inserted through the right atrium, or by exposing the cava through a right thoracotomy and incising the diaphragm, to allow enlargement of the caval diameter by venotomy and patching, or by the creation of an anastomosis of the cava to the azygos vein (Yamamoto *et al.*).

LYMPHATIC TRUNKS AND NODES

Three major lymphatic pathways of the abdomen terminate in the cisterna chyli. The two lateral para-aortic, or lumbar, trunks and their nodes drain the territory of the paired aortic branches, including the iliac vessels, and receive also the lymph from the inferior mesenteric pathway. The third, pre-aortic in position, stems from the structures supplied by the celiac and superior mesenteric arteries and makes up the intestinal trunk, which enters the cisterna directly or, more commonly, by joining the lumbar trunks (Jossifow, 1906) (Fig. 43). The para-aortic lymph nodes lie to the right and left of the aorta. Those of the right surround the vena cava. Those of the left lie mainly anterior to the aorta, but smaller nodes surround the aorta as well. All are

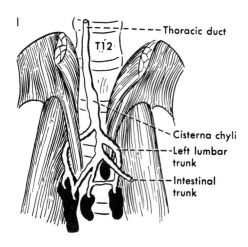

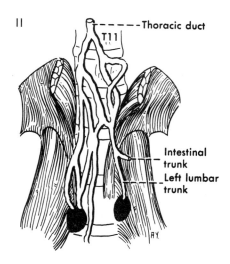

FIG. 43
The cisterna chyli and termination of the abdominal lymphatic trunks. I. The cisterna is saccular; the intestinal trunk joins it directly. II. The cisterna is plexiform; the intestinal trunk joins the left lumbar. (From Hollinshead, 1971, adapted from Jossifow, 1906.)

well interconnected. The iliac nodes and trunks are continuous with the inguinal nodes, as well as with the internal iliac and sacral (or rectal) lymphatics. Figure 44 shows this relationship in the male, and Figure 218 shows that in the female. Details of lymphatic drainage within the celiac territory are shown in Figure 57, and those of drainage of the large intestine, in Figure 146.

THE CISTERNA CHYLI AND THORACIC DUCT

The union of the three major trunks (the two lumbar and the intestinal) may or may not result in a single tubular structure about 5 mm. wide. It is convenient to call the

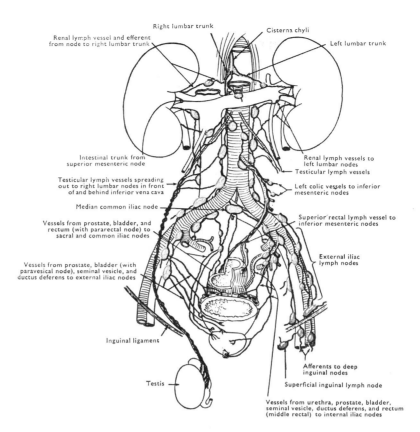

Right lumbar trunk

Cisterna chyli

Renal lymph vessel and efferent
from node to right lumbar trunk

Left lumbar trunk

Intestinal trunk from
superior mesenteric node

Renal lymph vessels to
left lumbar nodes

Testicular lymph vessels

Testicular lymph vessels spreading
out to right lumbar nodes in front
of and behind inferior vena cava

Left colic vessels to inferior
mesenteric nodes

Median common iliac node

Superior rectal lymph vessel to
inferior mesenteric nodes

Vessels from prostate, bladder, and
rectum (with pararectal node) to
sacral and common iliac nodes

External iliac
lymph nodes

Vessels from prostate, bladder (with
paravesical node), seminal vesicle, and
ductus deferens to external iliac nodes

Inguinal ligament

Afferents to deep
inguinal nodes

Testis

Superficial inguinal lymph node

Vessels from urethra, prostate, bladder,
seminal vesicle, ductus deferens, and rectum
(middle rectal) to internal iliac nodes

FIG. 44
Lymph vessels and nodes of male pelvis and abdomen. For clarity, only one node of the combined celiac and superior mesenteric pathway is shown. The junction of the cisterna chyli with its tributaries is actually located somewhat lower (see Fig. 45). (From Romanes, 1972.)

confluence of these ducts the cisterna even when it constitutes a plexiform structure. The cisterna lies on the anterior surface of the 1st and 2nd lumbar vertebrae to the right of the aorta, in the vicinity of origin of the superior mesenteric, renal, and gonadal arteries. Laterally it is covered by the right crus of the diaphragm above and the inferior vena cava below. Its lower end is crossed by the left renal vein and the right renal artery. It is here that the cisterna may be seen at the upper limit of aortic lymph node dissection (Fig. 45). Variations in location and formation are presented by Jossifow (1906).

At its upper end the cisterna receives two additional small posterior intercostal ('azygos') trunks descending from the lower posterior intercostal lymphatics. In most instances the cisterna extends upward to the right of the aorta as the thoracic duct. In some this extension is bilateral, to either side of the aorta, and rarely it is left sided (Edwards *et al.*, 1972).

Surgical exposures of the cisterna chyli to include the thoracic duct are generally by thoracotomy and section of

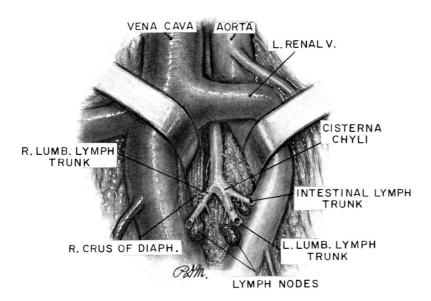

VENA CAVA | AORTA

L. RENAL V.

CISTERNA CHYLI

R. LUMB. LYMPH TRUNK

INTESTINAL LYMPH TRUNK

R. CRUS OF DIAPH.

L. LUMB. LYMPH TRUNK

LYMPH NODES

FIG. 45
Exposure of the cisterna chyli. The cisterna was unusually well formed in this anatomic specimen.

the posterior diaphragm. This may be accomplished extra-pleurally through the bed of the 12th rib (see Edwards *et al.,* 1972). As noted, the lower end of the cisterna can be seen abdominally between the vena cava and the aorta at the level of the left renal vein. It would be necessary to retract or divide the right crus of the diaphragm at the level of the celiac artery to gain further exposure of its upper part from an abdominal approach.

INGUINAL, ILIAC, AND AORTIC LYMPHADENECTOMY

Inguinal lymphadenectomy may be performed by itself or in continuity with removal of the iliac lymphatics. The inguinal lymph nodes and trunks are both superficial in proximity to the saphenous vein and deep in proximity to the femoral vein and artery. Both groups are removed in 'groin dissection,' a term applied to a procedure which may or may not include removal of the iliac lymphatics. Adequate removal of the superficial nodes and trunks requires excision of the subcutaneous fat from the lower abdominal wall from just above the inguinal canal, baring the external oblique aponeurosis and the inguinal ligament, down to the apex of the femoral triangle. The removal extends to the lateral border of the sartorius muscle, and to the medial border of the adductor longus (Fig. 46). Here, if the operation is done for carcinoma of the vulva or scrotum, the excision will be continued to remove parts of these structures. The superficial structures removed include the saphenous vein within this region, the superficial nerves (although the lateral femoral

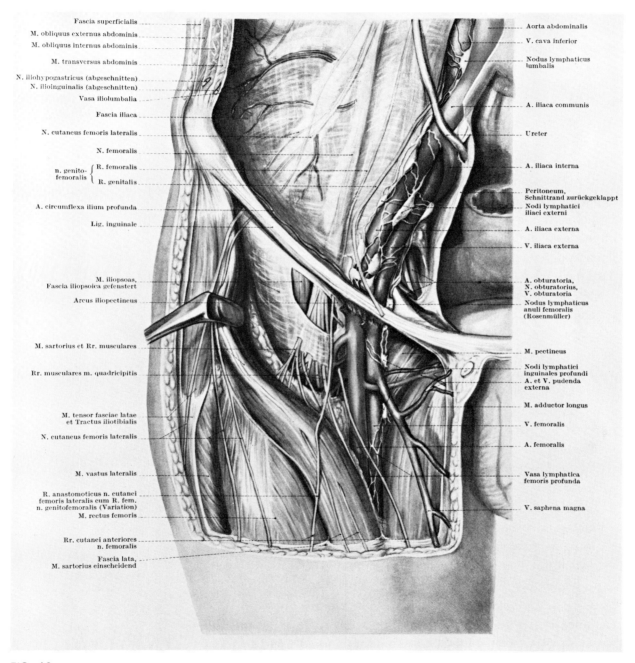

Fascia superficialis

M. obliquus externus abdominis

M. obliquus internus abdominis

M. transversus abdominis

N. iliohypogastricus (abgeschnitten)
N. ilioinguinalis (abgeschnitten)

Vasa iliolumbalia

Fascia iliaca

N. cutaneus femoris lateralis

N. femoralis

n. genito- { R. femoralis
femoralis { R. genitalis

A. circumflexa ilium profunda

Lig. inguinale

M. iliopsoas,
Fascia iliopsoica gefenstert

Arcus iliopectineus

M. sartorius et Rr. musculares

Rr. musculares m. quadricipitis

M. tensor fasciae latae
et Tractus iliotibialis

N. cutaneus femoris lateralis

M. vastus lateralis

R. anastomoticus n. cutanei
femoris lateralis cum R. fem.
n. genitofemoralis (Variation)
M. rectus femoris

Rr. cutanei anteriores
n. femoralis

Fascia lata,
M. sartorius einscheidend

Aorta abdominalis

V. cava inferior

Nodus lymphaticus
lumbalis

A. iliaca communis

Ureter

A. iliaca interna

Peritoneum,
Schnittrand zurückgeklappt
Nodi lymphatici
iliaci externi

A. iliaca externa

V. iliaca externa

A. obturatoria,
N. obturatorius,
V. obturatoria

Nodus lymphaticus
anuli femoralis
(Rosenmüller)

M. pectineus

Nodi lymphatici
inguinales profundi
A. et V. pudenda
externa

M. adductor longus

V. femoralis

A. femoralis

Vasa lymphatica
femoris profunda

V. saphena magna

FIG. 46
Iliac and inguinal blood vessels and nerves. (From Lang and Wachsmuth, 1972.)

cutaneous nerve is generally saved), the deep fascia, and the superficial branches of the femoral artery. The spermatic cord is laid bare. In the female the round ligament is removed to the internal ring. In either sex the nodes present in the inguinal canal are removed.

In the femoral region the deeper excision of fatty lymph-bearing tissue is carried beneath the sartorius muscle; the femoral arteries and veins are cleared, as are portions of the sartorius, adductor longus, iliopsoas, and pectineus muscles. In the course of this dissection the femoral cutaneous nerves encountered are excised to their origin from the femoral nerve. The node-bearing tissue of the femoral canal (Cloquet's node) is excised. Some surgeons transfer the sartorius muscle to cover the femoral vessels, during closure, by dividing the muscle from its origin and suturing it to the inguinal ligament, saving its blood supply from the superficial femoral vessels. The division of the superficial branches of the common femoral artery may cause necrosis of the skin flaps. For this reason the central part of these flaps may be excised and closure effected by rotation of the flaps or replacement by skin graft.

Iliac lymphadenectomy may be performed as an isolated procedure. Its scope is from either the aortic (Nathanson, 1954) or the iliac (Spratt *et al.,* 1965) bifurcation, above, to the inguinal ligament, below. The major internal iliac nodes are removed, but this removal does not go so far into the pelvis as when lymphadenectomy is done in continuity with removal of an organ for cancer, as of the cervix (see page 389) or the bladder (see page 328). Resection of the iliac nodes may be combined with aortic node dissection, as for cancer of the testis (see page 84). The iliac nodes are often removed as a routine part of the groin dissection, as for carcinomas of the lower limb or of the vulva (see page 388). Various clinical indications exist for and against extending groin dissections to the iliac nodes (Haagensen *et al.,* 1972).

When iliac lymphadenectomy is combined with inguinal lymphadectomy, exposure of the iliac nodes is accomplished by a suprainguinal division of the external oblique aponeurosis, after which the origin of the internal oblique and of the transversus muscle are detached from the inguinal ligament; the conjoined tendon and the inguinal ligament may also be divided (Fig. 46). Division of the inferior epigastric vessels and entry through the transversalis fascia allows a wide exposure of the extraperitoneal space. The ureter and the spermatic cord or round ligament are carried medially with the peritoneum and bladder as these structures are retracted. The round ligament is usually removed in the subsequent dissection, but the spermatic cord is usually saved.

Nathanson (1954) and Spratt *et al.* (1965) give excellent descriptions of the iliac procedure (Fig. 47). The fatty lymph-bearing tissue is removed from the iliac blood vessels, from the upper limit chosen to the inguinal ligament and obturator fossa, including the psoas and obturator fascia upon which these structures rest. The lateral limit of the dissection is the genitofemoral nerve. The medial limit within the pelvis generally lies beyond the obturator nerve to the arcus tendineus. To avoid ischemic injury to the ureter Nathanson advised saving its artery, which usually arises from the internal iliac, and leaving the ureter attached to the undersurface of the peritoneum. Injury is to be avoided to the fragile tributaries of the internal iliac vein.

Postoperative direct inguinal or femoral hernia is pre-

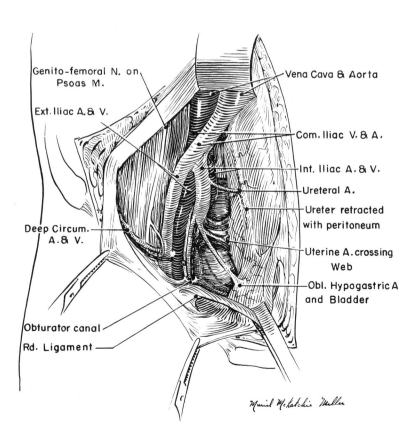

FIG. 47
Extraperitoneal iliac lymphadenectomy: The completed dissection. The surgeon has chosen not to remove the round ligament or the obliterated hypogastric artery. The ureteral branch of the internal iliac (somewhat exaggerated in size) is carefully maintained. The 'web' is the cardinal ligament of the uterus. (From Nathanson, I. T., in Surgical Treatment of Cancer of the Cervix, J. V. Meigs, Ed. New York, Grune & Stratton, 1954. By permission of the publisher.)

Genito-femoral N. on Psoas M.

Ext. Iliac A. & V.

Deep Circum. A. & V.

Obturator canal

Rd. Ligament

Vena Cava & Aorta

Com. Iliac V. & A.

Int. Iliac A. & V.

Ureteral A.

Ureter retracted with peritoneum

Uterine A. crossing Web

Obl. Hypogastric A and Bladder

vented by suturing the conjoined tendon to the pectineal (Cooper's) ligament medial to the femoral vessels, and to the inguinal ligament lateral to these vessels.

Exposure for aortic and iliac lymphadectomy may be transperitoneal, extraperitoneal, or thoracoabdominal (see page 14; Figs. 13, 170). Only the thoracoabdominal approach exposes the nodes above the renal level along with those below.

Stehlin and colleagues (1962) give a good account of the procedure as performed for cancer of the testis. They use a midline transperitoneal laparotomy, exposing the retroperitoneum by mobilizing the gut after incising the posterior peritoneum to the right of the ascending colon and around the cecum to the left of the mesentery (see Fig. 36). For left testis tumor it is necessary as well to mobilize the descending colon by incising the peritoneum to the left of this segment of bowel. The scope of the operation is to remove the testis and spermatic cord with the vas to the point where it leaves the pelvis, along with the testicular blood vessels and lymphatics and the areolar tissue around them; and the aorto-iliac lymph nodes and trunks from the inguinal ligament on the affected side and the iliac bifurcation on the opposite side, below, to the level of the renal veins, above. The lymphatic tissue is sought anterior to and around both the aorta and the vena cava; lumbar veins and occasionally lumbar arteries will need to be divided. Special attention is given to the upper end of this dissection, where the lower end of the cisterna chyli and lymphatic tissue, both behind and in front of the renal pedicles, are removed (Fig. 45).

REFERENCES

Batson, O. V.: The vertebral vein system. Amer. J. Roentgen. 78:195–212, 1957.

Breschet, G.: Récherches anatomiques, physiologiques et pathologiques sur le systeme veineux et speciálement sur les canaux veineux des os. Paris, Villaret, [1829–1830].

Edwards, E. A.: Clinical anatomy of lesser variations of the inferior vena cava; and a proposal for classifying the anomalies of this vessel. Angiology 2:85–99, 1951.

Edwards, E. A.: Diseases of the Veins. In Principles of Cardiovascular Diseases, Mason, D. T., Austen, W. G., Cohen, L. S., and Roberts, W. C., Eds. New York, Grune & Stratton. In Press, 1975.

Edwards, E. A., Dexter, L., and Donahue, W. C.: Recurrent pulmonary embolism as remediable cause of heart failure. Geriatrics 16:423–432, 1961.

Edwards, E. A., Malone, P. D., and Collins, J. J., Jr.: Operative Anatomy of Thorax. Philadelphia, Lea & Febiger, 1972.

Filler, R. M., and Edwards, E. A.: Collaterals of the lower inferior vena cava in man revealed by venography. Arch. Surg. 84:10–16, 1962.

Haagensen, C. D., Feind, C. R., Herter, F. P., Slanetz, C. A., Jr., and Weinberg, J. A.: The Lymphatics in Cancer. Philadelphia, W. B. Saunders, 1972.

Hirooka, M., and Kimura, C.: Membranous obstruction of the hepatic portion of the inferior vena cava. Surgical correction and etiological study. Arch. Surg. 100:656–663, 1970.

Hollinshead, W. H.: Anatomy for Surgeons, 2nd ed. Vol. 2. The Thorax, Abdomen, and Pelvis. New York, Harper & Row, 1971.

Jossifow, G. M.: Der Anfang des Ductus thoracicus und dessen Erweiterung. Arch. Anat. Physiol., Anat. Abt. Heft. I:68–76, 1906.

Lang, J., and Wachsmuth, W.: Praktische Anatomie. Vol. 1, Section 4. Bein und Statik. Berlin, Springer, 1972.

Moran, J. M., Kahn, P. C., and Callow, A. D.: Partial versus complete caval interruption for venous thromboembolism. Amer. J. Surg. 117:471–479, 1969.

Nathanson, I. T.: Retroperitoneal Lymph Node Dissection (Taussig). Chapter 7 in Surgical Treatment of Cancer of the Cervix, Meigs, J. V., Ed. New York, Grune & Stratton, 1954.

Romanes, G. J., Ed.: Cunningham's Textbook of Anatomy, 11th ed. London, Oxford, 1972.

Spratt, J. S., Jr., Shieber, W., and Dillard, B. M.: Anatomy and Surgical Technique of Groin Dissection. St. Louis, C. V. Mosby, 1965.

Stehlin, J. S., Jr., Jones, J. S., and Crigler, C. M.: Surgical Treatment of Cancer of the Testis. Chapter 2 in Treatment of Cancer and Allied Diseases, Pack, G. T., and Ariel, I. M., Eds. Vol. 4. The Male Genitalia and the Urinary Tract. New York, Harper & Row, 1962.

Yamamoto, S., Yokoyama, Y., Takeshige, K., and Iwatsuki, S.: Budd-Chiari syndrome with obstruction of the inferior vena cava. Gastroenterology 54:1070–1084, 1968.

6

AUTONOMIC NERVES

ABDOMINAL COMPONENTS OF THE AUTONOMIC NERVOUS SYSTEM

The organs of the abdomen and pelvis are supplied with both sympathetic and parasympathetic innervation. The plexuses containing the mixed fibers are located on or near the aorta and the iliac arteries (Fig. 48), their branches extending to each viscus via perivascular plexuses which are subsidiaries of the aortic or hypogastric (iliac) plexuses (Fig. 49). The ganglia of the plexuses, such as the celiac or renal, belong to the sympathetic system and contain the final neurons of this pathway. Ganglia such as the enteric, on or within the walls of the viscera, contain the last neurons of the parasympathetic pathway.

The sympathetic input for these plexuses is derived from the splanchnic nerves, stemming from the thoracic sympathetic trunks, plus aortic and iliac branches of the lumbosacral sympathetic trunks. The trunks receive outflow from the spinal nerves by the 'white' rami communicantes no lower than the second lumbar nerves. They nevertheless send postsynaptic fibers by the 'gray' rami to all the lumbar, sacral, and coccygeal nerves for distribution to their respective territories, as well as visceral branches to all the abdominal and pelvic organs.

The vagus nerves conduct the parasympathetic fibers for the upper abdominal organs. The right (posterior) vagus

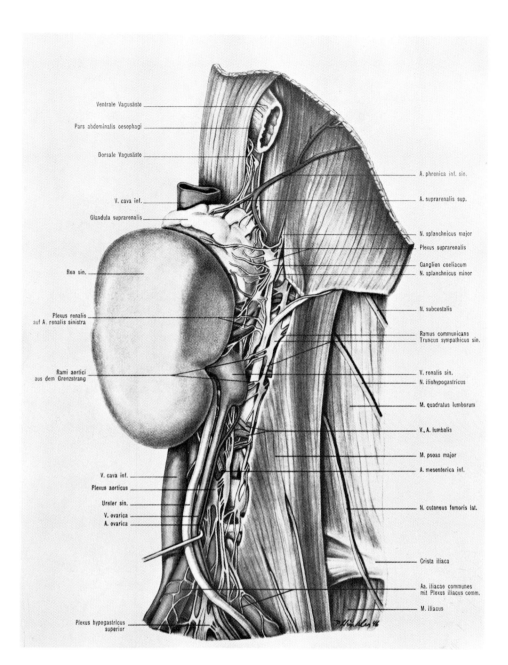

Ventrale Vagusäste

Pars abdominalis oesophagi

Dorsale Vagusäste

A. phrenica inf. sin.

A. suprarenalis sup.

V. cava inf.

Glandula suprarenalis

N. splanchnicus major
Plexus suprarenalis

Ren sin.

Ganglion coeliacum
N. splanchnicus minor

N. subcostalis

Plexus renalis
auf A. renalis sinistra

Ramus communicans
Truncus sympathicus sin.

Rami aortici
aus dem Grenzstrang

V. renalis sin.
N. iliohypogastricus

M. quadratus lumborum

V., A. lumbalis

M. psoas major

A. mesenterica inf.

V. cava inf.
Plexus aorticus
Ureter sin.
V. ovarica
A. ovarica

N. cutaneus femoris lat.

Crista iliaca

Aa. iliacae communes
mit Plexus iliacus comm.

M. iliacus

Plexus hypogastricus
superior

FIG. 48
Left lumbar sympathetic trunk, celiac plexus, and suprarenal gland. Note contributions of the right (posterior) vagus, and the greater and lesser splanchnic nerves to the celiac plexus. The left renal vein receives, as usual, the second lumbar and a communication from the hemiazygos vein (both unlabeled). (From Töndury, 1970.)

gives the greater contribution to the celiac and other pre-aortic plexuses; the left vagus is distributed more directly to the stomach and liver (see Vagotomy, in Chapter 7). Vagal distribution to the gut ends about the middle of the descending colon; the remainder of the gut and the other pelvic organs receive parasympathetic innervation from the inferior hypogastric plexus (Figs. 50, 51).

Viscerosensory fibers of posterior spinal root origin, with a few vagal contributions, course mainly through the

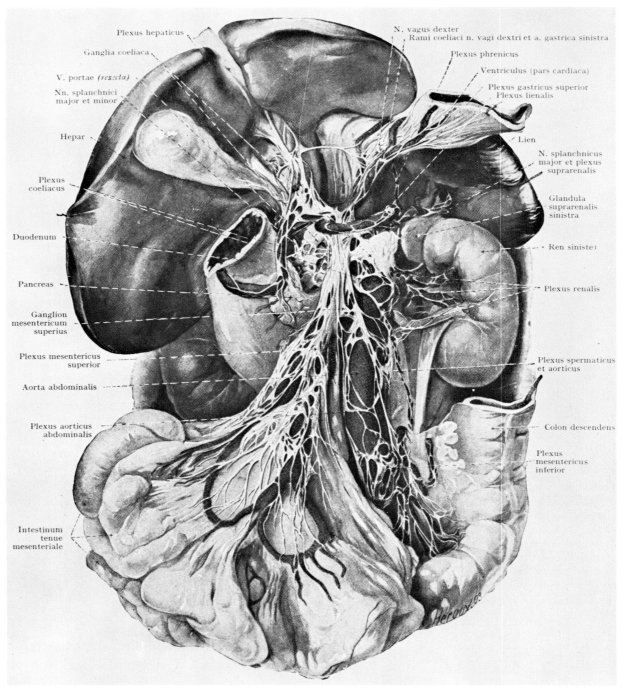

FIG. 49
The distribution of the celiac and mesenteric nerve plexuses. (From Spalteholz, 1954.)

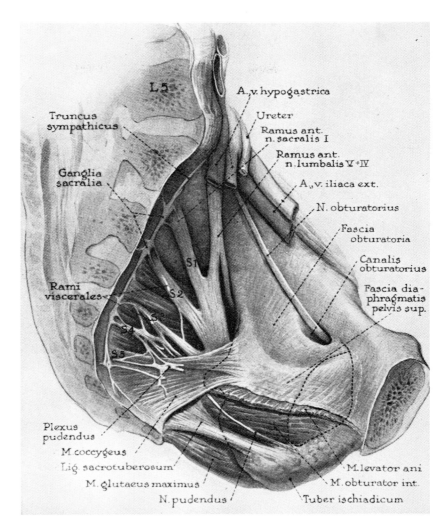

FIG. 50

Connections of the sacral and pelvic autonomic nerves. The dissection shows the anterior rami of sacral nerves, the sacral sympathetic trunk, and the pelvic splanchnic or para- sympathetic nerves, labeled 'plexus pudendus.' (This expression, no longer in use, originally referred to all branches of the lower anterior sacral rami.) The piriformis muscle lies be- hind the sacral nerves. The sciatic nerve is being formed from L-4,5 and S-1,2,3; the pudendal from S-(1),2,3,4,(5). Both leave the pel- vis through the greater sciatic fora- men above the ischial spine (dotted outline). The pudendal nerve is shown passing further below the ischial spine, thence in the opened canal in the obturator fascia. (From Curtis et al., 1942. By permission of Sur- gery, Gynecology & Obstetrics.)

splanchnic nerves and partly through other sympathetic branches. They are then conducted through the autonomic plexuses to the viscera. Some surgical implications of this course to the pancreas, and to the female pelvic organs, are considered in Chapters 7 and 24.

CELIAC GANGLIONECTOMY

The celiac plexus contains the majority of the terminal sympathetic ganglia for the abdominal viscera, as well as their sensory fibers. Celiac ganglionectomy has been per-

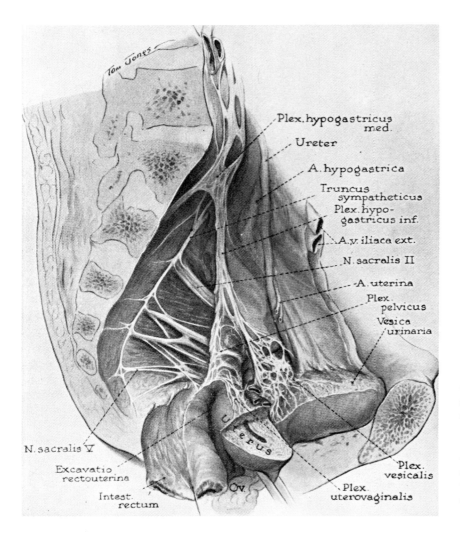

FIG. 51

The hypogastric nerve plexuses. The inferior hypogastric plexus ('plex. pelvicus') has received the sacral parasympathetic components and the sympathetic ('plex. hypogastricus med.' and 'plex. hypogastricus inf.'). Distribution to the pelvic organs by subsidiary plexuses is indicated. (From Curtis et al., 1942. By permission of Surgery, Gynecology & Obstetrics.)

formed to ablate the sensory fibers in painful conditions such as pancreatitis (Grimson *et al.,* 1947). The plexus is reached through the omental bursa, as for access to the celiac and superior mesenteric arteries. Although the ganglia are multiple, generally one large ganglion about 2 x 1 cm. will be found on either side of the celiac artery, overlain by celiac lymph nodes, and bound together by the stout nerves of the plexus. Their proximity to the suprarenal glands should be borne in mind. The splanchnic nerves enter the ganglia from behind (Fig. 48), where also lies the major source of their blood supply from the middle suprarenal arteries (see Fig. 152).

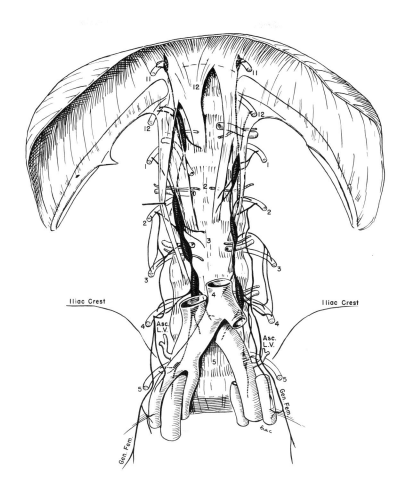

FIG. 52
Configuration and topography of the lumbar sympathetic trunks. Note the presence of an intermediate crus of the diaphragm on each side (retracted on the right)—usual incidence 50 per cent. The spinal nerves were exposed by removing the psoas muscles, thus allowing identification of the rami and trunk segments. Communications between some of the segmental rami or lumbar spinal nerves correspond to the 'connecting rami' of Kuntz. (From Edwards, 1951.)

THE LUMBAR SYMPATHETIC TRUNK: TOPOGRAPHY, BRANCHES, EFFECTS OF ABLATION

Each sympathetic trunk curves forward from the 12th thoracic ganglion, on the head of the 12th rib, to pierce the diaphragm and reach the front of the lumbar spine, where they descend on either side of the midline (Fig. 52). Both trunks lie anterior to the lumbar arteries, so that the left trunk is kept from approaching the midline of the body posteriorly by the take-off of these branches from the aorta. Although most lumbar veins lie behind the sympathetic trunks, the termination of right lumbar veins in the vena cava does not prevent the right trunk from being overlain by the cava. A lumbar vein may be found anterior to a trunk in about one third of dissections, somewhat oftener on the right than on the left. At the level of the 4th lumbar disc, the sympathetic trunk descends on each side behind the common iliac vein and its reception of the ascending lumbar and iliolumbar veins (Fig. 52). The sacral sympathetic trunk is shown in Figures 50, 51.

Of the branches of the trunk, the medial are the visceral, or peri-aortic, the lateral are the rami communicantes. Unlike the condition in the thoracic region, where one ganglion is usually present, with its rami visibly connected to each spinal nerve, the lumbar trunk exhibits three or four large ganglia, with a variable number of small additional ganglionic masses (Edwards, 1951) (Fig. 52). It is impossible at operation to be sure to which lumbar nerve segment each ganglion belongs, since the rami disappear in company with the lumbar vessels beneath small fibrous arches at the medial border of the psoas major muscle, their junction with the lumbar nerves being hidden by the overlying muscle. Within the substance of the psoas, too, a ramus may bifurcate to join adjacent lumbar nerves.

There nevertheless exists a usual topographic relationship between the lumbar vertebrae and the segments of the trunk and its rami which enables the operator to judge with fair accuracy the levels of the sympathetic components seen at operation (Table 5). The levels of lumbar vertebrae

TABLE 5
Vertebral Level of Origin of
*Rami from 40 Sympathetic Chains.**

Rami	Most Frequent Level of Origin	Range of Level of Origin
Twelfth thoracic	T-XII body to T-XII disc (24 instances)	T-XI disc to L-I disc
First lumbar	L-II body to L-II disc (32 instances)	L-I body to L-II disc
Second lumbar	L-II body to L-II disc (23 instances)	L-II body to L-III disc (uncommon)
Third lumbar	L-II body (31 instances)	L-II disc to L-III disc
Fourth lumbar	L-IV body (31 instances)	L-III body to L-V body
Fifth lumbar	L-V body to L-V disc (31 instances)	L-IV body to L-V disc

*From Edwards, 1951.

palpated at operation can be identified by their relationship to the top of the iliac crests. The line between these points generally crosses the 4th vertebral body in the male, and the 4th disc or 5th vertebral body in the female. In an occasional subject the intercristal line crosses the 3rd disc. A preoperative roentgenogram makes the relationship certain.

Since the exit of sympathetic fibers from the cord ceases below the L-2 level, it is apparent from the Table that, in most cases, a simple division of the trunk below the L-2 disc will produce sympathetic denervation of the entire sciatic distribution. The femoral and obturator nerves (L-2,3,4) will be deprived of their sympathetic fibers except for rami entering the 2nd lumbar nerve from a higher level in some instances. If one extended the sympathectomy above the body of L-2, even the femoral and obturator nerves would be totally deprived of sympathetic inflow.

The expected denervation may be incomplete because of the existence of certain anomalous sympathetic pathways. These include collaterals of the trunk, bifurcated rami, connecting rami (Fig. 52), and intermediate ganglia located in rami or anterior spinal nerve roots (Kuntz, 1949; Edwards, 1951). Theoretically, the removal of a considerable length of trunk, rather than simple division, may bring about a better denervation by removing some parts of such anomalous pathways. Ruberti and his co-workers (1960) could not attribute any effect to the presence of crossed communications between the two trunks.

The only constant effects of lumbar sympathectomy are vasodilatation and cessation of sweating in the lower limb, notably in the foot. Postural hypotension, gastrointestinal hypermotility, and some viscerosensory loss are unusual unless lower thoracic sympathectomy and splanchnicectomy have also been performed (Kuntz, 1949; White *et al.,* 1952). Irregularly, loss of external seminal ejaculation may occur in the male. White and his co-authors state: "Occasionally temporary, but never permanent, loss of ejaculation occurs in men submitted to extensive bilateral thoracic sympathectomy and splanchnicectomy, even though all the lumbar ganglia are left intact. . . . After bilateral lumbar sympathetic ganglionectomy the power of ejaculation is lost in 54 per cent if the three upper lumbar ganglia are resected on one side and two or more of these ganglia on the other."

Thus if sterility is to be avoided in the male, the first two lumbar ganglia on each side should be left intact. Impotence has been ascribed to thoracolumbar sympathectomy, and to the extensive peri-aortic dissection during aorto-iliac surgery. It is difficult to identify a precise mechanism in such a setting, in view of the constitutional state of patients for whom these operations are done, and the common uncertainty of establishing the cause of impotence in any individual.

ABDOMINAL SYMPATHECTOMIES

Sympathectomy in the abdomen may consist of removal of a lumbar trunk alone, in combination with removal of some portion of the thoracic sympathetic chain or with splanchnicectomy, or the removal of a subsidiary part—presacral neurectomy (considered in Chapter 24).

The lumbar trunks may be secured through anterolateral or posterolateral extraperitoneal approaches, or transperitoneally. In the anterolateral approach, the operator gains entry into the retroperitoneal fat after opening the transversalis fascia (Fig. 53). The peritoneum is retracted away from the psoas muscle and anterolateral surface of the spine. The ureter and gonadal vessels adhere to the peritoneum and are retracted with it. On the right the cava similarly rolls medially beneath the retractor. It is useful, by blunt dissection, to bare the psoas fascia as it crosses in a loose fashion upon the vertebrae over the sympathetic trunk, displacing medially the peri-aortic fat and lymph nodes. The trunk is best initially identified by palpating the hard consistency and the shape of a ganglion. The upper ganglia are larger, and one should search for them if a lower one is not encountered at once. The trunk may be partly overlain by a musculo-tendinous intermediate crus of the diaphragm (Fig. 52), which will require division. Rarely, 3 to 5 cm. of the trunk may be embedded within the edge of the psoas major muscle. The trunk need not be confused with the genitofemoral nerve running close by upon the psoas muscle rather than medial to it, nor with the tendon of the psoas minor muscle (incidence 60 per cent), which also lies anterior to the psoas major. Dissection posterior to the trunk should start over the convexity of a vertebral disc, since this place is devoid of

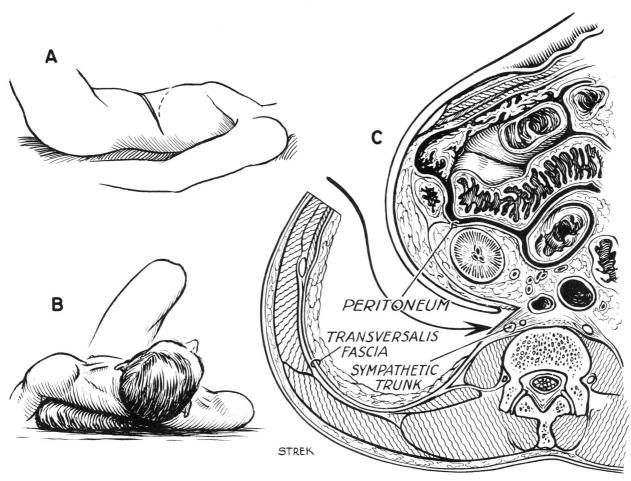

FIG. 53

Approach to the lumbar sympathetic trunk by anterolateral muscle-splitting retroperitoneal incision. A. Line of incision. B. Position of patient. C. The plane of approach lies within the extraperitoneal fat. The lower pole of the kidney within the renal fascia is shown retracted with the peritoneum. Lower down the ureter and gonadal vessels cling to and are retracted with the peritoneum. (From Edwards et al., in Surgical Treatment of Vascular Disease, Barker, W. F., Ed. Copyright 1962, McGraw-Hill Book Company, New York. Used with permission of McGraw-Hill Book Company.)

a lumbar artery and vein which course rather on the concave surface of the vertebral body. The identification of segments of the trunk and vascular relationships are described in the preceding pages.

A transabdominal approach has the advantage that bilateral sympathectomy can be done through one incision. Incising the posterior peritoneum lateral to the vena cava or the aorta endangers mesenteric blood vessels and the exposure cannot be extended much higher than the 2nd lumbar disc because of the presence of the renal pedicle. The peritoneum may instead be incised to the lateral side

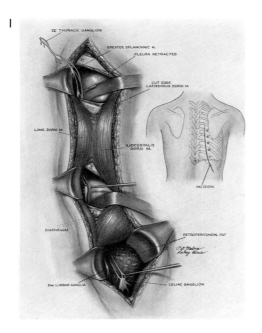

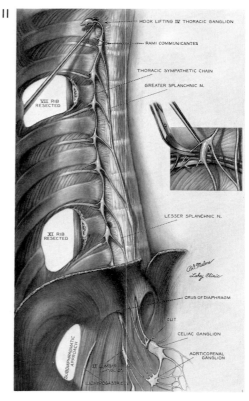

FIG. 54

Supra- and infradiaphragmatic sympathectomy and splanchnicectomy. I. Operative approach. II. Extent of the neurectomy. (From Poppen, 1947. By permission of Surgery, Gynecology & Obstetrics.)

of the ascending or descending colon and these parts be mobilized for a more extensive view of the sympathetic trunks.

A posterolateral or paravertebral extraperitoneal approach is rather cumbersome for most operators, but is useful when lumbar sympathectomy is combined with thoracic sympathectomy and splanchnicectomy as formerly done for hypertension (Fig. 54). The kidney and suprarenal gland can be examined simultaneously through the approach shown, or by the transthoracic transdiaphragmatic operation of Linton and his colleagues (1947) (see Edwards *et al.,* 1972).

REFERENCES

Curtis, A. H., Anson, B. J., Ashley, F. L., and Jones, T.: The anatomy of the pelvic autonomic nerves in relation to gynecology. Surg. Gynec. Obstet. 75:743–750, 1942.

Edwards, E. A.: Operative anatomy of the lumbar sympathetic chain. Angiology 2:184–198, 1951.

Edwards, E. A., Malone, P. D., and Collins, J. J., Jr.: Operative Anatomy of Thorax. Philadelphia, Lea & Febiger, 1972.

Edwards, E. A., Ruberti, U., and Ottinger, L.: Lumbar Sympathectomy. Chapter 8 *in* Surgical Treatment of Peripheral Vascular Disease, Barker, W. F., Ed. New York, McGraw-Hill, 1962.

Grimson, K. S., Hesser, F. H., and Kitchin, W. W.: Early clinical results of transabdominal celiac and superior mesenteric ganglionectomy, vagotomy, or transthoracic splanchnicectomy in patients with chronic abdominal visceral pain. Surgery 22:230–238, 1947.

Kuntz, A.: The Neuroanatomic Basis of Surgery of the Autonomic Nervous System. Springfield, Charles C Thomas, 1949.

Linton, R. R., Moore, F. D., Simeone, F. A., Welch, C. E., and White, J. C.: Thoracolumbar sympathectomy for hypertension. Improvements in paravertebral and transpleural routes to facilitate extensive neurectomy. Surg. Clin. N. Amer. 27:1178–1187, 1947.

Poppen, J. L.: Extensive combined thoracolumbar sympathectomy in hypertension. Surg. Gynec. Obstet. 84:1117–1123, 1947.

Ruberti, U., Edwards, E. A., and Ottinger, L.: Changes in the peripheral pulses after sympathectomy for arteriosclerosis. Surgery 47:105–114, 1960.

Spalteholz, W.: Hand Atlas of Human Anatomy, 15th ed. Revised by Spanner, R. Vol. III, Part II. Vascular System, Viscera, Nervous System, Sense Organs. Boston. Little, Brown, 1954.

Töndury, G.: Angewandte und topographische Anatomie, 4th ed. Stuttgart, Georg Thieme, 1970.

White, J. C., Smithwick, R. H., and Simeone, F. A.: The Autonomic Nervous System. Anatomy, Physiology, and Surgical Application, 3rd ed. New York, Macmillan, 1952.

SECTION 3

Stomach, Duodenum, Pancreas, Spleen

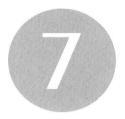

VASCULAR ANd NEURAL SUPRAMESOCOLIC RELATIONShIPS

It is useful to consider the close relationships of the supramesocolic viscera as regards their blood and nerve supply. Venous drainage is separately considered in Chapter 14.

EMBRYOLOGIC BASIS

Up to the fifth or sixth week the gastrointestinal tract is a midline structure. The stomach and duodenum, from which the other supramesocolic viscera will develop, are suspended by ventral and dorsal mesenteries (Fig. 55). The celiac artery, the main artery to this segment of the gut as well as to the derived viscera, reaches these organs through the dorsal mesogastrium.

The spleen develops from mesenchyme within the dorsal mesogastrium. The liver and biliary apparatus originate from a ventral diverticulum of the duodenum, whose connection with the gut remains as the bile duct. The pancreas has a dual origin. The ventral pancreas (not shown in Figure 55) buds out from the hepatic diverticulum. It gives rise to the head of the pancreas. Its duct (of Wirsung) usually remains as the termination of the main pancreatic duct. A larger

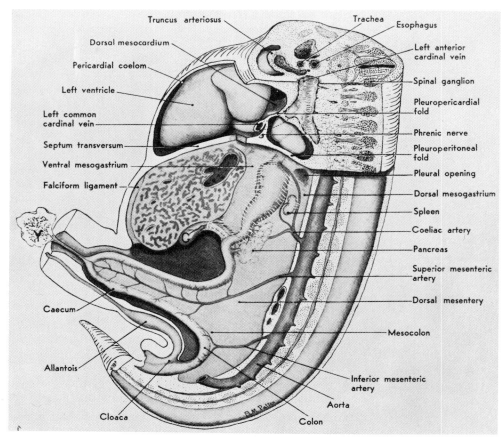

FIG. 55

The human embryo in the seventh week, in diagrammatic longitudinal section. (From Patten, B. M.: Human Embryology, 3rd ed. Copyright 1968, McGraw-Hill Book Company, New York. Used with permission of McGraw-Hill Book Company.)

dorsal bud ('pancreas' in Figure 55) originates from the duodenum. It gives rise to the body and tail of the pancreas. Its duct, the accessory pancreatic duct (of Santorini) is usually small since, after fusion of the two buds, the ventral duct more often becomes the major continuation of the pancreatic duct. Variations of the ducts are described in Chapter 13 (Fig. 110), and annular pancreas is described in Chapter 9 (Fig. 68).

As the stomach and duodenum develop, they are changed from the straight tube of the primitive gut to the S-shaped structure characterizing these organs in the postnatal state. As the foregut grows into this position the ventral mesogastrium and the anterior edge of the gastroduodenal tube turn to the right about the long axis; the dorsal mesogastrium and posterior edge turn to the left (see Fig. 122).

This also involves the terminal esophagus. The left vagus nerve comes to lie anterior to the terminal esophagus and the stomach, the right vagus, posterior. Within the ventral mesogastrium the liver grows from the ventrally located hepatic bud, but the duodenal end of the bud, becoming the bile and main pancreatic ducts, shifts farther to the right and then behind the duodenum. The budding head of the pancreas rotating in the same way with the other elements of the ventral hepatic bud can now fuse with the anlage of the body of the pancreas growing from the dorsal pancreatic bud.

As rotation of the gastroduodenal segment is concluded a final development, as for the rest of the gut, is fixation of these organs and their dorsal mesenteries to the posterior abdominal wall. Fixation occurs by a fusion of the mesothelium of these parts to adjacent portions of the posterior wall. In some places there is also fusion to already rotated parts of the gut, as where the great omentum is in contact with the transverse colon, or where the transverse mesocolon crosses the already rotated duodenum. Further considerations of the fusion process will be found in Chapter 15.

ARTERIES

The celiac is the main artery of supply of the supramesocolic viscera, assisted to a variable degree by the superior mesenteric artery. The two arteries communicate quite constantly by the junction of the superior and inferior pancreaticoduodenal arteries, shown in an anterior arcade in Figure 56 II (more accurately as a pair of arcades in Figure 70, and see also Figure 71). A second set of communications, irregular in their presence and size, exists behind the body of the pancreas and in front of the aorta. These include: (1) the rare common origin of the celiac and superior mesenteric arteries (incidence 1%); (2) anastomoses between pancreatic arteries and the middle colic and accessory left colic arteries; (3) the aberrant origin of a pancreatic artery from the superior mesenteric artery (see Fig. 76), or of a colic artery from the celiac (see page 235).

The stomach is the most richly vascularized part of the gut. Not only do the gastric and gastroepiploic arteries com-

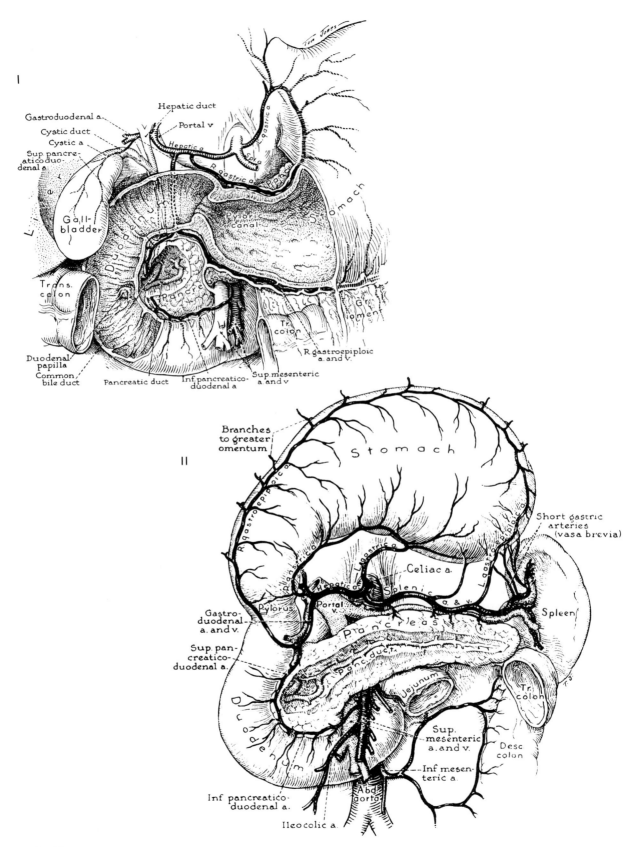

FIG. 56

Major branches of the celiac artery. I. Anterior view. II. Retrogastric view. (From Jones and Shepard, 1945.)

municate grossly in so-called inosculations, but communications also exist between small arteries within the wall of the organ. Numerous arteriovenous anastomoses are likewise present (Barlow *et al.,* 1951). However, the short gastric arteries supplying the fundus may be incapable of supplying distant portions of the stomach (see Chapter 8). It is generally considered safe, in mobilizing the stomach for anastomosis, as to the esophagus, to ligate all but one of the four major arteries. Nakayama (1954), however, as a result of extensive clinical experience and injection studies, concluded that, in order to maintain sufficient circulation in the proximal part of the mobilized stomach, it is essential to leave the arterial arches along the two curvatures ''completely untouched,'' in addition to preserving either the right gastric or the right gastroepiploic artery.

The richness of arterial anastomoses of the stomach abruptly gives way, beyond the pylorus, to a paucity of such arterial connections in the remainder of the gut until the lower rectum. The initial part of the duodenum is supplied by the usually single supraduodenal artery supero-anteriorly (see Fig. 64), and by one or more retroduodenal arteries posteriorly (see Fig. 70). The supraduodenal artery usually originates from the upper gastroduodenal, but may come from a hepatic or the cystic artery. Additional branches to the initial duodenum may stem from the right gastric, right gastroepiploic, or a superior pancreaticoduodenal artery. The remainder of the descending and transverse parts of the duodenum are supplied by vasa recta, branching from the anterior and posterior pancreaticoduodenal arcades. The close association of the duodenum and pancreas makes it hazardous to separate them, and leads to bypassing operations for benign duodenal disease, or to excision of both in malignant disease, such as cancer of the head of the pancreas (see Chapter 9).

LYMPHATICS

Just as the celiac and superior mesenteric arteries contribute to all the supramesocolic viscera, so do the lymphatics course to both celiac and superior mesenteric lymph nodes (Fig. 57). Their efferents join in the 'intestinal trunk' (Chapter 5).

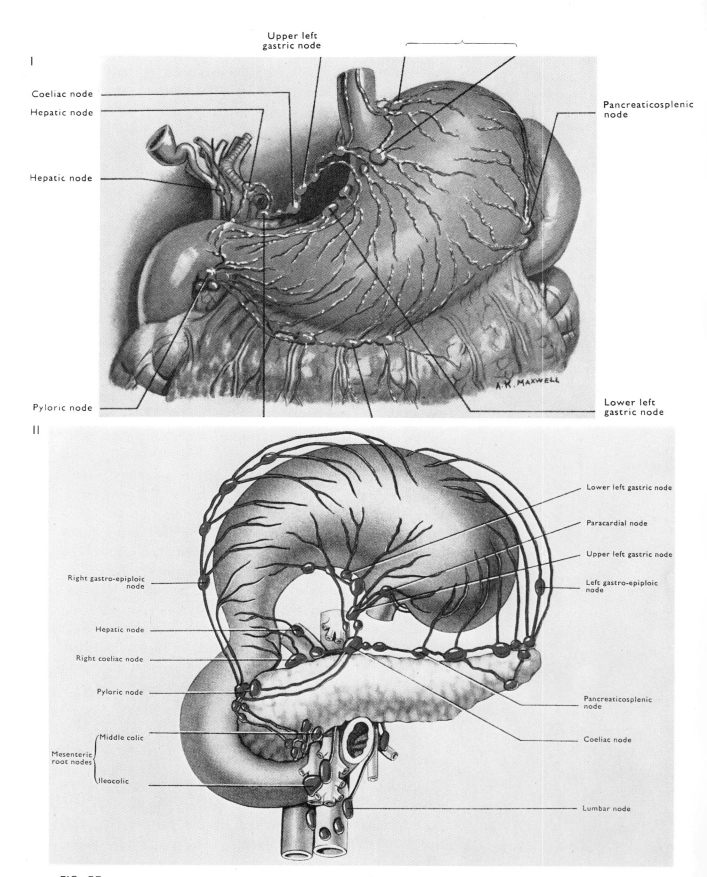

I

Coeliac node

Hepatic node

Hepatic node

Pyloric node

Upper left
gastric node

Pancreaticosplenic
node

Lower left
gastric node

A.K. MAXWELL

II

Right gastro-epiploic
node

Hepatic node

Right coeliac node

Pyloric node

Mesenteric
root nodes

Middle colic

Ileocolic

Lower left gastric node

Paracardial node

Upper left gastric node

Left gastro-epiploic
node

Pancreaticosplenic
node

Coeliac node

Lumbar node

FIG. 57

Supramesocolic lymphatics. I. Anterior view. II. Retrogastric view. (From Romanes, 1972.)

Three features of the lymphatics of this region interfere with an ideal outcome of resection for cancer. These are: (1) the interconnection of lymphatics of several organs, (2) the indispensable blood vessels passing through the field, and (3) the short distance the cancer cells need to travel from the primary site to escape into the thoracic duct.

NERVE PLEXUSES; CELIAC GANGLIONECTOMY

The general scheme of abdominal visceral sympathetic supply is described in Chapter 6. In the supramesocolic area, the sympathetic distribution is represented by the celiac and mesenteric ganglia and plexuses, and their peri-arterial distribution. The preganglionic input is mainly by the splanchnic nerves, aided by peri-aortic branches of the lumbar sympathetic trunks. The vagus nerves contribute the parasympathetic fibers which mingle with the sympathetic fibers (see Figs. 48, 59).

Sensory fibers also travel from the viscera through these autonomic nerves and plexuses. The splanchnic nerves are probably the greatest contributors of viscerosensory fibers. The somatic nerves of the posterior abdominal wall send sensory branches to the mesenteries of the organs. These branches may be involved in malignant infiltration. Sensory denervation for chronic abdominal pain has been attempted by resection of the vagi, splanchnic nerves, thoracolumbar sympathetic trunks, or the celiac plexus, all with variable results (Grimson et al., 1947; Bonica, 1953).

Celiac ganglionectomy (Grimson et al.) can be accomplished through the posterior wall of the omental bursa, as for access to the celiac and superior mesenteric arteries (see Fig. 151).

Denervation for relief of abdominal pain has probably been attempted most often for chronic pancreatitis. Yoshioka and Wakabayashi (1958) introduced an operation to divide the pancreatic plexus, which they showed extended to the uncinate process of the pancreas from the right celiac ganglion and from the superior mesenteric plexus. Generally nerve section in this disease has been superseded by pancreatectomy, or by drainage procedures.

VAGOTOMY

Vagotomy for abdominal disease, especially peptic ulcer, may be classified as supra- or infradiaphragmatic when total removal of the vagi is done, as 'selective' when only the gastric branches are divided, and as 'superselective' when the proximal gastric but not the pyloric branches are sectioned. The infradiaphragmatic is the more commonly used approach. Exposure may be improved by dividing the left triangular ligament and retracting the left portion of the liver to the right (Fig. 58) (see also page 13 and Fig. 8). The vagi are sought on the lowermost esophagus, where the trunks tend to be re-formed after having been broken up in the esophageal plexus at higher levels. There is variation in the completeness of the trunk formation, so that one must seek vagal branches about the entire circumference of the esophagus, in addition to the left (anterior) and the right (posterior) trunks. A vein usually accompanies each vagus (Butler, 1951). Griffith (1971) emphasizes that the vagal branches lie within the esophageal fascia, not in the deeper longitudinal muscle which becomes exposed on removing this fascia. Dissection through its muscular layers may perforate the esophagus.

In selective vagotomy (Fig. 59) the gastric branches are divided, while the hepatic and celiac branches are spared. The necessary identification of these components is made to the right of the esophagogastric junction. Here the anterior trunk divides into hepatic, gastric, and an occasional celiac branch. The posterior trunk gives a larger and more constant contribution to the right celiac ganglion, and smaller gastric branches (Mitchell, 1938). The anterior and posterior gastric branches run down the lesser curvature anterior and posterior, respectively, to the terminal part of the left gastric artery. Griffith (1971) advises dividing this vessel on the lesser curvature to ensure proper denervation.

In so-called 'superselective' (parietal cell, or proximal gastric) vagotomy the gastric vagal branches to the antrum (anterior and posterior nerves of Latarjet) are conserved, as described by Amdrup and Jensen (1970), to maintain gastric emptying (Goligher, 1974). The gastrohepatic omentum is detached from the stomach upward from the 'crow's foot' splay of the terminal anterior trunk branches 9 to 10 cm.

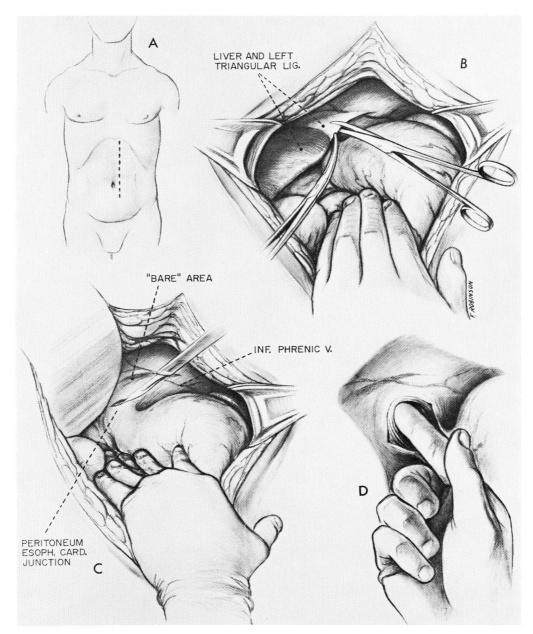

FIG. 58
Approach for infradiaphragmatic vagotomy. A. Left paramedian incision. B. Dividing the left triangular ligament. The left inferior phrenic vein is visible here, and in C and D. C. Incising the peritoneum about the esophagogastric junction. D. Mobilizing the esophagus. The fingertip lies in the esophageal hiatus. (From Madden, 1964.)

proximal to the pylorus (see Fig. 59). The dissection is continued to the lower esophagus above (Goligher). The addition of a drainage procedure is eliminated by maintaining antral innervation (Amdrup and Jensen). Further studies are necessary to determine the long-term results and place of this technique in ulcer surgery.

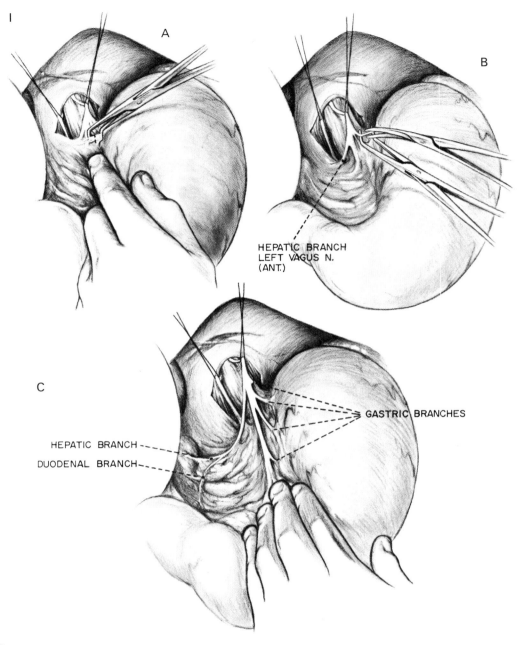

FIG. 59
Selective vagotomy.

I. Division of gastric branches of the left (anterior) vagus nerve. A. The vagal trunks are elevated. B. Identification of the left branches. The large hepatic branch is seen in the lesser omentum. A branch to the esophagogastric junction is about to be divided. C. Gastric branches run on the lesser curvature. A duodenal and an antral branch are not always identified.

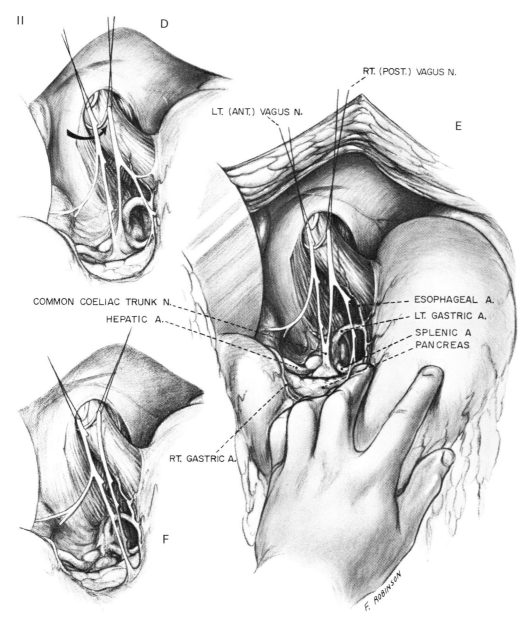

RT. (POST.) VAGUS N.

LT. (ANT.) VAGUS N.

COMMON COELIAC TRUNK N.

HEPATIC A.

ESOPHAGEAL A.

LT. GASTRIC A.

SPLENIC A

PANCREAS

RT. GASTRIC A.

F. ROBINSON

FIG. 59

Selective vagotomy (continued).

II. Division of gastric branches of the right (posterior) vagus nerve. D. The right vagus has been retracted to the patient's left. An unusual celiac branch of the left vagus joins the celiac branch of the right. E. All gastric branches have been divided except the terminal ones of the right vagus proceeding to the antrum. These are preserved in superselective proximal gastric vagotomy: The proximity of the vagal branching anterior and posterior to the left gastric artery is evident. F. The more usual branching is shown, with no celiac branch from the left vagus. The large lymph node usually overlying the origin of the common hepatic artery is seen in D, E, and F. (From Madden, 1964.)

REFERENCES

Amdrup, E., and Jensen, H.-E.: Selective vagotomy of the parietal cell mass preserving innervation of the undrained antrum. A preliminary report of results in patients with duodenal ulcer. Gastroenterology 59:522–527, 1970.

Barlow, T. E., Bentley, F. H., and Walder, D. N.: Arteries, veins, and arteriovenous anastomoses in the human stomach. Surg. Gynec. Obstet. 93:657–671, 1951.

Bonica, J. J.: The Management of Pain. With Special Emphasis on the Use of Analgesic Block in Diagnosis, Prognosis, and Therapy. Philadelphia, Lea & Febiger, 1953.

Butler, H.: The veins of the oesophagus. Thorax 6:276–296, 1951.

Goligher, J. C.: A technique for highly selective (parietal cell or proximal gastric) vagotomy for duodenal ulcer. Brit. J. Surg. 61:337–345, 1974.

Griffith, C. A.: Selective Gastric Vagotomy. Chapter 77 *in* The Craft of Surgery, Cooper, P., Ed., 2nd ed. Vol. II. Boston, Little, Brown, 1971.

Grimson, K. S., Hesser, F. H., and Kitchin, W. W.: Early clinical results of transabdominal celiac and superior mesenteric ganglionectomy, vagotomy, or transthoracic splanchnicectomy in patients with chronic abdominal visceral pain. Surgery 22:230–238, 1947.

Jones, T., and Shepard, W. C.: A Manual of Surgical Anatomy. Philadelphia, W. B. Saunders, 1945.

Madden, J. L.: Atlas of Technics in Surgery, 2nd ed. Vol. 2: Thoracic and Cardiovascular. New York, Appleton-Century-Crofts, 1964.

Mitchell, G. A. G.: The nerve supply of the gastro-oesophageal junction. Brit. J. Surg. 26:333–345, 1938.

Nakayama, K.: Approach to midthoracic esophageal carcinoma for its radical surgical treatment. Surgery 35:574–589, 1954.

Patten, B. M.: Human Embryology, 3rd ed. New York, McGraw-Hill, 1968.

Romanes, G. J., Ed.: Cunningham's Textbook of Anatomy, 11th ed. London, Oxford, 1972.

Yoshioka, H., and Wakabayashi, T.: Therapeutic neurotomy on head of pancreas for relief of pain due to chronic pancreatitis. A new technical procedure and its results. Arch. Surg. 76:546–554, 1958.

8

THE STOMACH

ANATOMIC FEATURES

Although the shape of the stomach varies among individuals it is possible to discern some fairly constant external features (Fig. 60). The angular notch, or incisura, on the lesser curvature separates the pyloric portion on the right from the body of the stomach on the left. The cardia is the zone adjacent to the esophagus; the fundus is the dome-shaped part to the left of the esophagogastric junction. The initial wider portion of the distal stomach is the antrum, and this term usually includes the adjacent pyloric canal ending at the pylorus, where the sphincter can be palpated. Heavily contracted muscle lying proximal to the sphincter and beneath an occasional indentation on the greater curvature may erroneously be taken to be the sphincter itself. The pyloric vein (Mayo, 1907), usually visible externally (Fig. 61), marks the gastric side of the pylorus. This vessel runs across the pylorus, connecting the veins of the two curvatures. It is larger and more constant at the greater curvature.

The arteries, lymphatics, and nerves of the stomach are considered in Chapter 7, the veins in Chapter 14.

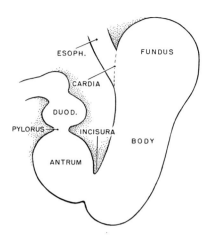

FIG. 60
External features of the stomach.

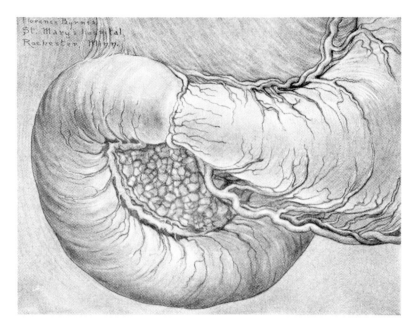

FIG. 61
The pyloric vein of Mayo. (From Mayo, 1907.)

GASTRECTOMY FOR BENIGN DISEASE

Duodenal ulcer remains the prototype indication for removal of the stomach. Gastrectomy was meant to lower gastric acidity by the removal of much of the acid-producing portion of the stomach (Moore, 1963). Berger, in 1934, mapped the location, by histologic means, of the acid-producing, or parietal, cells (Fig. 62). He found them most numerous in the body of the stomach and scanty or absent

FIG. 62

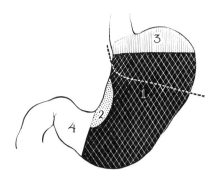

Distribution of parietal (acid-secret-
ing) cells in the human stomach. The
broken line shows the level for 75
per cent gastric resection.   1. Parie-
tal cells maximal in this area, and
rated 100 per cent.   2. Lesser cur-
vature, 75 per cent.   3. Fundus, 50
per cent.   4. Prepyloric area, 0 to 1
per cent. (From Shackelford, 1955;
modified from Berger, 1934.)

in the antrum. Surgeons agree that about three-quarters of the stomach should be removed to significantly lower gastric acidity.

In starting the gastrectomy it is desirable to locate the pyloric vein and the boundary between stomach and duodenum. Figure 63 shows the progress of dissection, in which the right gastric and gastroepiploic vessels are divided, three-quarters of the stomach is removed, the duodenal stump closed, and gastrointestinal continuity re-established. The gastrojejunal anastomosis shown is an example of the 'Billroth II' type. A gastroduodenostomy is termed a 'Billroth I' operation.

The commonest operative complications are those involved in the dissection of the ulcer or the closure of the duodenum. The commonest cause of death related to the operation is necrosis of the duodenum at the suture line when dissection has injured the supraduodenal or retroduodenal arteries, or the small arteries shared by the duodenum and pancreas (Wilkie, 1911; Shapiro and Robillard, 1946) (Fig. 64; see also Fig. 70).

Various maneuvers allow closure with minimal mobilization, as by leaving some of the antrum after removing its mucous membrane adjacent to the line of division of the duodenum (Cooper, 1971; Bennett, 1972). The ulcer is usually located in the initial duodenum. When it involves the posterior wall it may erode the gastroduodenal artery, or penetrate the pancreas. The mobilization necessary to obtain an adequate closure of the duodenum can precipitate pancreatitis or open a major pancreatic duct or the bile duct. Preliminary catheterization of the bile duct may allow easier location of this structure. Roe and his colleagues (1963) describe a fatality after partial gastrectomy due to failure to

I

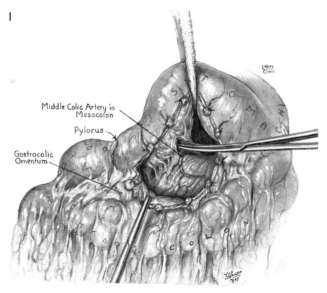

Middle Colic Artery in
Mesocolon

Pylorus

Gastrocolic
Omentum

II

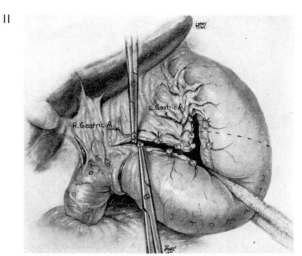

R. Gastric A.

L. Gastric A.

III

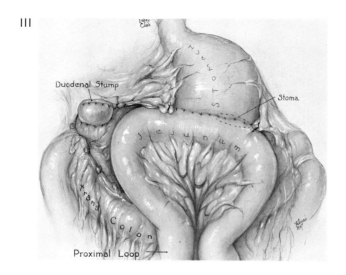

Duodenal Stump

Stoma

Proximal Loop

FIG. 63

*Partial gastrectomy for duodenal ulcer. I. The initial
dissection through the gastrocolic ligament, preserving
the gastroepiploic arterial arcades. The scissors are
dividing the adhesions of the posterior aspect of the
stomach, which are frequently present. Note the dangerous proximity of the middle colic artery. II. The
lesser omentum is divided, and branches of the gastric
arterial arcade are ligated. The bile duct has been exposed by dividing its peritoneal covering, making the
relationship of the duct to the ulcer easier to determine.
The dotted line shows the proximal extent of the gastric
resection. III. The completed duodenal closure and the
gastrojejunostomy. (From Lahey and Marshall, 1939.
By permission of Surgery, Gynecology & Obstetrics.)*

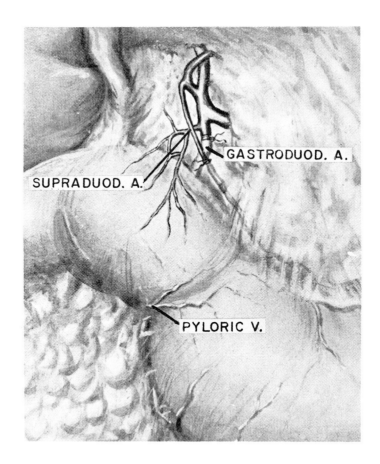

FIG. 64
The supraduodenal artery demonstrated by postmortem injection. (*From Wilkie, 1911.*)

recognize an anomalous entry of the bile and pancreatic ducts into the first part of the duodenum.

Another complication in gastrectomy is injury to the middle colic artery which lies behind the distal stomach and which may be obscured by adhesions across this part of the omental bursa (Figs. 63 and 65). Finally, necrosis of the gastric remnant can occur if the short gastric arteries or the gastroesophageal branch of the left gastric, on which the remnant must depend for its blood supply, is injured or is anatomically inadequate (Joseph, 1969). This necrosis may occur when splenectomy has to be performed because of inadvertent injury.

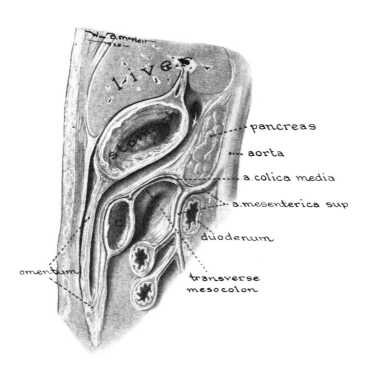

Labels on figure: pancreas, aorta, a. colica media, a. mesenterica sup, duodenum, transverse mesocolon, omentum

FIG. 65
Proximity of middle colic artery to stomach and greater omentum. (From Babcock, 1928.)

PYLOROPLASTY, HEMIGASTRECTOMY, ANTRECTOMY

Pyloroplasty, which enlarges the outlet of the stomach, is a frequent adjunct to vagotomy, when it is classified as a 'drainage procedure' to facilitate gastric emptying inhibited by total vagotomy. Procedures that remove the distal stomach, such as *hemigastrectomy* or *antrectomy,* are meant to serve an additional purpose, that of removing the antral mucosa which is the site of formation of gastrin. Thus, to the cancellation of the 'cephalic phase' of acid production by vagotomy is added a vitiation of the 'gastric phase.'

Pyloroplasty is generally accomplished in one of three ways. In the *Heineke-Mikulicz procedure,* a full-thickness longitudinal incision is made across the pylorus and the edges are then sutured transversely, enlarging the lumen. In the *Jaboulay technique,* incisions are made in adjacent faces of the stomach and duodenum and a gastroduodenostomy is performed. In the *Finney pyloroplasty,* the incisions are continuous at the pylorus, making one inverted U, and then are closed so as to enlarge the gastroduodenal passage.

The extent of the antral mucosa is pertinent in planning a hemigastrectomy or antrectomy. A general rule is to remove somewhat less than the distal half of the stomach, but most of the lesser curvature. The proximal level of the antral mucosa may be determined by the change in pH from the alkaline antral mucosa to the acid mucosa of the body of the stomach (Moe and Klopper, 1966; Kirk and Sussman, 1972). Some surgeons favor removal of only the mucosa of the antrum (Kirk and Sussman).

TOTAL GASTRECTOMY FOR CANCER OF THE STOMACH OR THE ABDOMINAL ESOPHAGUS

The lymphatic flow from the various parts of the stomach is primarily to adjacent groups of lymph nodes, thence to the celiac nodes and the intestinal trunk (see Fig. 57). This follows the usual rule that lymphatics trace the path of corresponding blood vessels. The retroperitoneal parts of this pathway are intimately connected with the lymphatics of the body and tail of the pancreas, but not with those of the pancreatic head (Grimes and Visalli, 1964).

If, indeed, the initial flow is to adjacent nodes, there is a valid basis for not removing the cardia if the cancer is prepyloric, or for leaving the antrum in place if the cancer is of the cardia or fundus. Some surgeons prefer total gastrectomy in all cases.

Reconstruction after total gastrectomy is usually by esophagojejunostomy. The anastomosis is made to the abdominal esophagus, unless the lesion has involved this structure or the cardia. In such cases the lower esophagus is also resected and the anastomosis is made at a higher level.

Operative access may be by abdominal incision alone, or by extension into the thorax, as through the 8th left intercostal space. Several maneuvers have been devised to increase exposure at the upper end of the abdominal incision to obviate the extension into the pleural cavity. These include removal of the xiphoid, or division or excision of part of the left costal arch below the pleura (see Chapter 1). After the abdomen is opened the left lobe of the liver is displaced to the right following division of the left portion of the coronary ligament ('triangular ligament') (see Figures 8 and 58).

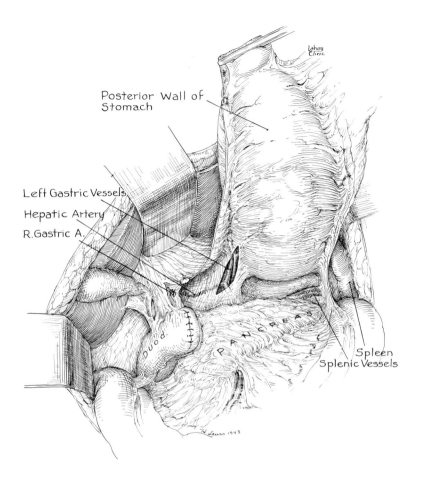

Posterior Wall of
Stomach

Left Gastric Vessels
Hepatic Artery
R. Gastric A.

Duod.

PANCREAS

Spleen
Splenic Vessels

FIG. 66
Total gastrectomy: mobilization of proximal stomach. (From Lahey and Marshall, 1944.)

The usual extent of resection in total gastrectomy is shown in Figure 66. All of the stomach and the duodenum to the line of the gastroduodenal artery are removed, along with all of the greater and lesser omenta. The blood supply to the liver is preserved. The left gastric artery is scrutinized for a potential origin of an aberrant hepatic artery (left hepatic in 18 per cent of all individuals, common hepatic in 0.5 per cent; see Fig. 97). Division of the vagus nerves facilitates mobilization of the distal esophagus and the stomach. The esophageal branch of the left gastric artery and the veins accompanying the vagus nerves are divided with them.

Lymph nodes removed in such a total gastrectomy include those lying on the two curvatures, the paracardial nodes, the nodes lying in the omenta, and the pyloric nodes. Splenectomy may be added in order to remove the pancreaticosplenic nodes.

An extended total gastrectomy carried out in the retrosplenic and retropancreatic planes includes more distal regional nodes. In this procedure, one seeks an *en bloc* removal of the stomach, spleen, the peritoneum and retroperitoneal tissues of the stomach bed, and the tail and body of the pancreas to the margin of the superior mesenteric artery (Fig. 67). At the conclusion of the procedure one has bared the left kidney and suprarenal gland, the duo-

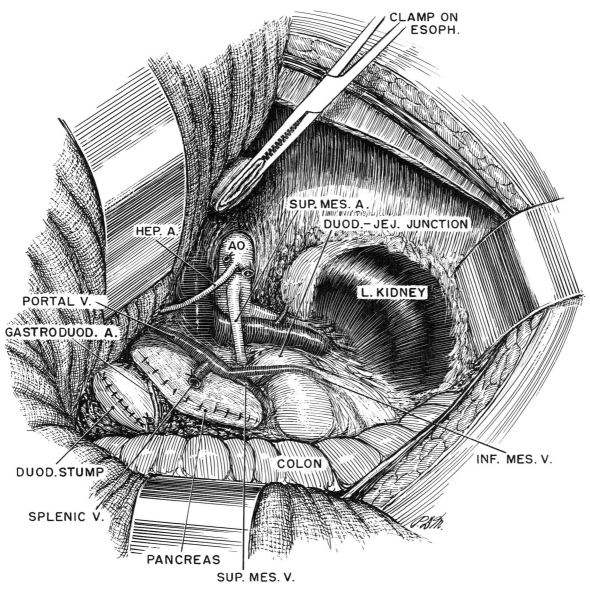

FIG. 67
Extended total gastrectomy. The incision is anterior thoracoabdominal with the diaphragm divided. (Modified from Grimes and Visalli, 1964.)

denojejunal junction, the crura of the diaphragm, and the aorta, vena cava, and portal vein. Appleby (1953), in presenting this operation, divided the celiac axis and origin of the hepatic artery, after ascertaining a separate origin from the aorta of the celiac and superior mesenteric arteries. He also removed the initial part of the duodenum to the line of the gastroduodenal artery. Grimes and Visalli (1964) preserve the origin of the hepatic artery and propose leaving the antrum when the carcinoma is of the 'proximal stomach'; indeed, they use the antrum for the concluding esophagogastrostomy.

REFERENCES

Appleby, L. H.: The coeliac axis in the expansion of the operation for gastric carcinoma. Cancer 6:704–707, 1953.

Babcock, W. W.: A Text-book of Surgery. Philadelphia, W. B. Saunders, 1928.

Bennett, J. M.: Modified Bancroft procedure for the difficult duodenal stump. Arch. Surg. 104:219–222, 1972.

Berger, E. H.: The distribution of parietal cells in the stomach: A histotopographic study. Amer. J. Anat. 54:87–114, 1934.

Cooper, P.: Duodenal Closure during Gastrectomy for Benign Ulcer. Chapter 82 in The Craft of Surgery, Cooper, P., Ed., 2nd ed. Vol. II. Boston, Little, Brown, 1971.

Grimes, O. F., and Visalli, J. A.: The embryologic approach to the surgical management of carcinoma of the upper stomach. Surg. Clin. N. Amer. 44:1227–1237, 1964.

Joseph, P. S.: Ischemic necrosis of the proximal gastric remnant. A complication of subtotal gastrectomy. Amer. J. Surg. 118:582–586, 1969.

Kirk, R. M., and Sussman, T.: Vagotomy and mucosal antrectomy in the elective treatment of duodenal ulcers. Amer. J. Surg. 123:323–328, 1972.

Lahey, F. H., and Marshall, S. F.: Technique of subtotal gastrectomy for ulcer. Surg. Gynec. Obstet. 69:498–507, 1939.

Lahey, F. H., and Marshall, S. F.: Indications for, and experiences with, total gastrectomy. Based upon seventy-three cases of total gastrectomy. Ann. Surg. 119:300–320, 1944.

Mayo, W. J.: The contributions of surgery to a better understanding of gastric and duodenal ulcer. Ann. Surg. 45:810–817, 1907.

Moe, R. E., and Klopper, P. J.: Demonstration of the functional anatomy of the canine gastric antrum. Operative technics not requiring gastrotomy. Amer. J. Surg. 111:80–88, 1966.

Moore, F. D.: Surgery in search of a rationale. Eighty years of ulcerogenic surgery. Amer. J. Surg. 105:304–312, 1963.

Roe, C. F., Gazzangia, A., McNamara, J., and Moore, F. D.:

Aberrant intrapancreatic ducts leading to fatality after gastrectomy. Amer. J. Surg. 105:685–690, 1963.

Shackelford, R. T.: Bickham-Callander Surgery of the Alimentary Tract. Vol. 1. Philadelphia, W. B. Saunders, 1955.

Shapiro, A. L., and Robillard, G. L.: Morphology and variations of the duodenal vasculature. Arch. Surg. 52:571–602, 1946.

Wilkie, D. P. D.: The blood supply of the duodenum. With special reference to the supraduodenal artery. Surg. Gynec. Obstet. 13:399–405, 1911.

тнε duodεnum,
pancreas, and spleen

THE DUODENUM AND HEAD OF THE PANCREAS AS A UNIT

Various surgical procedures can be performed separately on the duodenum or the pancreatic head, but these two organs are so bound by their embryonic origin, blood supply, lymphatic drainage, and the course of the bile and pancreatic ducts that resection of either—except for the most proximal or most distal portion of the duodenum, or of the distal pancreas—entails the removal of both.

In annular pancreas, the head of the pancreas lies in its usual position, but with two processes extending around the descending duodenum, usually fusing anteriorly (Fig. 68). Duodenal obstruction may result, and duodenal stenosis may also be present. A duct is usually present in the anterior portion running to the right, thence posteriorly to join the pancreatic duct (Cords, 1911; Théodoridès, 1964). Surgical division of the anterior part of the ring may open this duct and produce a fistula. Duodenojejunostomy is the favored treatment (Gross, 1953; Reemstma, 1960).

Duodenal diverticula almost always originate from the posteromedial wall of the descending duodenum, often

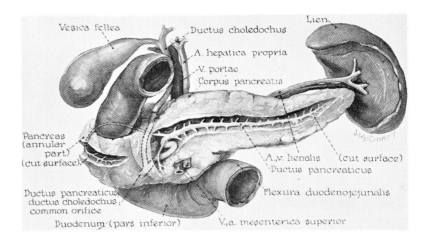

FIG. 68
Annular pancreas. (From Anson and McVay, 1971.)

Vesica fellea
Ductus choledochus
Lien.
A. hepatica propria
V. portae
Corpus pancreatis
Pancreas (annular part) (cut surface)
A., v. henalis (cut surface)
Ductus pancreaticus
Ductus pancreaticus, ductus choledochus; common orifice
Flexura duodenojejunalis
Duodenum (pars inferior)
V., a. mesenterica superior

pushing into the head of the pancreas near the bile and pancreatic ducts (Fig. 69). The duodenal papilla may be located within the diverticulum. The diverticula are approached surgically in the retroduodenal plane after performing the Kocher maneuver (see Fig. 73). Congenital stenosis of the duodenum is mentioned on page 223.

The arterial supply shared by the duodenum and pancreas has been referred to in Chapter 7 and is shown in Figure 56. Further detail on arteries to the first part of the duodenum is discussed with regard to gastrectomy (Chapter 8). Detail of the arteries to the pancreas are shown in Figure 70. The head and neck of the pancreas are supplied mainly by the anterior and posterior pancreaticoduodenal arteries. The anterior and posterior superior pancreaticoduodenal arteries usually arise separately from the gastroduodenal or the right gastroepiploic artery. The two inferior arteries most often possess a common stem. They may arise from a jejunal

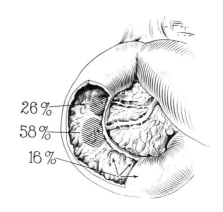

FIG. 69
Duodenal diverticula: Frequency of occurrence in various locations in 141 cases. (From Eusterman and Balfour, 1935.)

26 %
58 %
16 %

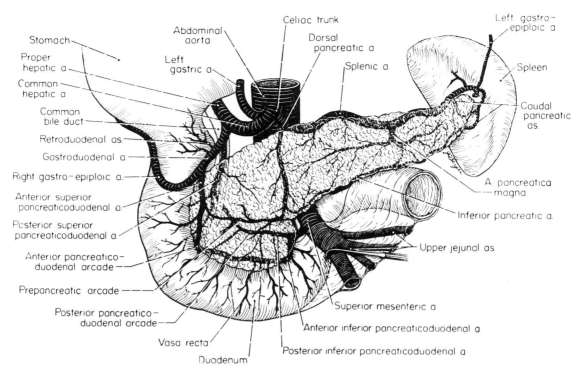

FIG. 70
Arteries of the pancreas and adjacent structures. (From Woodburne, 1973.)

artery; they then pass posterior to the superior mesenteric vessels and on to their arcades. The remainder of the pancreas is supplied by branches of the splenic artery, two of which are large and quite constant—the dorsal pancreatic and the pancreatica magna. Anomalously, the dorsal pancreatic may arise from the celiac, the common hepatic, or the superior mesenteric (see Fig. 76) or its middle colic or accessory left colic branch (see page 235, and Michels, 1962).

The veins of the head of the pancreas are arranged in anterior and posterior pancreaticoduodenal arcades accompanying the arteries. They are well shown by Descomps and de Lalaubie (1912) (Fig. 71). The posterior arcade ends in the portal vein above, and the superior mesenteric below. The posterior superior pancreaticoduodenal vein may follow its companion artery anterior to the bile duct, or it may run behind the duct. The inferior vein terminates on the left border of the superior mesenteric vein. Here it may be joined by a jejunal vein, or by the anterior inferior pancreaticoduodenal vein. Most of the anterior arcade is drained by the gastrocolic trunk through a vein termed 'inferior' by

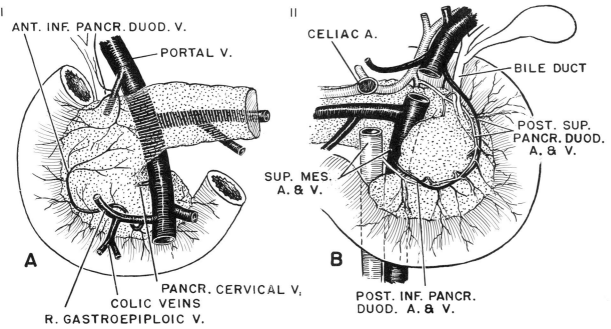

FIG. 71
Vessels about the head of the pancreas. A. Pancreaticoduodenal veins.   B. Posterior arterial and venous arcades.
(After Descomps and de Lalaubie, 1912.)

Descomps and de Lalaubie, 'superior' by Falconer and Griffiths (1950). The pancreatic cervical vein enters the right border of the lower portal vein. Several small pancreatic veins enter the major venous trunks of the portal system, but Falconer and Griffiths found that none entered the portal vein anteriorly as it lies behind the neck of the pancreas, allowing a safe separation here during resection across the neck.

The duodenum and pancreas are related to large blood vessels coursing to and from other structures (Figs. 72, 76, 115). The superior mesenteric vessels pass behind the neck of the pancreas and in front of the uncinate process and the third part of the duodenum. Here the mesenteric artery gives off significant branches (see Fig. 76), while the vein receives several tributaries (see Figs. 71, 115). The pancreas is in contact above with the celiac axis and the splenic artery; the splenic vein is partly embedded in it. Posterior to the pancreas lies the union of the splenic and the inferior and superior mesenteric in the portal vein (see Chapter 14). When the pancreas and these veins are turned up and to the right, one exposes the aorta and the celiac, superior

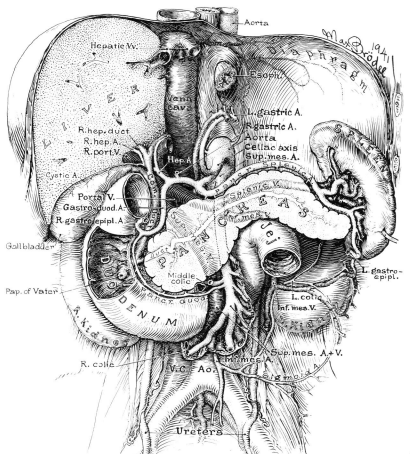

FIG. 72
Posterior relationships of the pancreas. (From Trimble et al., 1941. By permission of Surgery, Gynecology & Obstetrics.)

mesenteric, and renal arteries and the vena cava and renal veins (Fig. 73). On the right the descending duodenum and the head of the pancreas also overlie the hilum of the kidney, where they may be injured in operations on that organ. An anomalous hepatic artery arising from the superior mesenteric traverses or runs behind the head of the pancreas. When the anomalous artery is a right hepatic (incidence 18 per cent) it runs to the right, usually posterior to the portal vein and bile duct (Fig. 73); when the vessel is the common hepatic (incidence 4.5 per cent) it is most apt to run in front of the portal vein (Fig. 74). A very rare anomaly, the portal vein coursing anterior to the duodenum, is shown in Figure 114.

The relations of the pancreatic to the bile ducts are considered in Chapter 13. Variations of the pancreatic ducts are

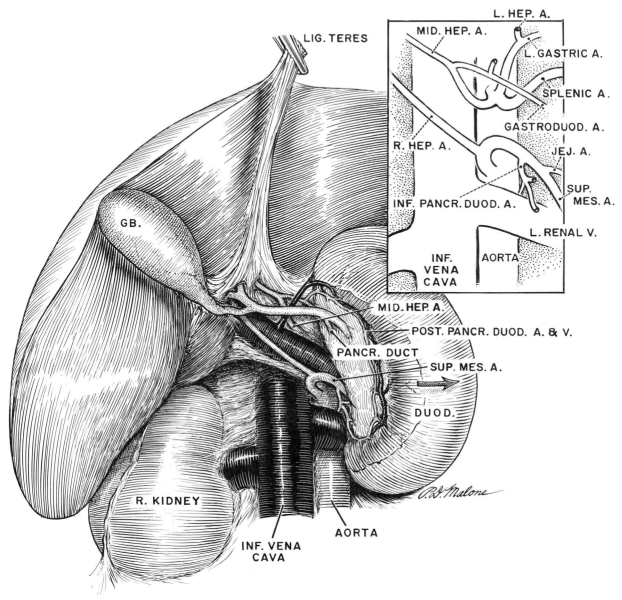

FIG. 73
Course of anomalous right hepatic artery arising from the superior mesenteric.

presented in Figure 110. The main and accessory pancreatic ducts lie close to the posterior surface of the gland, except in the tail, where the main pancreatic duct is approximately central. The duct is nevertheless sought by anterior section of the pancreas in creating an anastomosis between it and the jejunum in chronic pancreatitis (Puestow procedure) (Cattell and Warren, 1953; Howard, 1960; Puestow, 1964).

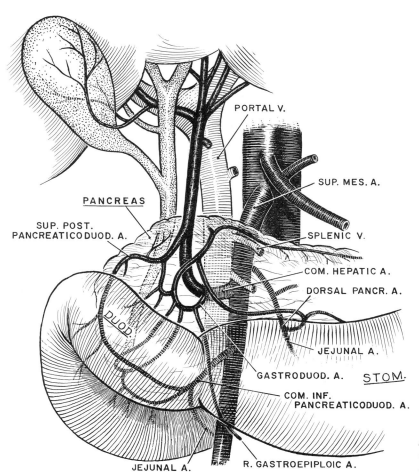

PORTAL V.

SUP. MES. A.

PANCREAS

SUP. POST.
PANCREATICODUOD. A.

SPLENIC V.

COM. HEPATIC A.

DORSAL PANCR. A.

DUOD.

JEJUNAL A.

GASTRODUOD. A.   STOM.

COM. INF.
PANCREATICODUOD. A.

JEJUNAL A.   R. GASTROEPIPLOIC A.

FIG. 74
Course of anomalous hepatic artery through pancreas and anterior to the portal vein. (After Michels, 1955.)

EXPOSURE OF THE DISTAL DUODENUM (Fig. 75)

The superior fold of the peritoneum above the para-duodenal fossa (p. 219) is often mistakenly termed the ligament of Treitz. In fact, the suspensory ligament of the duodenum lies retroperitoneally on the upper margin of the terminal duodenum (Fig. 76 II). Haley and Perry (1949) noted that the ligament is not invariably present. When it does exist, it is seen behind the pancreas and splenic vein, and in front of the left renal vein. It extends from the right crus of the diaphragm onto the duodenum and sometimes to the adjacent jejunum. Haley and Perry found that it was composed mainly of connective tissue, and, while some muscle was present in most cases, it was always of the smooth variety.

The third and fourth parts of the duodenum can be ex-

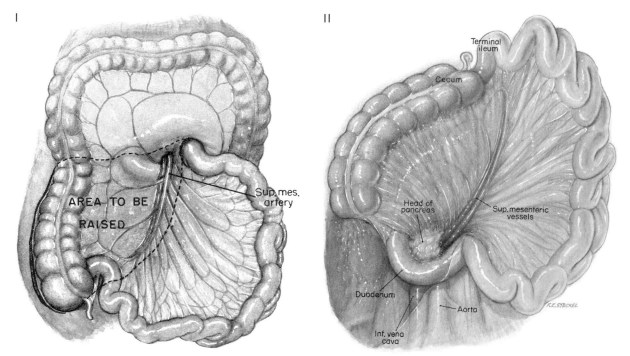

FIG. 75

Exposure of the distal duodenum. I. Planned retroperitoneal dissection. II. After mobilization of intestine and mesentery. (From Cattell and Braasch, 1960. By permission of Surgery, Gynecology & Obstetrics.)

posed by the method of Cattell and Braasch (1960), in which the mesentery of the small bowel and the cecum and ascending colon are freed retroperitoneally, and turned up (Fig. 75). The superior mesenteric vessels are clearly seen as they cross the duodenum. One can easily mobilize the duodenojejunal junction by dividing the usually tenuous suspensory ligament, remembering the proximity of the inferior mesenteric vein (Fig. 76). Once the suspensory ligament is divided, the terminal duodenum can be pushed to the right under the superior mesenteric vessels if desired. The blood supply for the duodenum to the left of the mesenteric artery is derived from that vessel and enters anteromedially. Although the duodenum here can be separated from the pancreas, the inferior pancreaticoduodenal vessels must be avoided.

In the condition known as arteriomesenteric duodenal obstruction, the third part of the duodenum is compressed by the overlying superior mesenteric vessels. A high anchorage of the duodenum by the suspensory ligament is postulated (Strong, 1958). The syndrome may be precipitated by

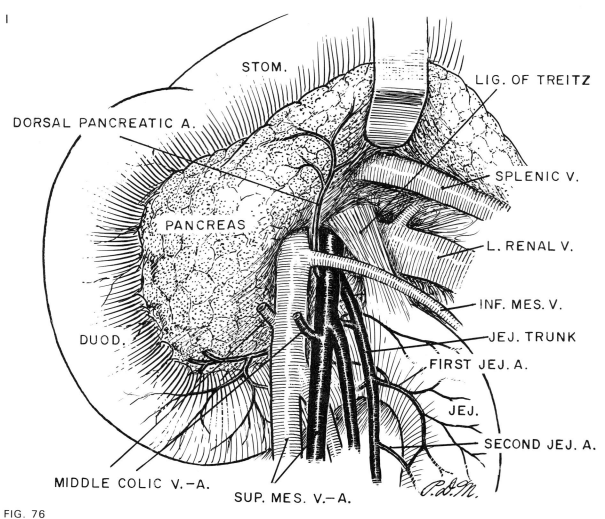

I

STOM.

LIG. OF TREITZ

DORSAL PANCREATIC A.

SPLENIC V.

PANCREAS

L. RENAL V.

INF. MES. V.

JEJ. TRUNK

DUOD.

FIRST JEJ. A.

JEJ.

SECOND JEJ. A.

MIDDLE COLIC V.—A.

SUP. MES. V.—A.

FIG. 76

The duodenojejunal junction. The pancreas is retracted upward.
I. The superior mesenteric vein is formed by two trunks, and is joined by the inferior mesenteric vein.

weight loss, as after severe burns (Ogbuokiri *et al.,* 1972), or by the application of a body cast (Puranik *et al.,* 1972). Relief may be obtained by turning the patient prone. Operative treatment consists either of dividing the suspensory ligament of the duodenum or of performing duodenojejunostomy.

APPROACHES TO THE PANCREAS

The anterior aspect of the pancreas can be approached by opening the omental bursa through the gastrohepatic

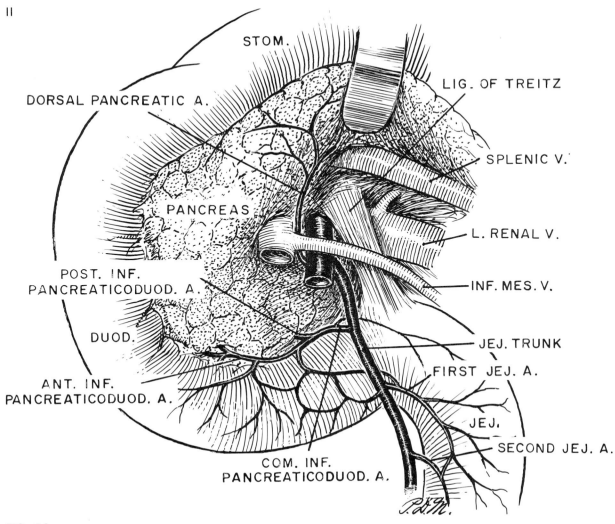

FIG. 76
The duodenojejunal junction (continued).
II. The superior mesenteric vein and artery have been removed to show the detail of arterial supply to the bowel. The artery gives off an anomalous branch to the pancreas and a special jejunal trunk.

ligament, the gastrocolic ligament, or the transverse meso-colon (Fig. 77). The gastrocolic ligament is incised above or below the course of the gastroepiploic vessels, depending on whether they lie closer to the stomach or the colon, and on the proposed operation; one divides branches of these vessels to the stomach or omentum accordingly. Near the spleen on the left, the left gastroepiploic and some short gastric vessels are often deliberately divided. Once the bursa is opened, the anterior surface of the entire gland is available through the posterior peritoneum except where the left half

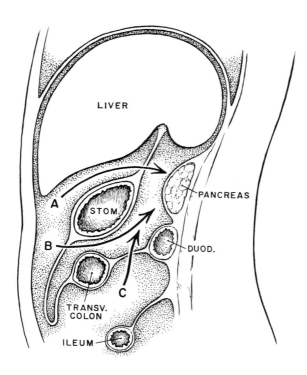

LIVER

A

STOM.

B

PANCREAS

DUOD.

C

TRANSV.
COLON

ILEUM

FIG. 77
Anterior approaches to the pancreas.

of the transverse mesocolon crosses and must be displaced downward. Certain blood vessels must be avoided. The middle colic artery may initially pass through the substance of the pancreas. Further on, it can arch upward within adhesions between the pyloric antrum and the neck of the pancreas (Fig. 63). Beneath the neck pass the superior mesenteric vessels, anterior to the uncinate process. The vein is here joined by tributaries passing anterior to the head of the pancreas (Fig. 71).

The posterior surface of the head of the pancreas is available on performing the Kocher maneuver (Fig. 73). The tail and body can also be exposed from behind by a retrosplenic and retropancreatic dissection (Fig. 78). A less extensive view is obtained by dissecting the tail off the splenic hilum; pancreatic branches of the splenic vessels then require division (see Fig. 83).

DISTAL SUBTOTAL PANCREATECTOMY

In distal subtotal pancreatectomy (Fig. 78), some or all of the head of the pancreas, with the terminations of the bile and pancreatic ducts, is allowed to remain in the duo-

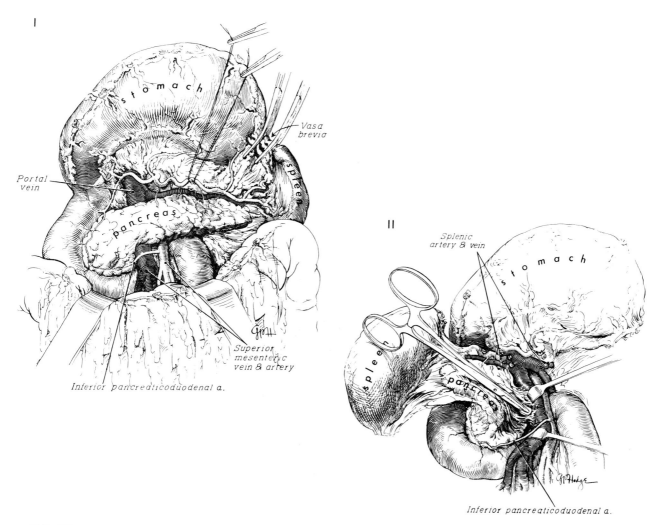

I

stomach

Vasa brevia

spleen

Portal vein

pancreas

Superior mesenteric vein & artery

Inferior pancreaticoduodenal a.

II

Splenic artery & vein

stomach

spleen

pancreas

Inferior pancreaticoduodenal a.

FIG. 78

Distal subtotal pancreatectomy. I. The omental bursa has been opened through the gastrocolic ligament. Structures behind the bursa are shown bare of their peritoneal covering. The anterior arcade of the pancreaticoduodenal arteries is evident. II. The splenic vessels have been divided, the spleen and pancreas are turned to the right, exposing the superior mesenteric vessels, the inferior mesenteric vein, and the beginning of the portal vein. III. A. The head of the pancreas is incised to leave a small portion within the duodenal curve. B. The bile duct (usually cannulated) is carefully preserved; the pancreatic duct is identified and ligated. (From Child, 1971.)

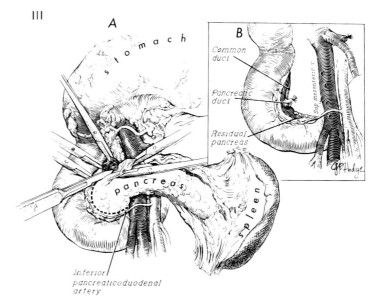

III

A

stomach

pancreas

B

Common duct

Pancreatic duct

Residual pancreas

Sup. mesenteric v.

spleen

Inferior pancreaticoduodenal artery

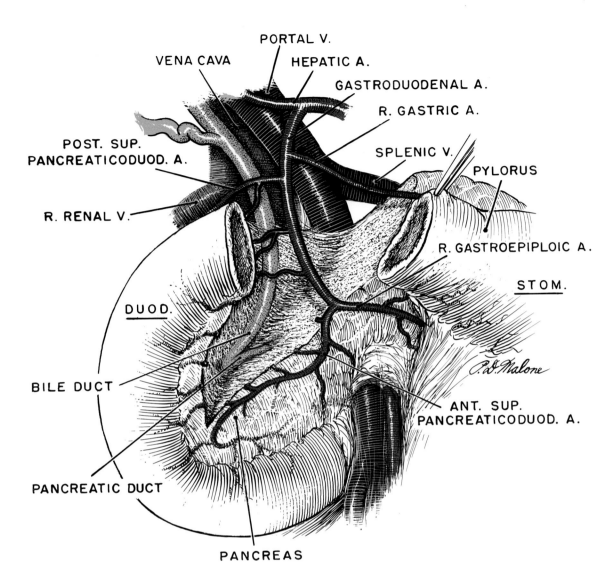

PORTAL V.

VENA CAVA

HEPATIC A.

GASTRODUODENAL A.

R. GASTRIC A.

POST. SUP.
PANCREATICODUOD. A.

SPLENIC V.

PYLORUS

R. RENAL V.

R. GASTROEPIPLOIC A.

STOM.

DUOD.

BILE DUCT

ANT. SUP.
PANCREATICODUOD. A.

PANCREATIC DUCT

PANCREAS

FIG. 79
Ducts and blood vessels in the head of the pancreas.

denal curve. The operation is simplified when the spleen is removed along with the resected pancreas if there is much pancreatic fibrosis. Entry to the retrosplenic and retropancreatic plane is gained after initial wide opening of the gastrocolic ligament, division of the splenocolic ligament, and downward displacement of the splenic flexure. The splenic artery is divided close to its origin. As previously noted, virtually no vessels enter the posterior aspect of the neck of the pancreas, so that a finger can start a separation between the neck and the anterior surface of the superior mesenteric vessels. Piedad and Wels (1972), intending to leave the spleen intact, start their dissection beneath the body, dividing the splenic vessels and elevating the pancreas toward the spleen. The three major components of the portal vein are readily disclosed. Pancreatic resection may end at the neck, or most of the head may also be removed (Fig. 79). In this event pancreatic veins, including the pancreatic cervical, will be divided on their course to the mesenteric vein (Fig. 71). One or preferably both of the pancreaticoduodenal arterial arcades are preserved, and care is taken not to injure the veins anterior to the head of the pancreas, mentioned previously.

PANCREATODUODENECTOMY

Pancreatoduodenectomy (Figs. 80, 81) is usually undertaken for cancer of the head of the pancreas, the duodenum, or the bile duct or the ampulla. It may be performed for chronic pancreatitis when there is much pathologic change in the head of the pancreas. Figure 80 shows the extent of resection. The gallbladder may be removed with the duodenum and the head and body of the pancreas (the tail remaining); the vagus nerves are sectioned to prevent gastrojejunal ulceration.

Child (1971) advises three initial steps which serve the dual purpose of displaying regional nodes to ascertain operability, and visualizing structures which must be dealt with if the resection proceeds. These are:

1. Mobilization of the duodenum and head of the pancreas (Fig. 81 I).

2. Exposure of structures in the hepatoduodenal and

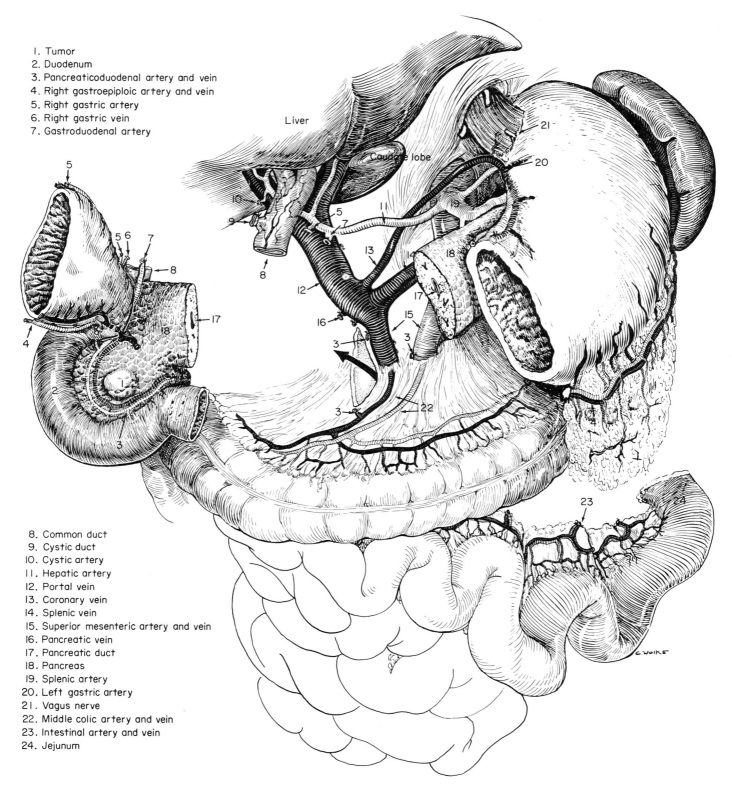

1. Tumor
2. Duodenum
3. Pancreaticoduodenal artery and vein
4. Right gastroepiploic artery and vein
5. Right gastric artery
6. Right gastric vein
7. Gastroduodenal artery

8. Common duct
9. Cystic duct
10. Cystic artery
11. Hepatic artery
12. Portal vein
13. Coronary vein
14. Splenic vein
15. Superior mesenteric artery and vein
16. Pancreatic vein
17. Pancreatic duct
18. Pancreas
19. Splenic artery
20. Left gastric artery
21. Vagus nerve
22. Middle colic artery and vein
23. Intestinal artery and vein
24. Jejunum

FIG. 80
Pancreatoduodenectomy: Extent of resection. (From Zollinger and Zollinger, 1967.)

gastrohepatic ligaments, removing the lymphatic tissue of the ligaments, and mobilizing the distal stomach (Fig. 81 II).

3. Exposure of the superior mesenteric vessels and nodes through the transverse mesocolon at the lower border of the neck of the pancreas (Fig. 81 III).

If resectability is confirmed, the common hepatic duct, stomach, and pancreas are divided; the duodenum and proximal pancreas, along with the gallbladder, are turned to the right, the pancreas being separated from the superior mesenteric vessels (Fig. 81 IV). The upper jejunum is then transected (Fig. 81 V). After division of the suspensory ligament, the duodenojejunal junction is pushed to the right behind the superior mesenteric vessels. The resected parts are now free. The concluding anastomoses of stomach, cut surface of the tail of the pancreas or the pancreatic duct, and the hepatic duct to the jejunum are shown in Figure 81 VI.

Total pancreatectomy has been advocated for diffuse tumor, rarely for chronic fibrosis and lithiasis, and for hyperinsulinism when the adenoma has otherwise not been located (Cattell and Warren, 1953). For total removal of the pancreas, resection of the spleen and tail of the pancreas is simply added to the procedure. The required dissection has been described previously under Distal Subtotal Pancreatectomy.

THE SPLENIC ARTERY

The splenic artery, instead of arising from the celiac, may stem from the aorta or the superior mesenteric artery. It may give off the following arteries: left inferior phrenic, left gastric, right gastroepiploic, left or right hepatic, superior mesenteric, middle colic, and dorsal pancreatic (Michels, 1942). The splenic artery may be divided without necrosis of the spleen. Collateral flow from gastric vessels is presumably the most significant.

Classically, five or six terminal splenic branches are said to arise at the hilum. Michels described the prehilar branching of the splenic artery as giving rise to 2 or 3 'terminal,' then to several 'penultimate,' and finally to 6 to 36 (average 17) 'ultimate' branches which enter the splenic substance

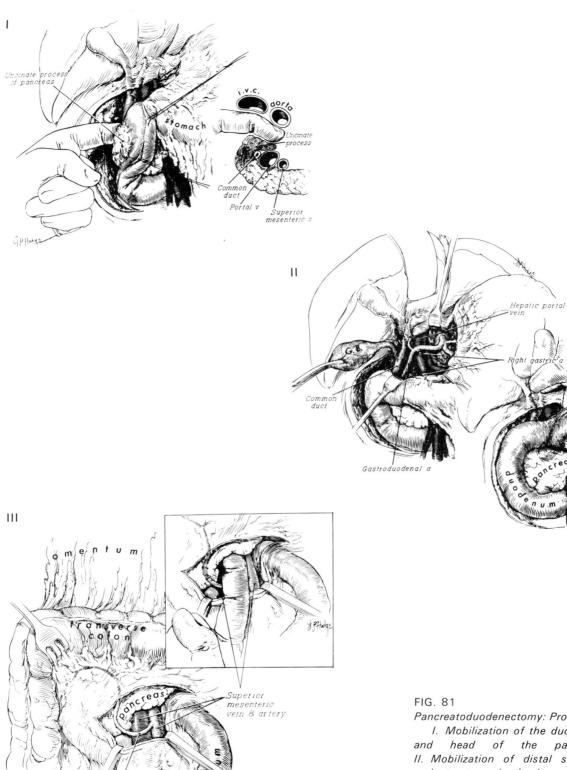

I

Uncinate process of pancreas

Stomach

I.V.C.

aorta

Uncinate process

Common duct

Portal v.

Superior mesenteric a.

II

Hepatic portal vein

Right gastric a.

Common duct

Gastroduodenal a.

Duodenum

Pancreas

III

o m e n t u m

Transverse colon

Pancreas

jejunum

Superior mesenteric vein & artery

Middle colic artery

FIG. 81

*Pancreatoduodenectomy: Procedure.
I. Mobilization of the duodenum and head of the pancreas.
II. Mobilization of distal stomach and structures in the lesser omentum. III. Identification of superior mesenteric vessels and mobilization of neck of pancreas.*

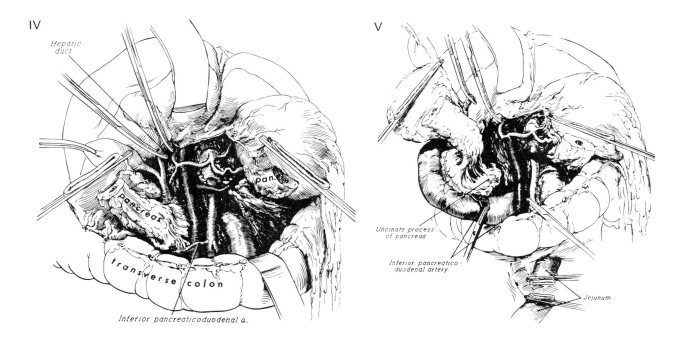

IV

Hepatic duct

pancreas

pan.

transverse colon

Inferior pancreaticoduodenal a.

V

Uncinate process of pancreas

Inferior pancreatico-duodenal artery

Jejunum

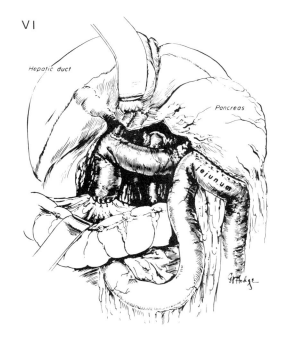

VI

Hepatic duct

Pancreas

jejunum

G.H.Hodge

FIG. 81
Pancreatoduodenectomy: Procedure (continued).

IV. Division of the stomach, pancreas, and common hepatic duct, and cholecystectomy. V. Division of jejunum and final mobilization of resected structures. VI. Anastomoses of cut end of jejunum to tail of pancreas; and side-to-end anastomoses to common hepatic duct and stomach. (From Child, 1971.)

(Fig. 82). He observed transverse hilar anastomoses (Fig. 82 I), but made no comment on anastomoses within the organ. Kyber (1870) found that each splenic branch goes to a 'lobe,' or segment, with no further communications with its neighbors. Gutierrez Cubillos (1969) confirmed the con-

I

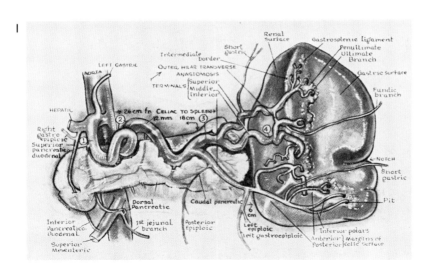

II

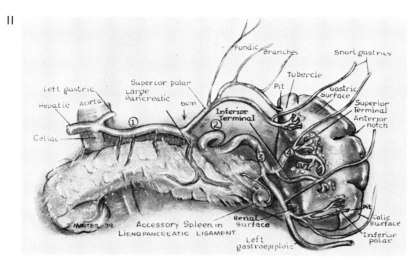

FIG. 82
Branching of the splenic artery in two specimens. Numbers 1, 2, 3, and 4 in both I and II indicate suprapancreatic, pancreatic, prepancreatic, and prehilar segments of the artery, respectively. I. There are three 'terminal' splenic branches, with one hilar transverse anastomosis. The inferior 'terminal' could as readily be called a polar artery. A caudal pancreatic branch is present. II. Two terminal and two polar arteries are identified. An accessory spleen is present. (From Michels, 1942.)

cept of circumscribed arterial segments in the spleen. 'Segmental' resection of the spleen has been performed by Campo Christo (1960) in three cases. Communications between segmental veins were noted by Kyber, and have been shown by injection by Braithwaite and Adams (1957).

SPLENECTOMY

Exposure of the spleen is usually adequate through an upper abdominal incision, often subcostal. With a very large spleen and vascular adhesions, a low left thoracoabdominal incision may be used. The spleen lies in the axis of the 10th rib, but such an incision is usually made through the 8th intercostal space.

The hilum of the spleen is approached anteriorly through the gastrocolic and gastrosplenic ligaments and the omental bursa (Fig. 83). This entails division of some short gastric arteries. The left gastroepiploic artery is also almost certainly divided, either in its course in the gastrosplenic ligament or in the hilum of the spleen where it has a variable origin (Fig. 82).

The peritoneal relationships of the spleen can now be seen. Its lower pole sits on the quite constant phrenicocolic ligament and the splenic flexure of the colon, to which it may be attached by the splenocolic ligament. Above this its convex surface is free on the diaphragm or can be freed of pathologic adhesions. The fingers slipped in behind the organ rest on the posterior leaf of the splenorenal ligament and the kidney surrounded by its fatty and fascial coverings. Anteriorly, the pancreas is seen through the anterior leaf of the splenorenal ligament, its tail folded about the lower half of the hilum. Injury to the tail of the pancreas is a well-known complication of splenectomy. The splenic artery proximal to

II

I

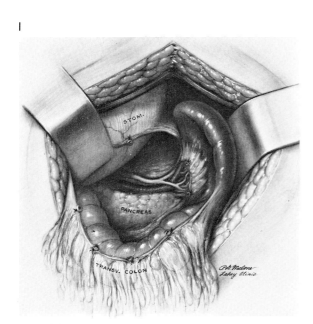
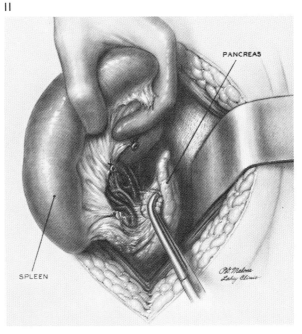

FIG. 83
Splenectomy. I. Anterior approach to the hilum. Note the substantial splenocolic ligament in this subject. II. Hilar dissection from behind. (From Lahey and Norcross, 1948.)

the hilum can usually be seen through the peritoneum above the pancreas, where it may be ligated prior to hilar dissection. The splenic vein is partly or wholly hidden by the upper edge of the pancreas.

A posterior view of the hilum is obtained after division of the peritoneum behind the spleen (posterior leaf of the splenorenal ligament). As the spleen is lifted up the tail of the pancreas will be seen in an inferior relationship to the hilar vessels, with more of the pancreas wrapped about the posterior aspect of the hilum than is usually present anteriorly (Fig. 83 II).

Accessory spleens usually measure only a few millimeters in size, but they may enlarge in hypersplenism and can continue the disease after splenectomy. Accessory spleens are common in infancy, but diminish in number with age, with an overall incidence of 10 per cent (Halpert and Eaton, 1951). With hypersplenism, an incidence of 50 per cent has been observed in the first decade, and 30 per cent for all ages (Curtis and Movitz, 1946). Curtis and Movitz found about half of these structures in the splenic hilum (Fig. 84), one fourth in relation to the pedicle and pancreas, and almost all the rest in the omentum near the greater curvature of the stomach. Some few were found elsewhere, in the female especially about the left ovary and tube. The acces-

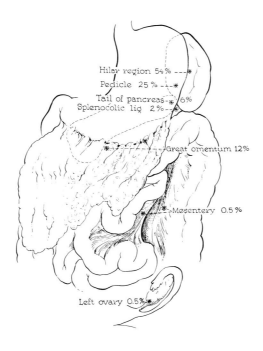

Hilar region 54%
Pedicle 25%
Tail of pancreas 6%
Splenocolic lig 2%
Great omentum 12%
Mesentery 0.5%
Left ovary 0.5%

FIG. 84
Location of accessory spleens. (From Anson and McVay, 1971; data from Curtis and Movitz, 1946.)

sory spleens were often multiple, up to eight in number, although all were grouped in one or two locations.

Either asplenia or polysplenia is often associated with partial situs inversus (see Chapter 2). Splenogonadal fusion is a very rare condition associated with ectromelia and micrognathism, but not with situs inversus. In this anomaly, splenic tissue or a fibrous cord extends from the spleen to the left gonad. The condition is more frequent in males, and the splenic mass in the inguinal region has been mistaken for a third testis (Gray and Skandalakis, 1972).

REFERENCES

Anson, B. J., and McVay, C. B.: Surgical Anatomy, 5th ed. Philadelphia, W. B. Saunders, 1971.

Braithwaite, J. L., and Adams, D. J.: The venous drainage of the rat spleen. J. Anat. 91:352–357, 1957.

Campo Christo, M.: Splénectomies partielles réglées. A propos de 3 cas operés. Presse Med. 68:485–486, 1960.

Cattell, R. B., and Braasch, J. W.: A technique for the exposure of the third and fourth portions of the duodenum. Surg. Gynec. Obstet. 111:378–379, 1960.

Cattell, R. B., and Warren, K. W.: Surgery of the Pancreas. Philadelphia, W. B. Saunders, 1953.

Child, G. C., 3rd: Subtotal Pancreatectomies. Chapter 99 in The Craft of Surgery, Cooper, P., Ed., 2nd ed. Vol. II. Boston, Little, Brown, 1971.

Cords, E.: Ein Fall von ringförmigem Pankreas, nebst Bemerkungen über die Genese dieser Anomalie. Anat. Anz. 39:33–40, 1911.

Curtis, G. M., and Movitz, D.: The surgical significance of the accessory spleen. Ann. Surg. 123:276–298, 1946.

Descomps, P., and de Lalaubie, G.: Les veines mésentériques. J. Anat. Phys. (Paris) 48:337–376, 1912.

Eusterman, G. B., and Balfour, D. C.: The Stomach and Duodenum. Philadelphia, W. B. Saunders, 1935.

Falconer, C. W. A., and Griffiths, E.: The anatomy of the blood-vessels in the region of the pancreas. Brit. J. Surg. 37:334–344, 1950.

Gray, S. W., and Skandalakis, J. E.: Embryology for Surgeons. The Embryological Basis for the Treatment of Congenital Defects. Philadelphia, W. B. Saunders, 1972.

Gross, R. E.: The Surgery of Infancy and Childhood. Its Principles and Techniques. Philadelphia, W. B. Saunders, 1953.

Gutiérrez Cubillos, C.: Segmentación esplénica. Rev. Esp. Enferm. Apar. Digest. 29:341–350, 1969.

Haley, J. C., and Perry, J. H.: Further study of the suspensory muscle of the duodenum. Amer. J. Surg. 77:590–595, 1949.

Halpert, B., and Eaton, W. L.: Accessory spleens: A pilot study of 600 necropsies (Abstract). Anat. Rec. 109:371, 1951.

Howard, J. M.: Treatment of Relapsing and Chronic Pancreatitis. Chapter 17 *in* Surgical Diseases of the Pancreas, Howard, J. M., and Jordan, G. L., Jr., Eds. Philadelphia, J. B. Lippincott, 1960.

Kyber, E.: Ueber die Milz des Menschen und einiger Säugethiere. Arch. mikr. Anat. 6:540–580, 1870.

Lahey, F. H., and Norcross, J. W.: Splenectomy: When is it indicated. Ann. Surg. 128:363–378, 1948.

Michels, N. A.: The variational anatomy of the spleen and splenic artery. Amer. J. Anat. 70:21–72, 1942.

Michels, N. A.: Blood Supply and Anatomy of the Upper Abdominal Organs. Philadelphia, J. B. Lippincott, 1955.

Michels, N. A.: The anatomic variations of the arterial pancreaticoduodenal arcades: Their import in regional resection involving the gallbladder, bile ducts, liver, pancreas and parts of the small and large intestines. J. Int. Coll. Surg. 37:13–40, 1962.

Ogbuokiri, C. G., Law, E. J., and MacMillan, B. G.: Superior mesenteric artery syndrome in burned children. Amer. J. Surg. 124:75–79, 1972.

Piedad, O. H., and Wels, P. B.: Retrograde distal pancreatectomy. Amer. J. Surg. 124:431–432, 1972.

Puestow, C. B.: Surgery of the Biliary Tract, Pancreas, and Spleen, 2nd ed. Chicago, Year Book Medical Publishers, 1964.

Puranik, S. R., Keiser, R. P., and Gilbert, M. G.: Arteriomesenteric duodenal compression in children. Amer. J. Surg. 124:334–339, 1972.

Reemstma, K.: Embryology and Congenital Anomalies of the Pancreas. Chapter 3 *in* Surgical Diseases of the Pancreas, Howard, J. M., and Jordan, G. J., Jr., Eds. Philadelphia, J. B. Lippincott, 1960.

Strong, E. K.: Mechanics of arteriomesenteric duodenal obstruction and direct surgical attack upon etiology, Ann. Surg. 148:725–730, 1958.

Théodoridès, T.: Pancréas annulaire. J. Chir. (Paris) 87:445–462, 1964.

Trimble, I. R., Parsons, J. W., and Sherman, C. P.: A one stage operation for the cure of carcinoma of the ampulla of Vater and of the head of the pancreas. Surg. Gynec. Obstet. 73:711–722, 1941.

Woodburne, R. T.: Essentials of Human Anatomy. 5th ed. New York, Oxford, 1973.

Zollinger, R. M., and Zollinger, R. M., Jr.: Atlas of Surgical Operations. Vol. II. New York, Macmillan, 1967.

SECTION 4
The Liver; Biliary and Portal Systems

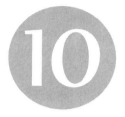

poRTAl lobulATioN;
iNTERNAL disTRibuTioN
of poRTAl TRiAd
ANd THE HEpATic vEiNS

LOBES, SEGMENTS, AND SUBSEGMENTS

No consideration of the operative anatomy of the liver can be attempted until the internal distribution of its blood vessels and ducts has been described. The pattern of branching of the portal structures was examined by several workers in the last century, especially by Rex (1888). The lobulation of the liver based on this branching was firmly established by Cantlie (1897), who stated ''. . . the gall-bladder occupies a central position in the liver; that on either side of it lie the true right and left lobes of the liver, and that a line from the fundus of the gall-bladder to the exit of the hepatic veins [Fig. 85] divides the liver into equal portions, as shown by injections, by weighings, by developmental, by pathological, and by clinical observations.'' We adopt his suggestion, calling these halves of the liver the right and left lobes. For the gross anatomical portions located to the right and left of the falciform and teres liga-

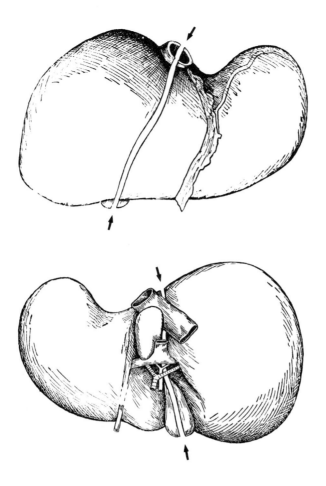

FIG. 85
The sagittal fissure: Cantlie's inter-
lobar line. (From Cantlie, 1897.)

ments, heretofore called 'lobes,' we propose the expression
''major and minor portions'' (portio major and portio minor).

Numerous injection experiments (Sérégé, 1901; Segall,
1923; and McIndoe and Counseller, 1927) established that
there is no communication between the branches of the
portal triad (Fig. 86) across Cantlie's line. Hepatic arteriolar
communications do exist in the liver capsule, and perhaps
within the liver, which are capable of re-establishing lobar
arterial flow following ligation (Mays, 1972). These studies
culminated in those of Healey and Schroy (1953) and of
Michels (1955), who found that the lobes are divisible into
segments and subsegments ('areas') of delimited blood supply and duct drainage (Fig. 87). Table 6 shows the relation
of their nomenclature for the subdivisions with those of
Hjortsjö and Couinaud, whose writings on this subject are
of importance. The expressions 'quadrate lobe' and 'caudate
lobe' are generally maintained. The quadrate lobe constitutes

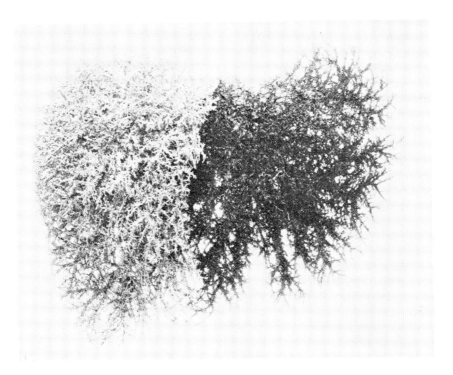

FIG. 86
Limitation of distribution of lobar branches of the portal vein shown by celloidin injection and corrosion. (From McIndoe and Counseller, 1927.)

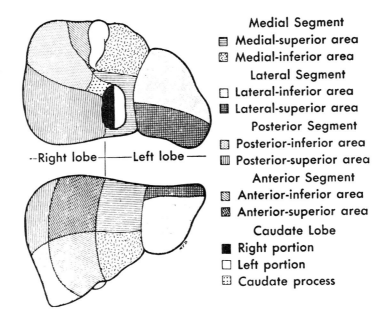

Medial Segment
⊞ Medial-superior area
▨ Medial-inferior area
Lateral Segment
☐ Lateral-inferior area
▦ Lateral-superior area
Posterior Segment
▨ Posterior-inferior area
▥ Posterior-superior area
Anterior Segment
▨ Anterior-inferior area
▨ Anterior-superior area
Caudate Lobe
■ Right portion
☐ Left portion
⊞ Caudate process

--Right lobe——Left lobe——

FIG. 87
Hepatic lobes, segments, and areas (subsegments). (From Healey, Schroy, and Sorensen, 1953.)

TABLE 6

TABLE 6
Designation of Hepatic Segments and Subsegments

Hjortsjö (1951) 'Segments' and 'Portions'	Healey, Schroy, and Sorensen (1953) 'Segments' and 'Subsegments' ('Areas')	Couinaud (1955) 'Segments'
	RIGHT LOBE	
Intermediate and Ventrocranial segments	Anterior Segment	
	Superoanterior subsegment	VIII
	Inferoanterior subsegment	V
Dorsocaudal Segment	Posterior Segment	
	Superoposterior subsegment	VII
	Inferoposterior subsegment	VI
	LEFT LOBE	
Medial Portion	Medial Segment	IV
	Superomedial subsegment	
	Inferomedial subsegment ("Quadrate Lobe")	
Lateral Portion	Lateral Segment	
	Superolateral subsegment	II
	Inferolateral subsegment	III
	CAUDATE LOBE	I
	Right Portion	
	Left Portion	
	Caudate Process	

the inferomedial subsegment (left lobe); the caudate lobe belongs to both right and left lobes.

Three internal fissures are recognized: The median sagittal (main, interlobar fissure), unmarked on the surface, follows Cantlie's line. The right, or segmental, fissure, also unmarked, separates the anterior from the posterior segment. The left lateral, or segmental, fissure is marked on the inferior surface by the umbilical fissure, containing the ligamentum teres, or umbilical vein, and the fissure for the ligamentum venosum, or ductus venosus (see Fig. 121).

INTRAHEPATIC DISTRIBUTION OF THE PORTAL STRUCTURES

Of the three components of the portal triad, the branching of the portal vein is the most prominent and subject to the least variation (Fig. 88). The vein divides at the porta hepatis into right and left branches. These primary branches and their subdivisions maintain a position within the liver posterior to the bile ducts, and generally anterior to the branches of the hepatic artery (pp. 177; Figs. 99 III, 102 II, 103, 104, 105). The right branch of the portal vein shortly divides into the anterior and posterior segmental veins, which further divide into subsegmental branches. The left portal vein is long. Its transverse portion reaches the umbilical fissure, giving off branches to the caudate lobe. The umbilical portion, within the fissure, gives off medial and lateral segment veins, often as separate subsegmental

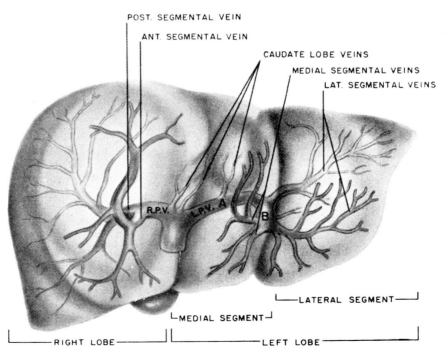

FIG. 88
Intrahepatic portal vein branching. (From Healey and Schwartz, 1964.)

branches. The left portal vein also receives the ligamentum teres anteriorly, and the ligamentum venosum posteriorly (Fig. 121).

The proper hepatic artery usually reaches the porta anterior to the portal vein and divides into the right and left hepatic arteries for the corresponding lobes (Fig. 89). The medial segment, or quadrate lobe, artery, named the middle hepatic by Rex (1888), is a branch of the left hepatic in about 75 per cent of cases. It stems from that artery in the porta, directly or via the inferolateral subsegment branch (Fig. 90). In about 25 per cent of subjects the middle hepatic arises from the proper hepatic, the right hepatic, or from a replaced left hepatic coming from the left gastric (Fig. 90). Its subsegmental branches may arise separately in various combinations. The lateral segment artery runs either anterior or posterior to the left hepatic duct. Its division into subsegment arteries usually takes place in the umbilical fissure

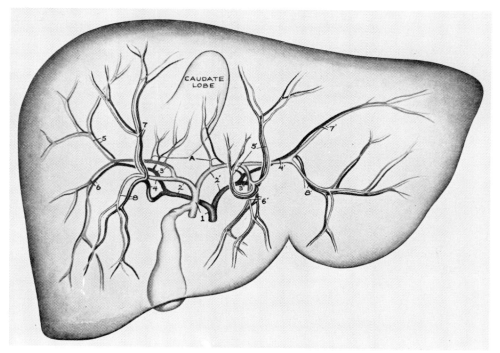

FIG. 89

Intrahepatic arteries and ducts. Numbers refer to artery and duct of each part. 1. Common hepatic duct and artery. A. Branches to caudate lobe. Branches to right lobe: 2. Lobar. 3. Posterior segment. 4. Anterior segment. 5. Superoposterior subsegment. 6. Inferoposterior subsegment. 7. Superoanterior subsegment. 8. Inferoanterior subsegment. Branches to left lobe: 2'. Lobar. 3'. Medial segment. 4'. Lateral segment. 5'. Superomedial subsegment. 6'. Inferomedial subsegment. 7'. Superolateral subsegment. 8'. Inferolateral subsegment. (From Healey, Schroy, and Sorensen, 1953.)

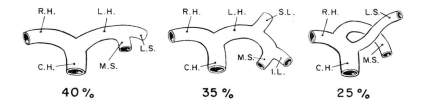

(see Fig. 102 I), but division to the right of the fissure occurs in about one third of livers.

The right hepatic artery usually passes behind the common hepatic duct (Fig. 99 II), and terminates in the anterior and posterior segment arteries. Initially, the anterior segment artery runs inferior to the posterior segment artery. Its tortuous course, especially when it originates prematurely, places it close to the gallbladder, where it may be injured (Fig. 99 II). Exceptionally, a branch supplying an anterior subsegment may come off the posterior segment artery, or one supplying a posterior subsegment may come off the anterior segment artery.

Supernumerary arteries or ducts each supply some well-circumscribed subdivision of the liver, and are not accessory in the sense of compensating for loss of an artery or duct.

The intrahepatic biliary ducts parallel the branches of the hepatic artery and portal vein (Healey and Schroy, 1953) (Fig. 89). The prevailing pattern shown in Figure 89 exists in 72 per cent for the right lobe and 67 per cent for the left (Fig. 91). Johnston and Anson (1952) found an accessory right duct of undetermined origin terminating in the cystic duct almost as frequently as in the common duct. Healey and Schroy describe a "subvesical duct" in the gallbladder bed in 35 per cent of their specimens (Fig. 99 II), terminating in either the anterior segmental or the right hepatic duct. Neither pair of workers ever found a biliary duct entering the gallbladder, but Sachs (1952) reported a case in which the two hepatic ducts terminated in the gallbladder. Left-sided ductal variations include a frequent union of the left segmental or subsegmental ducts to the right of the umbilical fissure.

Small aberrant ducts other than those seen at the portal hilum have been found in the fossa for the vena cava, the umbilical fissure, and the hepatogastric and the coronary and triangular ligaments. Aberrant ducts in the left triangular

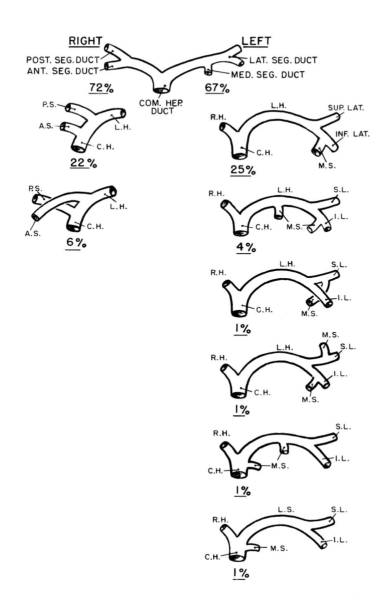

FIG. 91
Variations in termination of hepatic segmental ducts. (From Healey and Schroy, 1953.)

ligament are of special interest. Here the appendix fibrosa hepatica (the fibrous tapering end of the left lobe of the liver) attaches to the diaphragm. Small aberrant biliary ducts and bits of liver tissue may be seen within this appendage (Rapant and Hromada, 1950; Hobsley, 1958). These ducts are also described by Michels (1955) and Tôn (1962). They are said to be more numerous after infancy, incident to a relative shrinkage of the liver parenchyma. Healey and Schroy (1953) found them in 5 per cent of their preparations, extending from the superolateral subsegment duct. These aberrant ducts are subject to injury, with resultant bile leakage, during detachment of the left triangular ligament (see Fig. 8), as occurred in two cases of Rapant and Hromada. Tôn also reported such an event occurring during the performance of a left lobectomy for intrahepatic calculus. He points out that these aberrant ducts are specially significant because the duct of the superolateral subsegment is a frequent site of intrahepatic calculi.

THE HEPATIC VEINS

The hepatic veins constitute a second hilar system for the liver. Three major hepatic veins—right, middle, and left—terminate in the inferior vena cava adjacent to the inferior surface of the diaphragm (Fig. 92), and four or more small hepatic veins end in the cava as it lies in its groove

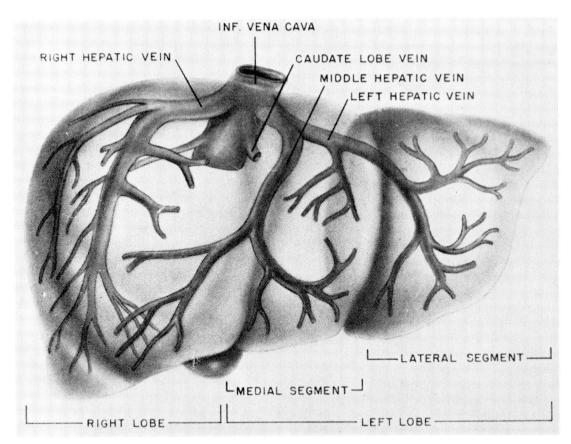

FIG. 92

Intrahepatic course of the major hepatic veins. (From Healey and Schwartz, in Surgical Diseases of the Liver, by S. I. Schwartz. Copyright 1964, McGraw-Hill Book Company, New York. Used with permission of McGraw-Hill Book Company.)

in the liver (see Fig. 101). In the anomaly which one of us has termed azygos continuation (see Fig. 40), the inferior vena cava fails in its formation above the renal veins, the blood returning from the renal level via the azygos system. In this condition, the hepatic veins converge on the caval orifice of the diaphragm and pass as one vessel through the orifice to enter the right atrium. What replaces the usual connections of the umbilical vein and the inferior vena cava in this condition has not been described. Each major hepatic vein traverses one of the major fissures of the liver, receiving tributaries from adjacent lobes or segments, an arrangement comparable to that in the lung.

The middle hepatic vein, in the interlobar fissure, is formed by union of the inferior subsegment veins of the (right) anterior segment and the (left) medial segment. This union lies anterior to the primary bifurcation of the portal structures (see Fig. 99 III). The middle hepatic joins the left hepatic vein just prior to its termination in the cava, or the two veins enter the cava immediately adjacent to each other.

The right hepatic vein runs in the right segmental fissure, draining the entire posterior segment, and the superoanterior subsegment (Fig. 92). Its two component veins may fail to join until just prior to its termination.

The left hepatic vein is formed by the union of the two subsegment veins of the lateral segment in the upper part of the left segmental fissure; then it turns to the right, receiving the superomedial subsegment vein prior to ending in the cava. In their terminal course the right and left hepatic veins lie close to the diaphragmatic surface of the bare area, and each receives a small superior hepatic vein which parallels this surface (Fig. 93). The superior hepatic veins may end separately in the cava. At its termination, the left hepatic is not covered by liver tissue on its superior surface; here it may receive the left inferior phrenic vein. The vena cava or the left hepatic, left superior hepatic, or the left inferior phrenic vein may be torn in the detachment of the left triangular and coronary ligaments in upper abdominal exposures (see Fig. 8).

Variations of the major hepatic veins hinge mainly on the completeness with which the middle hepatic vein drains the adjacent medial and anterior segments. From the figures of Elias and Sherrick (1969), it appears that most commonly

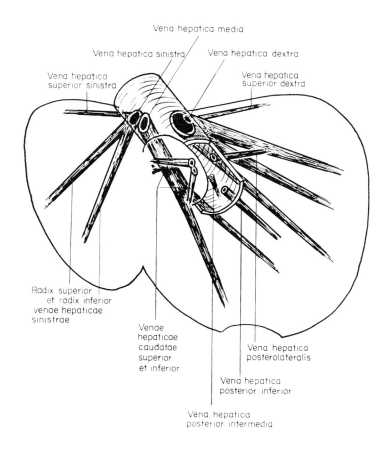

Vena hepatica media

Vena hepatica sinistra / Vena hepatica dextra

Vena hepatica
superior sinistra

Vena hepatica
superior dextra

Radix superior
et radix inferior
venae hepaticae
sinistrae

Venae
hepaticae
caudatae
superior
et inferior

Vena hepatica
posterolateralis

Vena hepatica
posterior inferior

Vena hepatica
posterior intermedia

FIG. 93
*Caval termination of major and minor
hepatic veins. The liver is viewed
from behind. (From Elias and Sherrick, 1969.)*

this vein drains both the upper and the lower medial subsegment, although Healey and Schwartz (Fig. 92) indicate that
the upper subsegmental vein usually enters the left hepatic.
This distinction is blurred when the middle and left hepatic
veins join much proximal to their termination, with the
superomedial segment vein entering the angle between the
two. On the right, the middle hepatic vein generally drains
only the inferior part of the anterior segment. Elias and
Sherrick show one liver in which the entire anterior segment
is drained by the middle hepatic vein.

Several small hepatic veins (Fig. 93) are described by
Elias and Sherrick (1969) as constant. The right and left
hepatic veins usually receive a right and a left superior
hepatic vein draining the posterosuperior margins of the
liver. The other small veins terminate in the inferior vena
cava as it lies in its groove in the liver: (1) Superior and
inferior caudate hepatic veins drain the caudate lobe. (2) The
posterior intermediate hepatic vein drains the caudate process. (3) The posterior inferior hepatic drains a territory to

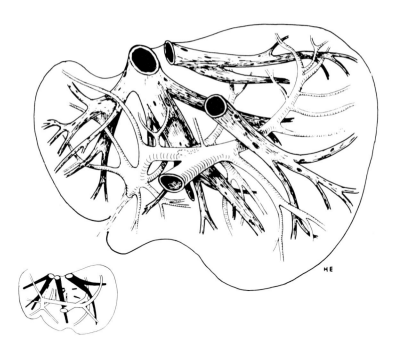

FIG. 94
Unusual large posterior inferior hepatic vein replacing the posterior tributary of the right hepatic vein. The liver is viewed from behind. The small figure shows the prevailing pattern of the major hepatic and the portal veins. (From Elias and Sherrick, 1969.)

the right of the gallbladder. (4) The posterolateral drains the ridge between the renal and duodenal impressions of the right lobe. Occasionally one of the small hepatic veins appropriates an unusually large tributary. Thus Elias and Sherrick show one case in which the posterior inferior vein is augmented by taking over much of the drainage usually coursing to the right hepatic vein (Fig. 94).

REFERENCES

Cantlie, J.: On a new arrangement of the right and left lobes of the liver. Proc. Anat. Soc. Gr. Brit. and Ireland, June 1897, pp. iv–ix. (Bound with J. Anat. Physiol. [London], vol. 32, 1898.)

Couinaud, C.: Recherches sur la chirurgie du confluent biliaire supérieur et des canaux hépatiques. Presse Med. 63:669–674, 1955.

Elias, H., and Sherrick, J. C.: Morphology of the Liver. New York, Academic Press, 1969.

Healey, J. E., Jr., and Schroy, P. C.: Anatomy of the biliary ducts within the human liver. Analysis of the prevailing pattern of branchings and the major variations of the biliary ducts. Arch. Surg. 66:599–616, 1953.

Healey, J. E., Jr., Schroy, P. C., and Sorensen, R. J.: The intrahepatic distribution of the hepatic artery in man. J. Int. Coll. Surg. 20:133–148, 1953.

Healey, J. E., Jr., and Schwartz, S. I.: Surgical Anatomy. Chapter

1 *in* Surgical Diseases of the Liver, Schwartz, S. I., Ed. New York, McGraw-Hill, 1964.

Hjortsjö, C.-H.: The topography of the intrahepatic duct systems. Acta Anat. 11:599–615, 1951.

Hobsley, M.: Intra-hepatic anatomy. A surgical evaluation. Brit. J. Surg. 45:635–644, 1958.

Johnston, E. V., and Anson, B. J.: Variations in the formation and vascular relationships of the bile ducts. Surg. Gynec. Obstet. 94:669–686, 1952.

McIndoe, A. H., and Counseller, V. S.: The bilaterality of the liver. Arch. Surg. 15:589–612, 1927.

Mays, E. T.: Lobar dearterialization for exsanguinating wounds of the liver. J. Trauma 12:397–407, 1972.

Michels, N. A.: Blood Supply and Anatomy of the Upper Abdominal Organs. Philadelphia, J. B. Lippincott, 1955.

Rapant, V., and Hromada, J.: A contribution to the surgical significance of aberrant hepatic ducts. Ann. Surg. 132:253–259, 1950.

Rex, H.: Beitrage zur Morphologie der Säugerleber. Morph. Jahr. 14:517–617, 1888.

Sachs, A. E.: Absence of common bile duct. J.A.M.A. 149:1462–1463, 1952.

Segall, H. N.: An experimental anatomical investigation of the blood and bile channels of the liver. Surg. Gynec. Obstet. 37:152–178, 1923.

Sérégé, H.: Recherches expérimentales sur la distribution du sang porté dans le foie. J. Med. Bordeaux 31:208, 271–275, 291–295, 1901.

Tôn That Tung: Chirurgie d'exérèse du foie. Hanoi, Editions en Langues Étrangères, 1962.

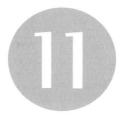

EXTERNAL ANATOMY and ATTACHMENTS of THE liver; elements of THE portal pedicle

VARIATIONS IN FORM AND LOCATION OF THE LIVER

There is considerable variation in the extent of the normal liver seen below the costal arch, and in its occupancy of the right and left hypochondria. This is based on differences in size of the entire organ, on variation in the relative size of its major and minor portions (portions to either side of the falciform ligament, as explained in Chapter 10), and on variations in the curvature of the spine and in the position of the diaphragm.

Anomalously lobed or accessory livers are quite rare. They are well described by Poirier and Charpy (1901) and by Cullen (1925). Probably the commonest of these anomalies is Riedel's 'lobe,' a linguiform projection from the inferior border on the right of the gallbladder (Fig. 95 I). 'Mul-

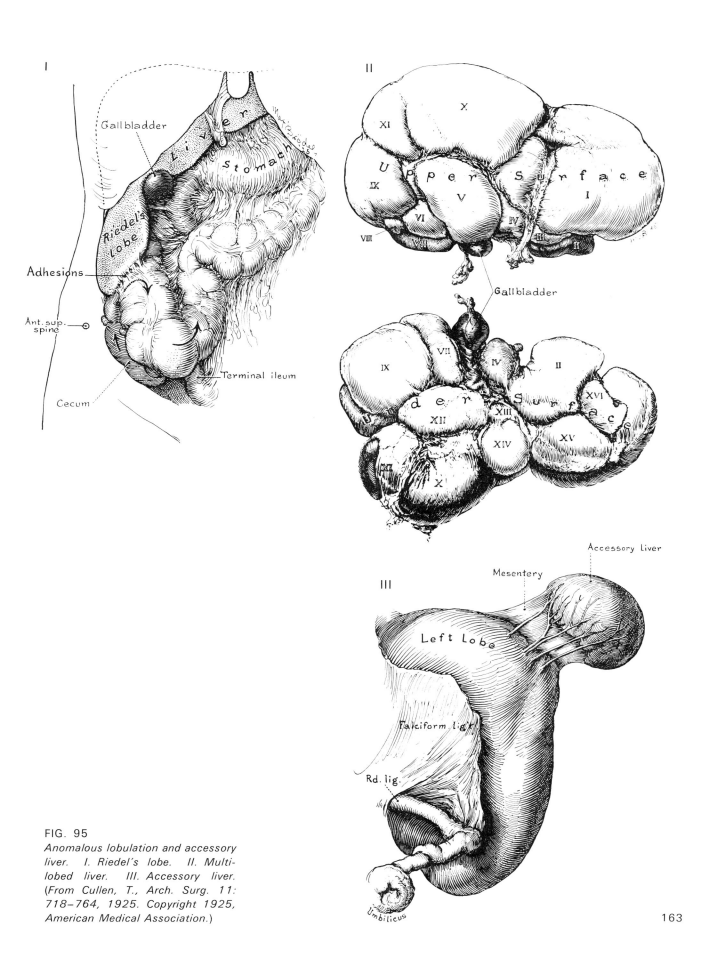

I

Gallbladder

Liver

Stomach

Riedel's
Lobe

Adhesions

Ant. sup.
spine

Cecum

Terminal ileum

II

X

XI

U p p e r   S u r f a c e

IX

V

I

VI

IV

VIII

VII

III

II

Gallbladder

VII

IV

II

IX

XVI

d e r   S u r f a c e

XII

XIII

XV

XIV

XI

X

Accessory liver

Mesentery

III

Left Lobe

Falciform lig.

Rd. lig.

Umbilicus

FIG. 95

*Anomalous lobulation and accessory
liver. I. Riedel's lobe. II. Multi-
lobed liver. III. Accessory liver.
(From Cullen, T., Arch. Surg. 11:
718–764, 1925. Copyright 1925,
American Medical Association.)*

163

tilobed' livers (Fig. 95 II) may represent a separation into segments or subsegments, but only more recently, in the simplest of examples, have attempts been made to identify the subdivisions represented (Tôn, 1962; and Couinaud, 1955). The same is true of the excessively rare 'accessory' livers (Fig. 95 III) (Llorente and Dardik, 1971). The identification of these normal variations by radioactive scanning is described by Feist and Lasser (1959).

PERITONEAL ATTACHMENTS

The liver develops in the ventral mesentery of the stomach and duodenum, growing upward to the junction of that mesentery with the peritoneum covering the diaphragm. The liver thus spreads the leaves of the junction so that its more central upper surface is bare where it rests upon the diaphragm. The bare area and the surrounding ligaments constitute a major zone for the passage of lymphatics from the liver to intrathoracic nodes, for collateral hepatic artery flow and portasystemic venous communications, and for some innervation from the phrenic nerves. The reflection of peritoneum from the under surface of the diaphragm upon the liver is the coronary ligament (Fig. 96); the right and left extremes of the coronary ligament constitute the triangular ligaments. While the liver ascends in its growth, its portal pedicle remains within its path of ascent—the ventral mesogastrium, called in the adult the lesser omentum (see Fig. 55). The right lateral border of the lesser omentum, containing the portal pedicle, is the hepatoduodenal ligament. The remainder may be called the hepatogastric ligament.

The upper attachment of the lesser omentum is to the hilum of the liver. To the left is the lesser curvature of the stomach and the abdominal esophagus. Posterior to the omentum lies the upper recess of the omental bursa, open to the right through the epiploic foramen. Here, with the index finger in the foramen and the thumb anterior, one can compress the hepatic artery and portal vein in the classic maneuver used to control hemorrhage during cholecystectomy and other procedures (see Fig. 107). The bursa is closed above and to the left by the reflection of the posterior peritoneum to the esophagus and cardia of the stomach. The

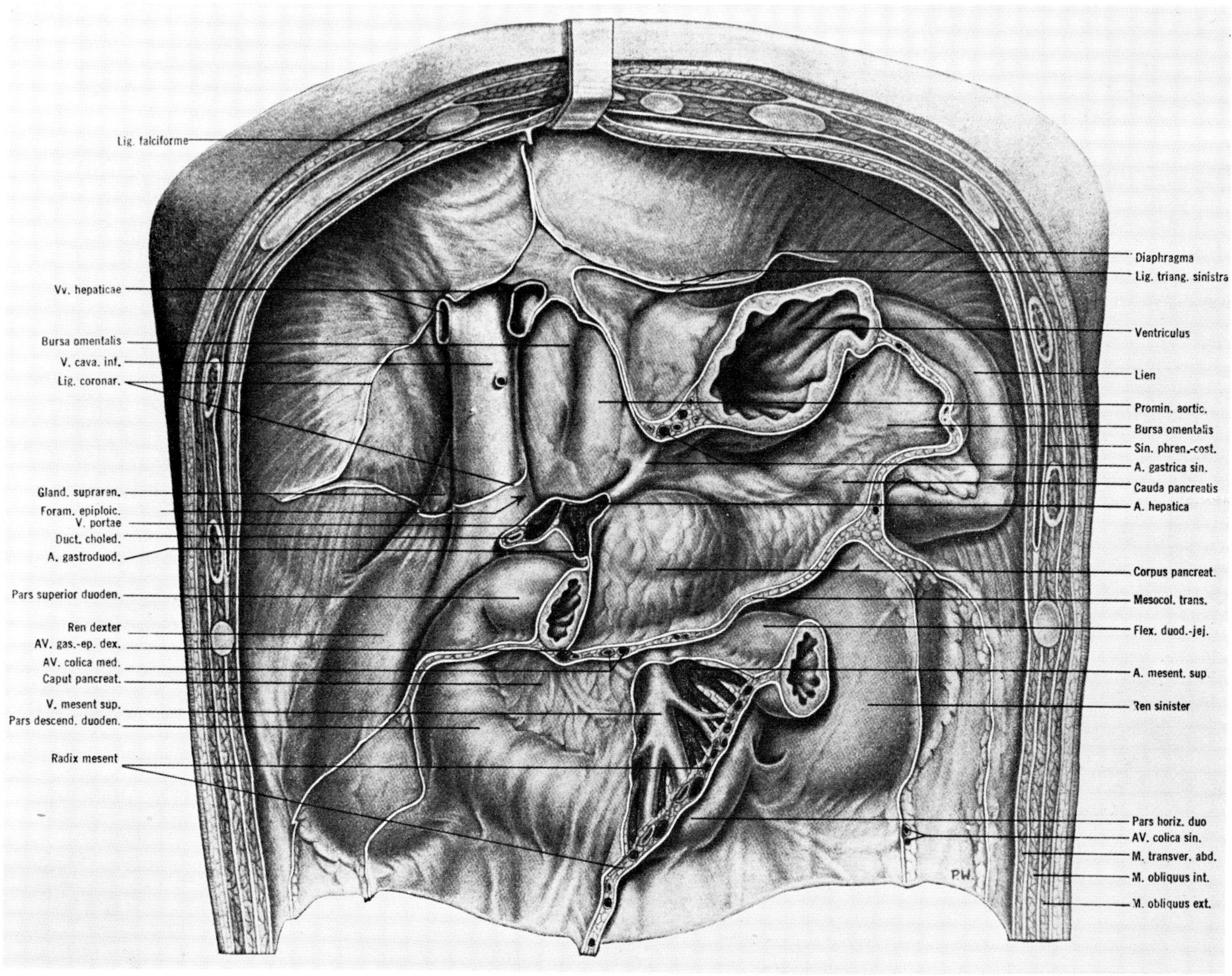
Lig. falciforme
Vv. hepaticae
Bursa omentalis
V. cava. inf.
Lig. coronar.
Gland. supraren.
Foram. epiploic.
V. portae
Duct. choled.
A. gastroduod.
Pars superior duoden.
Ren dexter
AV. gas.-ep. dex.
AV. colica med.
Caput pancreat.
V. mesent sup.
Pars descend. duoden.
Radix mesent
Diaphragma
Lig. triang. sinistra
Ventriculus
Lien
Promin. aortic.
Bursa omentalis
Sin. phren.-cost.
A. gastrica sin.
Cauda pancreatis
A. hepatica
Corpus pancreat.
Mesocol. trans.
Flex. duod.-jej.
A. mesent. sup
Ren sinister
Pars horiz. duo
AV. colica sin.
M. transver. abd.
M. obliquus int.
M. obliquus ext.
PW.

FIG. 96
Peritoneal relationships of the liver and other subdiaphragmatic structures. (From Töndury, 1970.)

posterior peritoneum of the upper bursa is lifted up in the fold known as the left gastropancreatic fold, in which the left gastric artery courses upward to the esophagogastric junction, and branches of the right vagus nerve course downward to the celiac plexus (Fig. 96). The elevation of the floor of the bursa caused by the course of the common hepatic artery is termed the right gastropancreatic fold.

EXTRAHEPATIC VARIATIONS OF THE HEPATIC ARTERY; HEPATIC ARTERY COLLATERALS

In only 55 per cent of individuals does the entire blood supply of the liver derive from a single vessel arising from the celiac artery. In the remainder, either the right or the left hepatic artery is aberrant (Fig. 97).

The course of the usual common hepatic artery is from the celiac to the right in the right gastropancreatic fold to reach the left anterior surface of the portal vein. Giving off the gastroduodenal, it continues as the proper hepatic artery, and ascends on the portal vein to the left of the (common) bile duct, or the main hepatic duct. Near the hilum, the right hepatic artery turns right, usually behind the main hepatic duct.

In about 9 per cent of subjects a hepatic artery will be found behind the portal vein (Grant, 1972). This is most

---

FIG. 97

Sources of the hepatic arteries. A. Entire hepatic artery from the celiac (55%). B. Replaced left hepatic from left gastric (10%). C. Replaced right hepatic from superior mesenteric (11%). D. Accessory left hepatic from left gastric (8%). E. Accessory right hepatic from superior mesenteric (7%). F. Entire hepatic from superior mesenteric (4.5%). Anomalous hepatic arteries arose from both the superior mesenteric and the left gastric artery (4%), and the entire hepatic from the left gastric (0.5%). The entire hepatic may stem from the aorta.

(Michels uses the term "replaced" for a separate right, left, or middle hepatic artery, and the expression "accessory" for a supernumerary artery supplying other segments or subsegments.)

AcHD, accessory hepatic duct; AcLG, accessory left gastric artery; AcLH, accessory left hepatic artery; AcRH, accessory right hepatic artery; C, cystic artery; CBC, common bile duct; CD, cystic duct; CE, cardio-esophageal branches; CL, caudate lobe; DP, dorsal pancreatic artery (superior pancreatic); Fis, fissured area; GD, gastroduodenal artery; H, hepatic artery; HD, hepatic duct; LG, left gastric artery; LGE, left gastroepiploic artery; LH, left hepatic artery; MCol, middle colic artery; MH, middle hepatic artery; P, inferior phrenic artery; RD, retroduodenal artery (post. sup. pancreaticoduodenal in official nomenclature); ReLH, replaced left hepatic artery; ReRH, replaced right hepatic artery; RG, right gastric artery; RGE, right gastroepiploic artery; RH, right hepatic artery; S, splenic artery; SD, supraduodenal artery of Wilkie; SM, superior mesenteric artery; SPD, superior pancreaticoduodenal artery, (anterior); TP, transverse pancreatic artery (inferior pancreatic). (Figure modified from Michels in Schaeffer (1966); incidences from Michels, 1955.)

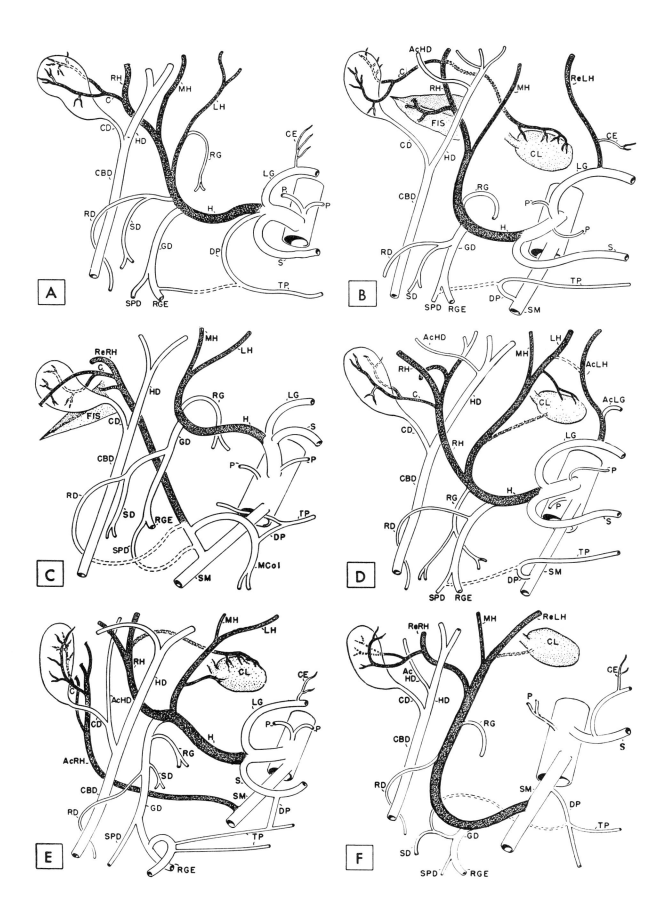

often an aberrant right hepatic artery stemming from the superior mesenteric (see Fig. 73), but an aberrant left hepatic artery may also take this posterior course. Michels' dissections show an occasional right hepatic artery of superior mesenteric origin coursing anterior to the portal vein. The rare common hepatic of superior mesenteric origin more often courses anterior to the portal vein (see Fig. 74). A hepatic artery derived from the left gastric reaches the liver hilum via the left gastropancreatic fold and the lesser omentum.

The hepatic artery has been accidentally ligated during cholecystectomy, in pancreatectomy (with anomalous origin from the superior mesenteric), and in gastrectomy (with anomalous origin from the left gastric), or occluded during infusion for cancer chemotherapy. Intentional ligation has been performed for cirrhosis, hepatic malignancy, hepatic artery aneurysm, and liver injury. The celiac artery at its origin has been intentionally ligated in radical gastrectomy. The older figure for mortality was about 30 per cent following hepatic artery ligation in cirrhosis (Mays, 1967), but 60 per cent after ligation of either the proper hepatic or a lobar artery in other clinical situations (collected series of Graham and Cannell, 1933; Alessandri, 1937; Michels, 1953; Monafo et al., 1966; and Karasewich and Bowden, 1967). However, reviewing their own and reported cases, Brittain and his associates (1964) concluded that the ligation was not ordinarily fatal in the absence of prior hepatic or other disease. More recent reports of intentional ligation are also encouraging, in cases where the indication has been liver trauma (Mays, 1972; Madding and Kennedy, 1972), or carcinoma of the liver (Balasegaram, 1972). Better general support of the patient is undoubtedly responsible for the better results.

As a rule the mortality after hepatic artery obstruction is lessened when a ligation is done at levels proximal to the portal pedicle. This is attributed to the greater availability of collaterals for the hepatic artery at this level. Michels (1953) (see also Bengmark and Rosengren, 1970) divides the collaterals into three categories: (1) Hepatic arteries arising from sources other than the celiac–common hepatic trunk. (2) Pathways outside the hepatic arteries but capable of connecting with them—mainly vessels of the pancreas, stomach, and esophagus. (3) Pathways outside the celiac blood supply—including arteries of the pancreas, diaphragm, and of the falciform and round ligaments.

Ligation of the portal vein, while usually well tolerated, does induce morbidity from the effects of portal obstruction, plus encephalopathy in patients with poor liver function. Child (1954) states that concomitant ligation of the portal vein and the hepatic artery is always fatal.

Temporary occlusion of the portal pedicle, as by a vascular clamp, is reported to be well tolerated for 15 minutes under normothermic conditions, and for at least 30 minutes with hypothermia (Albo *et al.,* 1969; Yellin *et al.,* 1971).

OTHER STRUCTURES OF THE PORTAL PEDICLE

The extrahepatic bile ducts and the gallbladder are considered in Chapter 13 and the portal vein in Chapter 14. Here we may take note of the lymphatics and nerves of the liver.

The largest lymphatic pathway extends from the hilum to the celiac nodes, passing mainly through the portal pedicle, where intercalary nodes are quite constant (see Fig. 57), but also via the lesser omentum and gastric nodes, and posteriorly along an inferior phrenic pathway. A portion of the lymph leaves the upper parts of the liver through the diaphragm to retrosternal and posterior mediastinal nodes.

The nerves enter the liver through the portal pedicle, except for some sensory innervation from the phrenic nerves superiorly. As in other viscera, motor or autonomic innervation is by way of perivascular plexuses. The main contribution is from the celiac plexus, where sympathetic fibers arrive through the splanchnic nerves, probably with some contribution from the upper lumbar sympathetic trunks. Hepatic vagal fibers reach the celiac plexus from the right (posterior) vagus (see Fig. 59). The left (anterior) vagus supplies hepatic branches which run more horizontally through the upper lesser omentum to the portal pedicle. The hepatic plexus, as it passes up the pedicle, is divisible into an anterior portion along the hepatic artery, and a posterior portion on the posterior aspect of the portal vein (Alexander,

1940; Shafiroff and Hinton, 1950). Sensory fibers are said to run through the splanchnic nerves, but the extent of denervation offered by splanchnicectomy is debatable.

REFERENCES

Albo, D., Jr., Christensen, C., Rasmussen, B. L., and King, T. C.: Massive liver trauma involving the suprarenal vena cava. Amer. J. Surg. 118:960–963, 1969.

Alessandri, A.: Aneurysm of hepatic artery. *In* Nelson Loose-Leaf Surgery. Vol. V. Chapter 10A, p. 608A. New York, T. Nelson, 1937.

Alexander, W. F.: The innervation of the biliary system. J. Comp. Neurol. 72:357–370, 1940.

Anson, B. J.: Morris' Human Anatomy, 12th ed. New York, Blakiston, 1966.

Balasegaram, M.: Complete hepatic dearterialization for primary carcinoma of the liver. Report of twenty-four patients. Amer. J. Surg. 124:340–345, 1972.

Bengmark, S., and Rosengren, K.: Angiographic study of the collateral circulation to the liver after ligation of the hepatic artery in man. Amer. J. Surg. 119:620–624, 1970.

Brittain, R. S., Marchioro, T. L., Hermann, G., Waddell, W. R., and Starzl, T. E.: Accidental hepatic artery ligation in humans. Amer. J. Surg. 107:822–832, 1964.

Child, C. G.: The Hepatic Circulation and Portal Hypertension. Philadelphia, W. B. Saunders, 1954.

Couinaud, C.: Le foie. Paris, Masson, 1955.

Cullen, T. S.: Accessory lobes of the liver. An accessory hepatic lobe springing from the surface of the gallbladder. Arch. Surg. 11:718–764, 1925.

Feist, J. H., and Lasser, E. C.: Identification of uncommon liver lobulations. J.A.M.A. 169:1859–1862, 1959.

Graham, R. R., and Cannell, D.: Accidental ligation of the hepatic artery. Report of one case with a review of the cases in the literature. Brit. J. Surg. 20:566–579, 1933.

Grant, J. C. B.: An Atlas of Anatomy, 6th ed. Baltimore, Williams & Wilkins, 1972.

Karasewich, E. G., and Bowden, L.: Hepatic artery injury. Surg. Gynec. Obstet. 124:1057–1063, 1967.

Llorente, J., and Dardik, H.: Symptomatic accessory lobe of the liver associated with absence of the left lobe. Arch. Surg. 102:221–223, 1971.

Madding, G. F., and Kennedy, P. A.: Hepatic artery ligation. Surg. Clin. N. Amer. 52:719–728, 1972.

Mays, E. T.: Observations and management after hepatic artery ligation. Surg. Gynec. Obstet. 124:801–807, 1967.

Mays, E. T.: Lobar dearterialization for exsanguinating wounds of the liver. J. Trauma 12:397–407, 1972.

Michels, N. A.: Collateral arterial pathways to the liver after ligation of the hepatic artery and removal of the celiac axis. Cancer 6:708–724, 1953.

Michels, N. A.: Blood Supply and Anatomy of the Upper Abdominal Organs. Philadelphia, J. B. Lippincott, 1955.

Monafo, W. W., Jr., Ternberg, J. L., and Kempson, R.: Accidental ligation of the hepatic artery. Arch. Surg. 92:643–652, 1966.

Poirier, P., and Charpy, A.: Traité d'anatomie humaine. Vol. IV. Paris, Masson, 1901.

Shafiroff, B. G. P., and Hinton, J. W.: Surgical anatomy of the choledochal nerves. Arch. Surg. 60:944–952, 1950.

Tôn That Tung: Chirurgie d'exérèse du foie. Hanoi, Editions en Langues Étrangères, 1962.

Töndury, G.: Angewandte und topographische Anatomie, 4th ed. Stuttgart, Georg Thieme, 1970.

Yellin, A. E., Chaffee, C. B., and Donovan, A. J.: Vascular isolation in treatment of juxtahepatic venous injuries. Arch. Surg. 102:566–573, 1971.

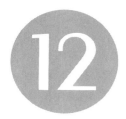

RESECTiONS;
AppRoAchES TO poRTAl
ANd hEpATic vENOUS
pEdiclES

PLANES FOR TRANSHEPATIC DISSECTION

Resection of a portion of the liver was put on a logical basis by the demonstration of the delimitation of lobes, segments, and subsegments, and the relationship of these parts to the course of the hepatic veins (Chapter 10). ". . . there can be no doubt that any surgical interference with the liver will be much more readily tolerated as it approaches that line, which I have termed the mid-line of the liver, and that the haemorrhage has less to be dreaded as the liver is incised or torn in the neighbourhood of that line" (Cantlie, 1897). Cantlie's suggestion has been nicely extended by Goldsmith and Woodburne (1957) (Fig. 98).

It should be noted that the three major fissures of the liver through which the surgeon separates the portal territories and reaches the major hepatic veins are variously angled toward the horizontal of the patient's back. Thus, while the depth of the interlobar fissure reaches a line be-

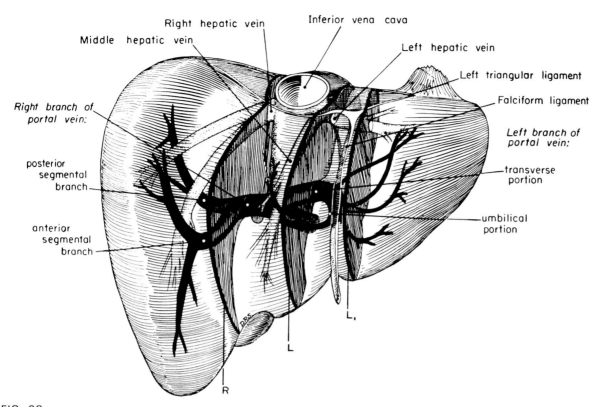

Right hepatic vein

Middle hepatic vein

Inferior vena cava

Left hepatic vein

Left triangular ligament

Falciform ligament

Right branch of portal vein:

posterior segmental branch

anterior segmental branch

Left branch of portal vein:

transverse portion

umbilical portion

L₁

L

R

FIG. 98

Planes of operative transhepatic dissection. R, to the right of the interlobar fissure and middle hepatic vein for a right lobectomy. L, to the left of the fissure and the middle hepatic vein for a left lobectomy. L$_1$, to the left of the umbilical fissure for resection of the lateral segment. The hepatic veins are here shown diagrammatically (cf. Fig. 92). (From Goldsmith and Woodburne, 1957. By permission of Surgery, Gynecology & Obstetrics.)

tween the gallbladder and inferior vena cava, it starts on the anterior surface of the liver 3 or 4 cm. to the left, so as to cut the liver at an angle of about 75 degrees, open to the left (Fig. 99 I). The left intersegmental fissure forms an angle of about 45 degrees, also open to the left. The right intersegmental fissure is most variable, with an angle of about 30 degrees, open to the right.

Transhepatic dissection is done as a stage in resection for cancer (Lortat-Jacob and Robert, 1952; Couinaud, 1955; Reifferscheid, 1957; Tôn, 1962; Schwartz, 1964; Taylor *et al.,* 1969; Brasfield *et al.,* 1972); as a means of controlling hemorrhage after trauma to the liver or the inferior vena cava (Schrock *et al.,* 1968; Albo *et al.,* 1969; Ackroyd *et al.,* 1969; Madding and Kennedy, 1971); or as a means of approach to the biliary duct system, when the extrahepatic ducts have been obscured (Waddell, 1967). The alternative procedures of ligation of the lobar artery in trauma and of the common hepatic artery in cancer are mentioned on page 168.

Operation for membranous obstruction of the terminal inferior vena cava and of the orifices of the hepatic veins, well known in Japan, is considered on page 77.

RIGHT HEPATIC LOBECTOMY

The basic plan for a right lobectomy described by Lortat-Jacob and Robert has been widely adopted. A right thoraco-abdominal incision is generally made through the 8th intercostal space with section of the costal arch. The diaphragm is cut to the inferior vena cava. This allows control of the cava and displacement of the liver to permit good exposure of the portal pedicle and hepatic veins, and has the added effect of minimizing air embolism by equalizing the right thoracic and abdominal pressures (Taylor *et al.,* 1969). The addition of a median sternotomy to an exploratory abdominal incision also gives satisfactory exposure of the liver and the vena cava, in cases of trauma.

Hemorrhage is further guarded against by adopting the suggestion of Heaney and his colleagues (1966) to insert a shunt in the cava (Fig. 99 I). They point out that if the thorax is not opened the supradiaphragmatic cava can still be approached by incising the central part of the diaphragm and the pericardium from below. Division of the round and the right triangular and the adjacent coronary ligament allows the liver to be displaced anteriorly and upward, to gain exposure of the hilum, where the appropriate portal structures can be divided (Fig. 99 II, III).

The sheath about the portal structures is notably heavy (Fig. 100). It is the "capsule" Glisson was emphasizing (1654). Couinaud calls it the hilar "plaque." The portal vein and hepatic artery will be found free within the portal sheath, but the sheath joins the thin-walled bile duct. Portal elements pertaining to the right lobe may now be ligated. If there is doubt as to their identity enough of the transhepatic dissection can be done to establish their destination.

The extrahepatic termination of the right hepatic vein is

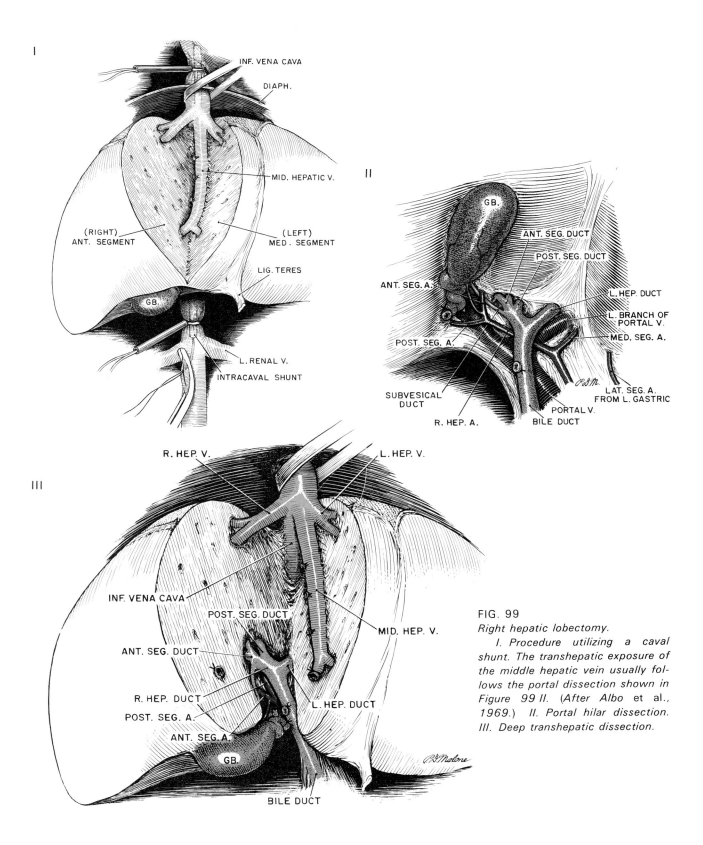

I

INF. VENA CAVA

DIAPH.

MID. HEPATIC V.

(RIGHT)
ANT. SEGMENT

(LEFT)
MED. SEGMENT

LIG. TERES

GB.

L. RENAL V.

INTRACAVAL SHUNT

II

GB.

ANT. SEG. DUCT

POST. SEG. DUCT

L. HEP. DUCT

L. BRANCH OF
PORTAL V.

MED. SEG. A.

ANT. SEG. A.

POST. SEG. A.

LAT. SEG. A.
FROM L. GASTRIC

SUBVESICAL
DUCT

PORTAL V.

R. HEP. A.

BILE DUCT

III

R. HEP. V.

L. HEP. V.

INF. VENA CAVA

POST. SEG. DUCT

MID. HEP. V.

ANT. SEG. DUCT

R. HEP. DUCT

POST. SEG. A.

L. HEP. DUCT

ANT. SEG. A.

GB.

BILE DUCT

FIG. 99
Right hepatic lobectomy.
I. Procedure utilizing a caval shunt. The transhepatic exposure of the middle hepatic vein usually follows the portal dissection shown in Figure 99 II. (After Albo et al., 1969.) II. Portal hilar dissection. III. Deep transhepatic dissection.

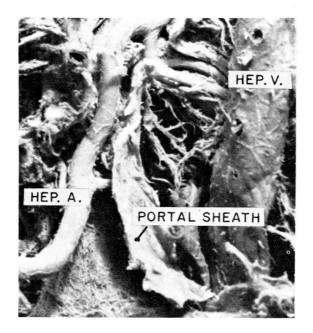

FIG. 100
The portal sheath within the liver, from a fixed specimen. The sheath has been opened on its inferior aspect exposing branches of the hepatic artery and portal vein. The bile duct lies above, and is not visible. Note the lack of a sheath about an adjacent hepatic vein. (Photograph by Dr. Arlan Fuller.)

approached, and that vessel is ligated. The capsule of the liver is now incised slightly to the right of the line of the interlobar fissure, which will have been indicated by a blanching of the right lobe incident to ligation of the artery. Blunt dissection reveals the right tributaries of the middle hepatic vein, which are to be ligated, leaving intact the tributaries from the medial segment (Fig. 99 III). The portal structures will become evident deeply, in the inferior part of the interlobar fissure, the lobar duct being anterior to the portal vein. In 10 per cent some hepatic arterial branch will lie most anteriorly (Elias and Petty, 1952). The inferior vena cava is seen in the deepest part of the dissection and several small hepatic veins (Fig. 101 I, II) will require division.

RESECTION OF THE LATERAL HEPATIC SEGMENT

Steps for a segmental resection are comparable to those for a lobectomy. The initial division of hepatic ligaments, in this case the round, falciform, and the left triangular and coronary ligaments, allows a rotation of the liver downward and to the right (see Fig. 8). The portal structures to the left segment can now be divided (Fig. 102 I). Structures endan-

gered in the initial subdiaphragmatic division of these ligaments are mentioned on pages 156 and 158. Incision of
the upper surface of the liver to the left of the intersegmental
plane, identified by the termination of the left hepatic vein
and the umbilical fissure, allows further transhepatic dissection with division of the left tributaries of the left hepatic
vein until the portal structures are divided and the posterior
limit of the organ is gained (Fig. 102 II).

The relationship of the portal structures to each other,
when seen through the liver, deserves explanation. The portal vein is flexed at the hilum, the lobar ducts coursing in
the crotch of the vein to gain an anterior relationship (Fig.
103). This flexion of the portal vein bifurcation is not evident
in dissections from below when the liver is pulled up anteriorly. The hepatic artery branches course on the same surface of the portal vein branch as on the main portal vein,
thus usually lying behind a portal branch when viewed
transhepatically.

EXTENDED RIGHT LOBECTOMY

The term extended right lobectomy describes a resection
of the entire portio major of the liver, *i.e.,* all of the right
lobe plus the medial segment of the left. The hilar dissection
divides the portal structures to the right lobe and the medial
segment (Fig. 102 I). The line of liver resection starts to the
right of the falciform ligament, uncovering a varying length
of the left hepatic vein (Fig. 104). The right, middle, and
small hepatic veins are divided, plus those tributaries of the
left hepatic vein draining the medial segment.

RESECTION OF THE POSTERIOR
HEPATIC SEGMENT

The posterior segment may be resected for trauma or
cancer of this part. The dissection first discloses the right
hepatic vein (Fig. 105). Division of its tributaries from the
posterior segment brings one to the portal elements for this
segment.

FIG. 101
The hepatic portion of the inferior vena cava.
I. Relationships at the epiploic foramen. The insert shows the veins of the caudate lobe.

TOTAL HEPATECTOMY AND LIVER TRANSPLANTATION

The removal of the diseased liver in its entirety is a preliminary to orthotopic transplantation. Figure 106 shows the operative field, with the vessels and bile duct awaiting anastomosis to those of the donor liver. Suturing of the

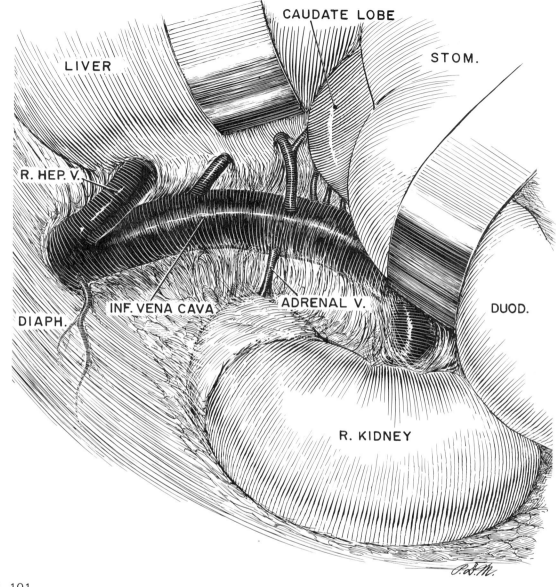

FIG. 101
The hepatic portion of the inferior vena cava (continued).
II. Hepatic and other tributaries.

coronary and triangular ligaments of the new liver secures it in place.

Experimentally it was found essential in the dog to provide exit of the blood from the portal vein and distal cava, by appropriate shunting, until the venous anastomoses were completed (Moore *et al.,* 1960). In the human, collaterals for these two beds appear to be sufficient to make shunting unnecessary (Starzl, 1969).

I

GB.

MED. SEG. DUCTS
AND ARTERY

LAT. SEG. DUCT

ANT. SEG. A.

INF. LAT. SUBSEG. A.
AND PORTAL V.

POST. SEG. A.

SUP. LAT. SUBSEG. A.
AND PORTAL V.

HEPATIC A.

BILE DUCT

PORTAL V.

FIG. 102
Resection of the lateral hepatic segment.
  I. Portal hilar dissection.

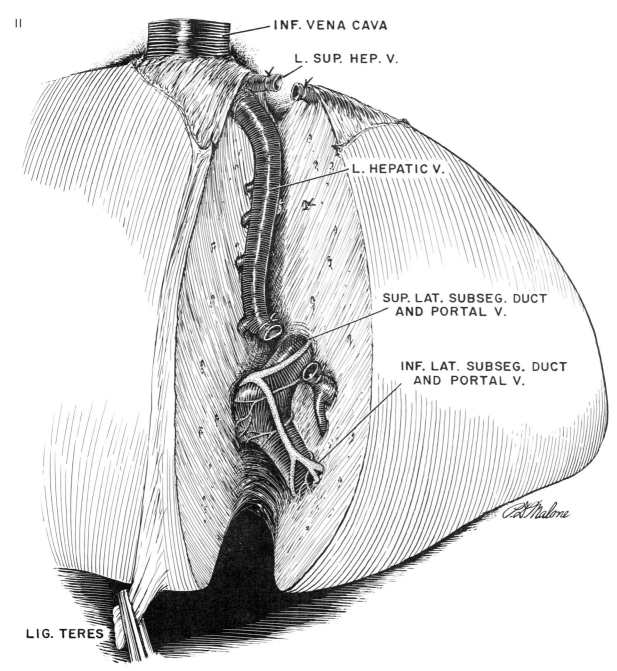

II

INF. VENA CAVA

L. SUP. HEP. V.

L. HEPATIC V.

SUP. LAT. SUBSEG. DUCT AND PORTAL V.

INF. LAT. SUBSEG. DUCT AND PORTAL V.

LIG. TERES

FIG. 102
Resection of the lateral hepatic segment (continued).
    II. Transhepatic dissection.

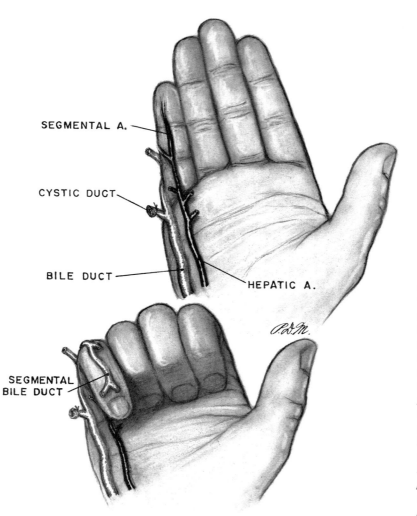

SEGMENTAL A.

CYSTIC DUCT

BILE DUCT

HEPATIC A.

SEGMENTAL
BILE DUCT

FIG. 103
The flexed-finger model of portal triad relationships. The hypothenar border represents the duodenohepatic ligament. The left branch of the portal vein is represented by the fifth finger, flexed at the porta. With fingers extended, the hand represents the parts during portal dissection. The portal vein is extended by upward liver retraction. The hand with fingers flexed represents the structures during transhepatic dissection. The previously extended portal vein is allowed to return to its normally flexed position at the hilum. The common hepatic duct, within the bifurcation of the vein, sends the left duct onto the anterior aspect of the lobar vein. The hepatic artery branch continues on the same surface of the portal vein branch as on the main portal vein (90 per cent of instances) so that within the liver it lies on the posterior aspect of the vein.

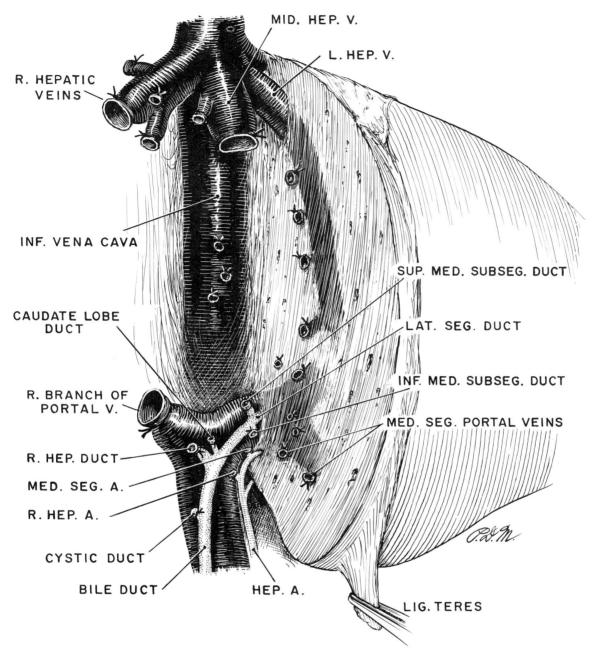

MID. HEP. V.

L. HEP. V.

R. HEPATIC VEINS

INF. VENA CAVA

CAUDATE LOBE DUCT

R. BRANCH OF PORTAL V.

R. HEP. DUCT

MED. SEG. A.

R. HEP. A.

CYSTIC DUCT

BILE DUCT

HEP. A.

SUP. MED. SUBSEG. DUCT

LAT. SEG. DUCT

INF. MED. SUBSEG. DUCT

MED. SEG. PORTAL VEINS

LIG. TERES

FIG. 104
Extended right lobectomy: transhepatic dissection. The liver shown is the same as in Figure 102 I and II.

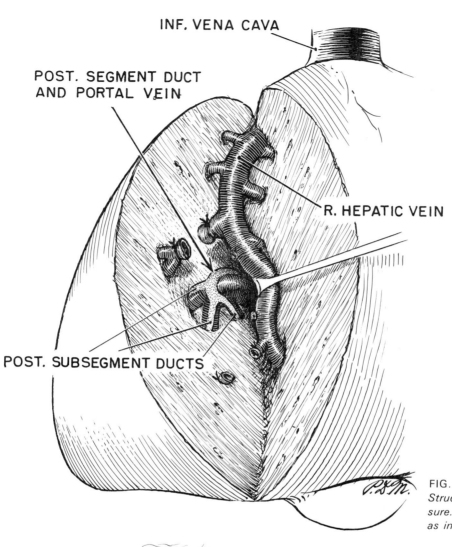

INF. VENA CAVA

POST. SEGMENT DUCT
AND PORTAL VEIN

R. HEPATIC VEIN

POST. SUBSEGMENT DUCTS

FIG. 105
Structures in the right segmental fissure. The liver shown is the same as in Figure 99 I, II, and III.

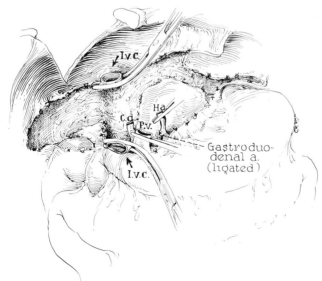

I.v.C.

Hₐ
C.d.
P.V.

I.v.C.

Gastroduodenal a.
(ligated)

FIG. 106
Operative field after total hepatectomy anticipating liver transplantation. (From Starzl et al., 1963. By permission of Surgery, Gynecology & Obstetrics.)

REFERENCES

Ackroyd, F. W., Pollard, J., and McDermott, W. V., Jr.: Massive hepatic resection in the treatment of severe liver trauma. Amer. J. Surg. 117:442–448, 1969.

Albo, D., Jr., Christensen, C., Rasmussen, B. L., and King, T. C.: Massive liver trauma involving the suprarenal vena cava. Amer. J. Surg. 118:960–963, 1969.

Brasfield, R. D., Bowden, L., and McPeak, C. J.: Major hepatic resection for malignant neoplasms of the liver. Ann. Surg. 176:171–177, 1972.

Cantlie, J.: On a new arrangement of the right and left lobes of the liver. Proc. Anat. Soc. Gr. Brit. and Ireland, June, 1897, pp. iv–ix. (Bound with J. Anat. and Physiol. [London], vol. 32, 1898.)

Couinaud, C.: Le foie. Paris, Masson, 1955.

Elias, H., and Petty, D.: Gross anatomy of the blood vessels and ducts within the human liver. Amer. J. Anat. 90:59–111, 1952.

Glisson, F.: Anatomia Hepatis. London, Pullein, 1654.

Goldsmith, N. A., and Woodburne, R. T.: The surgical anatomy pertaining to liver resection. Surg. Gynec. Obstet. 105:310–318, 1957.

Heaney, J. P., Stanton, W. K., Halbert, D. S., Seidel, J., and Vice, T.: An improved technic for vascular isolation of the liver: Experimental study and case reports. Ann. Surg. 163:237–241, 1966.

Lortat-Jacob, J.-L., and Robert, H.-G.: Hépatectomie droite réglée. Presse Med. 60:549–551, 1952.

Madding, G. F., and Kennedy, P. A.: Trauma to the Liver, 2nd ed. Vol. III in the Series, Major Problems in Clinical Surgery, Dunphy, J. E., Ed. Philadelphia, W. B. Saunders, 1971.

Moore, F. D., Wheeler, H. B., Demissianos, H. V., Smith, L. L., Balankura, O., Abel, K., Greenberg, J. B., and Dammin, G. J.: Experimental whole organ transplantation of the liver and of the spleen. Ann. Surg. 152:374–387, 1960.

Reifferscheid, M.: Chirurgie der Leber. Stuttgart, Georg Thieme, 1957.

Schrock, T., Blaisdell, F. W., and Mathewson, C., Jr.: Management of blunt trauma to the liver and hepatic veins. Arch. Surg. 96:698–704, 1968.

Schwartz, S. I.: Surgical Diseases of the Liver. New York, McGraw-Hill, 1964.

Starzl, T. E.: Experience in Hepatic Transplantation. Philadelphia, W. B. Saunders, 1969.

Starzl, T. E., Marchioro, T. L., Von Kaulla, K. N., Hermann, G., Brittain, R. S., and Waddell, W. R.: Homotransplantation of the liver in humans. Surg. Gynec. Obstet. 117:658–676, 1963.

Taylor, P. H., Filler, R. M., Nebesar, R. A., and Tefft, M.: Experience with hepatic resection in childhood. Amer. J. Surg. 117:435–441, 1969.

Tôn That Tung: Chirurgie d'exérèse du foie. Hanoi, Éditions en Langues Étrangères, 1962.

Waddell, W. R.: Exposure of intrahepatic bile ducts through interlobar fissure. Surg. Gynec. Obstet. 124:491–500, 1967.

gallbladder; biliary and pancreatic ducts

CONGENITAL ANOMALIES OF THE GALLBLADDER

The incidence of major anomalies of the gallbladder is under 1 per cent. Reported cases were reviewed by Gross in 1936, and by Flannery and Caster in 1956. Hollinshead (1971) offers an excellent description. The anomalies include absence, doubling, left-sidedness, "floating" (with free pedicle), or intrahepatic lodgment. A cul-de-sac at the neck, called "Hartmann's pouch," may hide the position of the bile duct (see Fig. 108 K). Michels (1955) pointed out that two cystic arteries are common, a deep cystic being added to the usual more superficial vessel. The lymphatics and nerves join those of the portal pedicle. Most of the venous drainage penetrates the bed of the gallbladder to enter branches of the portal vein. Other veins drain to the portal vein in the portal pedicle (Johnston and Anson, 1952). The flow of bile that may be observed following cholecystectomy is apparently due to the opening of small bile ducts in the bed of the organ. The presence of large ducts entering the gallbladder or cystic duct is rare (Chapter 10).

CHOLECYSTECTOMY

The cystic duct and artery are secured in simple cholecystectomy in the vicinity of the cystohepatic triangle, or triangle of Calot, bounded by the quadrate lobe of the liver above, the common hepatic duct on the left, and the neck of the gallbladder and cystic duct to the right (Fig. 107). Ordinarily the right hepatic artery turns right deep to the hepatic duct and gives off the cystic artery within the triangle (Fig. 108 A). The right hepatic artery may, however, course anterior to the hepatic duct (Fig. 108 B), lie close to the gallbladder, or give off a second cystic artery. Not shown in Figure 108 is the frequent variation of the cystic artery arising to the left of the hepatic duct from the right hepatic or common hepatic artery and crossing anterior to that duct. Variations in the gallbladder or the cystic or hepatic ducts may be confusing if dissection is inadequate (Fig. 108 G, H, I, K). Accessory ducts, as in J, have been commented on in Chapter 10. If exploration of the common duct is added to cholecystectomy other hazards are introduced, as in E or F. This will be expanded below.

The spiral fold (valves of Heister) within the cystic duct

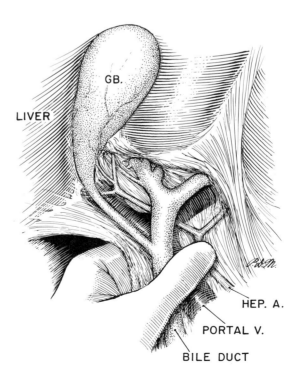

FIG. 107
The portal pedicle and its digital control. The index finger is in the epiploic foramen.

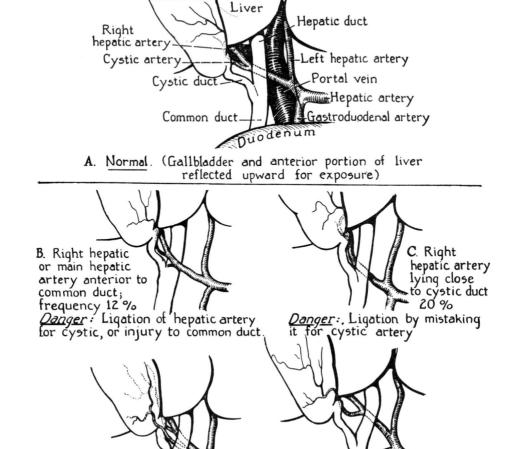

A. Normal. (Gallbladder and anterior portion of liver reflected upward for exposure)

B. Right hepatic or main hepatic artery anterior to common duct; frequency 12%
Danger: Ligation of hepatic artery for cystic, or injury to common duct.

C. Right hepatic artery lying close to cystic duct 20%
Danger: Ligation by mistaking it for cystic artery

D Two cystic arteries; 15%
Danger: After ligation of one, the second may be cut and common duct injured while controlling bleeding.

E. Gastroduodenal artery anterior to common duct; 10%
Danger: Injury to artery or or to common duct.

FIG. 108
Usual relationships (A) and anatomic hazards (B-K) in cholecystectomy and bile duct exploration. (From Cole, 1955.)

renders cannulation difficult, as in an attempt to introduce contrast media for cholangiography via the cystic duct.

SUPRADUODENAL BILIARY DUCTS

The right and left hepatic ducts join to become the common hepatic duct, which, when joined by the cystic, is then designated the common bile duct, or simply the bile duct.

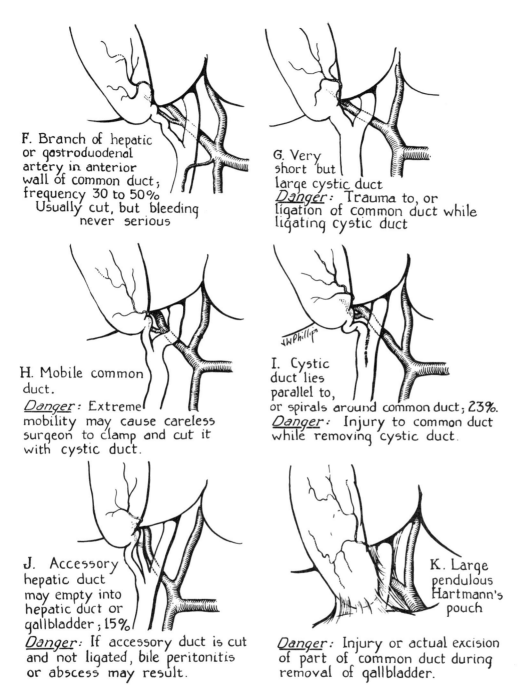

F. Branch of hepatic or gastroduodenal artery in anterior wall of common duct; frequency 30 to 50% Usually cut, but bleeding never serious

G. Very short but large cystic duct
Danger: Trauma to, or ligation of common duct while ligating cystic duct

H. Mobile common duct.
Danger: Extreme mobility may cause careless surgeon to clamp and cut it with cystic duct.

I. Cystic duct lies parallel to, or spirals around common duct; 23%.
Danger: Injury to common duct while removing cystic duct.

J. Accessory hepatic duct may empty into hepatic duct or gallbladder; 15%
Danger: If accessory duct is cut and not ligated, bile peritonitis or abscess may result.

K. Large pendulous Hartmann's pouch
Danger: Injury or actual excision of part of common duct during removal of gallbladder.

FIG. 108
Anatomic hazards in cholecystectomy and bile duct exploration (continued).

Johnston and Anson (1952) noted that the right and left hepatic ducts emerge from the liver usually below the quadrate lobe or, less commonly, to its right, closer to the gallbladder. Only rarely do the two ducts merge within the liver, but frequently the tip of the quadrate lobe must be retracted

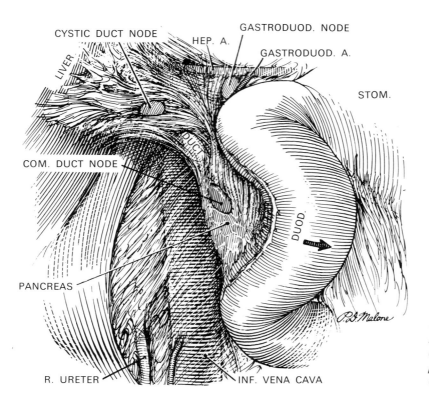

CYSTIC DUCT NODE
GASTRODUOD. NODE
HEP. A.
GASTRODUOD. A.
LIVER
STOM.
COM. DUCT NODE
DUCT.
DUOD.
PANCREAS
R. URETER
INF. VENA CAVA

P.D. Malone

FIG. 109
Lymph nodes related to the bile duct. (From Cattell and Braasch, 1959. By permission of Surgery, Gynecology & Obstetrics.)

to see their junction. The frequent existence of a right accessory extrahepatic duct has been mentioned in Chapter 10.

The bile duct courses near the free edge of the lesser omentum, or hepatoduodenal ligament, until it reaches the upper border of the initial duodenum, whereupon it turns gently toward the right in its further extent. Within the hepatoduodenal ligament the bile duct usually lies to the right of the proper hepatic artery and, lower down, to the right of the portal vein. The portal vein lies behind both duct and artery, and the epiploic foramen lies posterior to all three structures.

The length of the bile duct varies according to the level at which the cystic duct joins the common hepatic duct. Rarely this junction is delayed until the common hepatic has run behind the duodenum. Johnston and Anson emphasize that mobilization may uncover a long parallel course of the two ducts, the length of the bile duct being less than was first apparent.

The nerves and lymphatics of the portal pedicle are intimately related to the bile duct, hepatic artery, and the portal vein. Lymph nodes are numerous in the portal pedicle, draining the liver and biliary system (p. 169). Certain nodes are of special interest because of their large size and constancy (Fig. 109). These include: (1) The cystic duct node, lying anterior and to the left of the neck of the gallbladder. (2) A node posterior to the bile duct just above the duodenum—the 'common duct node' (Cattell and Braasch, 1959); this node lies adjacent to a group of small posterior pancreaticoduodenal nodes behind the retroduodenal and retropancreatic course of the bile duct. (3) The 'gastroduodenal node' lying above the first part of the duodenum at the site of origin of the gastroduodenal from the common hepatic artery.

TERMINAL COURSE OF THE BILE DUCT;
THE PANCREATIC DUCTS

Kune (1964) found that a groove in the pancreas for lodgment of the bile duct could always be palpated, although the duct was actually bare on its posterior aspect in only 12 per cent. Posteriorly the duct here lies against the inferior vena cava. When, as usual, the main pancreatic duct (of Wirsung) ends at the major duodenal papilla, it lies alongside the bile duct for some millimeters (see Fig. 79). The terminal bile duct itself lies adjacent to the wall of the descending duodenum and is adherent to it by fibrous tissue for 8 to 22 mm. (Kune).

The frequency with which the bile and pancreatic ducts join in the hepatopancreatic ampulla (of Vater) is disputed, probably because of the difficulty of definition when the common channel is short. The ducts open separately in the duodenum on the same or on separate papillae in about 5 per cent. Even when a common ampulla is present it is often 2 mm. or less in length (Rienhoff and Pickrell, 1945).

The duodenal termination of the main pancreatic duct is rudimentary in about 10 per cent. In these instances the accessory duct, entering the duodenum through the minor papilla (Fig. 110 A), carries the pancreatic secretion. The main pancreatic duct lacks its own duodenal termination, as in Figure 110 C, with exceeding rarity. The minor papilla, however, is lacking, or the accessory duct is insignificant (Fig. 110 B), in more than half of all subjects (Grant, 1972).

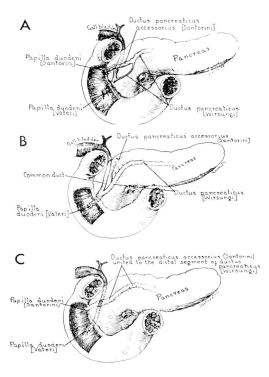

FIG. 110
Some variations of the pancreatic ducts. A. Both ducts are present, but the accessory is the major duct (incidence about 10 per cent). B. The accessory joins the pancreatic duct, with absence of the minor papilla (incidence about 50 per cent). C. The entire pancreatic duct terminates via the minor papilla (exceedingly rare). (From Anson and McVay, 1971.)

Rienhoff and Pickrell noted a higher proportion of communication between the two pancreatic ducts than have most workers. Thus, in two thirds of their cases, there were separate duodenal openings of the ducts, as well as some interductal communication, versus less than one third cited by Grant (1972) and by Kasugai and colleagues (1972). How frequently the communication is adequate to overcome obstruction of one duct is uncertain. Kasugai and his co-workers found the diameter of the normal main pancreatic duct as seen by endoscopic pancreatocholangiography to average 3 mm. in the head of the gland, 2.4 mm. in the body, and 1.4 mm. in the tail. The accessory duct was usually smaller, averaging 1.4 mm. in the head.

The sphincter musculature about the termination of the bile and pancreatic ducts is, collectively, the hepatopancreatic sphincter (of Oddi). According to Boyden (1941), the sphincter fibers are stronger about the bile duct, just proximal to the ampulla, than about the ampulla itself. Occasionally there will be a recognizable sphincter about the terminal pancreatic duct proximal to the ampulla. Kune points out that the external diameter of the bile duct is enlarged as it lies against the duodenum, but that its lumen is normally reduced and that the term 'ampulla' is a misnomer. There is general agreement that the duct narrows sharply as it traverses the duodenal wall and papilla.

ATRESIA OF THE BILIARY DUCT SYSTEM

Atresia may affect the intrahepatic or the extrahepatic course of the biliary system, or both. Gross (1953) analyzed 146 cases, finding that in only 18 per cent was there adequate development of a lobar or common hepatic duct to make possible a surgical anastomosis to the duodenum or jejunum (Fig. 111). Suruga and his colleagues (1972) have had some success when no extrahepatic duct was present, by dissecting within the liver adjacent to the porta hepatis, and, on discovering some bile duct, anastomosing the jejunum to the cut surface of the liver and the opened duct.

EXPOSURES OF THE HEPATIC DUCTS AFTER BILE DUCT DIVISION OR STRICTURE

When possible, the surgeon prefers to anastomose the two ends of a scarred or divided bile duct; when that is not possible the end of the proximal portion, or a hepatic duct, is anastomosed to the duodenum or jejunum (Lahey and Pyrtek, 1950). The proximal duct may be easily identified. If not, a commonly used maneuver is to seek a hepatic duct by removing the tip of the quadrate lobe overlying the usual

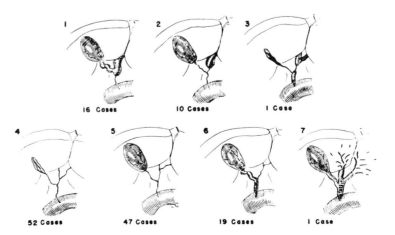

FIG. 111
Biliary atresia of variable extent.
(From Gross, 1953.)

confluence of the ducts. The portal sheath adherent to the ducts should not be removed, for without this tissue the duct wall is too thin to withstand suturing. The occasional presence of a hepatic artery anterior to the ducts (incidence 10 per cent) should be kept in mind.

Two alternative plans are available for finding a hepatic duct within the liver substance. The first is that of Longmire and Sanford (1948). A wedge resection of a portion of the lateral segment is done to find a dilated intrahepatic bile duct, often the inferolateral subsegment duct. A second approach, introduced by Waddell (1967), is to dissect through the lower part of the interlobar fissure of the liver to uncover the junction of the lobar ducts. Hobsley (1958) similarly suggests dissecting upward along the ligamentum teres (in the umbilical fissure) to find the lateral segmental duct anterior to the portal vein (see Fig. 102 II).

EXPOSURE OF THE BILE DUCT

Exposure of the bile duct accompanying cholecystectomy requires only simple extension of the dissection in the hepatoduodenal ligament below the cystic duct and artery.

The more extensive exposure needed in operations for correction of stenosis or division of the bile duct usually begins by incising the peritoneum lateral to the descending duodenum and below its third portion. This allows the necessary mobilization of the duodenum and pancreas. Fixation of the hepatic flexure of the colon by adhesions to the under surface of the liver may necessitate prior mobilization of the flexure. The duodenal and pancreatic mobilization is extensive enough to expose the vena cava at the level of termination of the right renal and gonadal veins, and the aorta (Braasch, 1960).

The epiploic foramen is identified. The pulsation of one or more hepatic arteries is sought on the left and right aspects of the hepatoduodenal ligament prior to its dissection. Cattell and Braasch (1959) noted that the common duct node (Fig. 109), often 2 cm. in diameter, lies posterolateral to the duct as it enters the pancreatic groove. Kune emphasized that the duct is either bare on its posterior aspect or so lightly covered by pancreas that the groove can be palpated. When necessary, Lahey and Pyrtek advised splitting the pancreas posteriorly to find the bile duct. Current opinion tends toward identifying the duct by retrograde probing after duodenotomy.

Hazards connected with exposures of the bile duct relate especially to adjacent vessels. Above the duodenum the duct may be crossed by the right or the proper hepatic artery, or occasionally by the right gastric. At the upper edge of the duodenum it is regularly crossed by the supraduodenal (see Fig. 64). To its left here lie the common hepatic and the gastroduodenal artery. In 38 per cent (Johnston and Anson, 1952) the latter descends anterior to the bile duct. The posterior superior pancreaticoduodenal artery crosses anterior to the duct in at least 80 per cent (Johnston and Anson), to wind around its lateral border, thence continuing in the posterior pancreaticoduodenal arcade. The accompanying vein similarly crosses the duct to reach the portal vein (Fig. 71). A right hepatic or proper hepatic artery of superior mesenteric origin may travel in close apposition to the duct (p. 166) (Fig. 73). Finally, the vessels to the duct itself may be injured. The duct is supplied mainly by a branch of the posterior superior pancreaticoduodenal artery as it crosses anteriorly. The vessel makes up a periductal plexus with descending branches from the cystic artery (Shapiro and Robillard, 1948; Parke *et al.,* 1963). As with other long structures similarly vascularized, excessive removal of this external plexus may produce ischemia of the duct.

TRANSDUODENAL SPHINCTEROTOMY OF BILE AND PANCREATIC DUCTS

An extensive Kocher maneuver (Fig. 73) is a usual preliminary. The duodenal papilla lies on the posteromedial wall of the second part of the duodenum, about 10 cm. from the pylorus. Palpation of the papilla, although difficult, may locate it prior to the duodenotomy; after duodenotomy scrutiny of the mucous membrane discloses the longitudinal fold atop which lies the papilla (Fig. 112). The minor, or accessory, papilla lies 1.5 cm. higher and somewhat anterior.

With extreme rarity, the bile and pancreatic ducts may

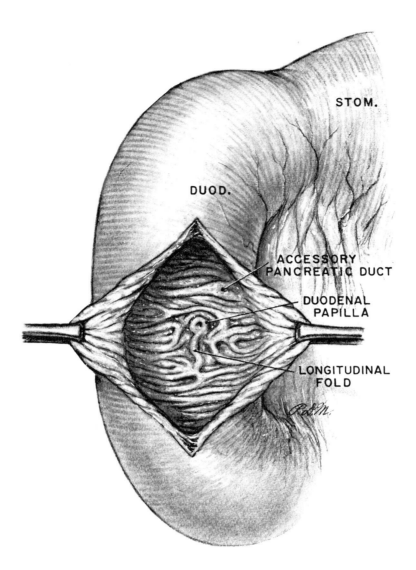

STOM.

DUOD.

ACCESSORY
PANCREATIC DUCT

DUODENAL
PAPILLA

LONGITUDINAL
FOLD

FIG. 112
The major and minor duodenal papill-
lae.

together terminate in the third, or transverse, part of the duodenum (Wood, 1966). As noted previously (p. 191) a common ampulla, when present, is short, so that the opening of the pancreatic duct can be seen on its lower lip. The diameter of the duct varies considerably, according to the data of Kune. Bartlett and Nardi (1960) considered the orifice of the bile duct stenotic if it resisted an instrument of 4 mm. diameter; that of the main pancreatic duct, one of 3 mm.; and that of the accessory, when acting as the main duct, one of 2 mm. diameter (see p. 192).

The bile duct opens on the upper lip of the papilla, where sphincterotomy of this duct is performed (Fig. 113). The incision is continued from the ampulla into the bile duct

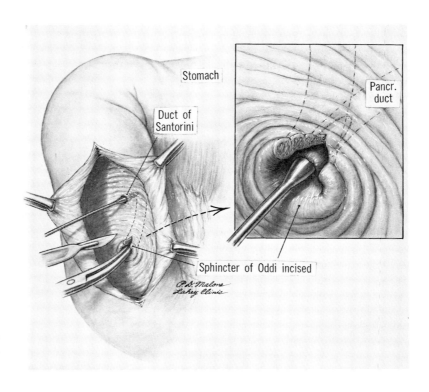

Stomach

Duct of
Santorini

Pancr.
duct

Sphincter of Oddi incised

FIG. 113
*Transduodenal biliary sphincterot-
omy. (From Warren and Veidenheimer, 1966.)*

itself, where the sphincter is strongest (Boyden). Although
many advise an incision 15 mm. long, Kune counseled
against it being longer than 5 mm. He found that the extent
of intimate contact of the duct to the duodenum, proximal
to the termination, varied from 8 to 22 mm. A long incision
requires approximation of the duodenal mucosa to the open
duct, to prevent a duodenal or bile-duct fistula.

REFERENCES

Anson, B. J., and McVay, C. B.: Surgical Anatomy, 5th ed. Philadelphia, W. B. Saunders, 1971.

Bartlett, M. K., and Nardi, G. L.: Treatment of recurrent pancreatitis by transduodenal sphincterotomy and exploration of the
pancreatic duct. New Eng. J. Med. 262:643–648, 1960.

Boyden, E. A.: Hypertrophy of the sphincter choledochus. A cause
of internal biliary fistula. Surgery 10:567–571, 1941.

Braasch, J. W.: Secondary biliary tract procedures. Surg. Clin. N.
Amer. 40:705–710, 1960.

Cattell, R. B., and Braasch, J. W.: Primary repair of benign strictures of the bile duct. Surg. Gynec. Obstet. 109:531–538,
1959.

Cole, W. H.: The Gallbladder and Bile Ducts. Chapter 14 *in* Operative Technic in General Surgery, Cole, W. H., Ed., 2nd ed.
Vol. I. New York, Appleton-Century-Crofts, 1955.

Flannery, M. G., and Caster, M. P.: Congenital abnormalities of the gallbladder; 101 cases. Int. Abstr. Surg. 103:439–457, 1956.

Grant, J. C. B.: An Atlas of Anatomy, 6th ed. Baltimore, Williams & Wilkins, 1972.

Gross, R. E.: Congenital anomalies of the gallbladder. A review of one hundred and forty-eight cases, with report of a double gallbladder. Arch. Surg. 32:131–162, 1936.

Gross, R. E.: The Surgery of Infancy and Childhood. Its Principles and Techniques. Philadelphia, W. B. Saunders, 1953.

Hobsley, M.: Intra-hepatic anatomy. A surgical evaluation. Brit. J. Surg. 45:635–644, 1958.

Hollinshead, W. H.: Anatomy for Surgeons, 2nd ed. Vol. 2. The Thorax, Abdomen, and Pelvis. New York, Harper & Row, 1971.

Johnston, E. V., and Anson, B. J.: Variations in the formation and vascular relationships of the bile ducts. Surg. Gynec. Obstet. 94:669–686, 1952.

Kasugai, T., Kuno, N., Kobayashi, S., and Hattori, K.: Endoscopic pancreatocholangiography. I. The normal endoscopic pancreatocholangiogram. Gastroenterology 63:217–226, 1972.

Kune, G. A.: Surgical anatomy of common bile duct. Arch. Surg. 89:995–1004, 1964.

Lahey, F. H., and Pyrtek, L. J.: Experience with the operative management of 280 strictures of the bile ducts. With a description of a new method and a complete follow-up study of the end results in 229 of the cases. Surg. Gynec. Obstet. 91:25–56, 1950.

Longmire, W. P., Jr., and Sanford, M. C.: Intrahepatic cholangiojejunostomy with partial hepatectomy for biliary obstruction. Surgery 24:264–276, 1948.

Michels, N. A.: Blood Supply and Anatomy of the Upper Abdominal Organs. Philadelphia, J. B. Lippincott, 1955.

Parke, W. W., Michels, N. A., and Ghosh, G. M.: Blood supply of the common bile duct. Surg. Gynec. Obstet. 117:47–55, 1963.

Rienhoff, W. F., Jr., and Pickrell, K. L.: Pancreatitis. An anatomic study of the pancreatic and extrahepatic biliary systems. Arch. Surg. 51:205–219, 1945.

Shapiro, A. L., and Robillard, G. L.: The arterial blood supply of the common and hepatic bile ducts with reference to the problems of common duct injury and repair. Surgery 23:1–11, 1948.

Suruga, K., Nagashima, K., Kohno, S., Miyano, T., Kitahara, T., and Inui, M.: A clinical and pathological study of congenital biliary atresia. J. Pediat. Surg. 7:655–659, 1972.

Waddell, W. R.: Exposure of intrahepatic bile ducts through interlobar fissure. Surg. Gynec. Obstet. 124:491–500, 1967.

Warren, K. W., and Veidenheimer, M. C.: Surgery of chronic relapsing pancreatitis. Postgrad. Med. 40:465–478, 1966.

Wood, MacD.: Anomalous location of the papilla of Vater. Amer. J. Surg. 111:265–268, 1966.

14

ThE poRTAl vENOUS SYSTEM

VARIATIONS OF COURSE AND
TRIBUTARIES OF PORTAL VEIN

Major variations of the portal vein are extremely rare.
They include the reception by the portal vein of anomalous
pulmonary veins (Woodwark *et al.,* 1963; Edwards, 1968),
termination in an abdominal systemic vein, especially the
vena cava, duplication (Marks, 1969), and location anterior to the duodenum and head of the pancreas (Fig. 114).
Bower and Ternberg (1972) reviewed 32 cases of preduodenal portal vein, including 3 of their own. The abnormal
position of the vein often caused duodenal obstruction.

The mode of union of the three main components of the
portal vein is of surgical interest (Fig. 115). Falconer and
Griffiths (1950) note that the superior mesenteric vein is
usually formed by two trunks—a larger, lying to the right
of the superior mesenteric artery, and a smaller, left trunk
receiving proximal jejunal veins. In most instances the left
trunk passes behind the artery to join the right. In one third
of their cases it passed anterior to the artery. The inferior
mesenteric vein joins the splenic in approximately one third
of subjects, the angle of union of the splenic and superior
mesenteric in another third, and the superior mesenteric vein
in the remainder. In the latter instances, the inferior mesenteric vein runs anterior to the superior mesenteric artery, to

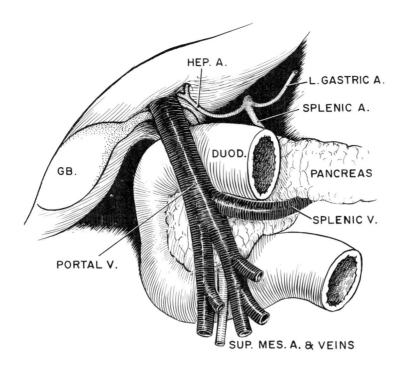

FIG. 114
Anomalous pre-duodenal portal vein.
(After Knight, 1921.)

enter the superior mesenteric vein on its medial border (see Fig. 76).

The veins about the stomach are arranged in two parallel arcades. The first of these, the coronary vein of the stomach, parallels the arteries on the lesser curvature. The arcade is small on its right, or pyloric, end (right gastric vein), and

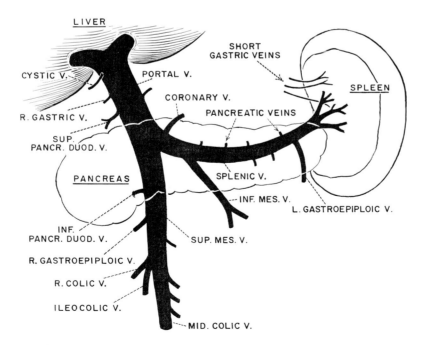

FIG. 115
Termination of tributaries of the portal system. (After Douglass et al., 1950.)

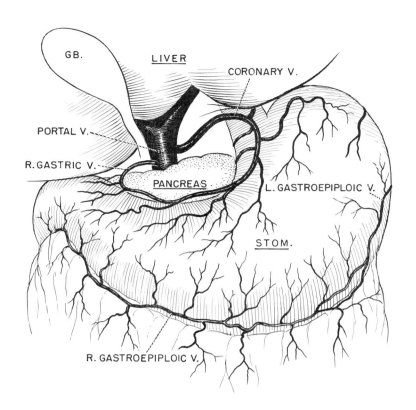

FIG. 116
The coronary and other veins of the stomach. (After Walsham, 1880.)

becomes progressively larger as it courses to the left (left gastric vein). After receiving esophageal tributaries, the coronary vein courses through the lesser omentum, usually joining the portal; less often it runs to the splenic vein (Fig. 116). Retrograde flow through the coronary vein is involved in the hemorrhage of gastroesophageal varices in portal hypertension.

The term 'pyloric vein' had been used by Winslow in 1732, according to Petrén (1929), to denote the right extremity of the arcade mentioned above, which terminates in the portal vein. The term is better employed for a vein described by Mayo (1907), which runs vertically across the pylorus, connecting the veins of the greater and lesser curvatures (see Fig. 61). The pyloric vein is small but quite constant, especially in its lower part. In its upper part it lies near the supraduodenal artery. Mayo noted that the vein indicates accurately the gastric side of the pylorus, and is therefore helpful in differentiating a gastric from a duodenal ulcer.

The second venous arcade, on the greater curvature, ends in the two gastroepiploic veins, the left joining the splenic, the right the portal, vein. In more than half of individuals the right gastroepiploic receives the middle and right colic and anterior inferior pancreaticoduodenal veins (see Fig. 71). Falconer and Griffiths (1950) found that various colic veins also empty into the terminal superior mesenteric itself, the portal, or the terminal splenic vein.

The veins parallelling the pancreaticoduodenal arteries are described on page 126.

PORTASYSTEMIC COMMUNICATIONS

The normal patency of the portasystemic connections was confirmed by postmortem injection (Edwards, 1951). The deep communications—about the esophagus and diaphragm, at the retroperitoneal faces of the abdominal viscera, and in the pelvis—were found to be more significant than those of the anterior abdominal wall reached by umbilical and parumbilical veins (Fig. 117). The portal system is well supplied with valves at birth, but the valves soon become incompetent (Wilkie, 1911), so that the communi-

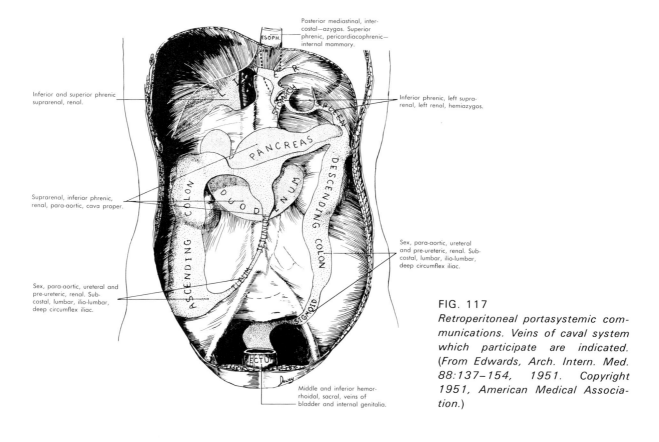

FIG. 117
Retroperitoneal portasystemic communications. Veins of caval system which participate are indicated. (From Edwards, Arch. Intern. Med. 88:137–154, 1951. Copyright 1951, American Medical Association.)

cations can transmit blood in either direction. Thus the systemic veins can carry away portal blood, and the portal system can act as a collateral in instances of high obstruction of the inferior vena cava (Edwards, 1951). The effectiveness of the portasystemic collaterals in man obviates the necessity of temporary shunting during occlusion of the portal vein and inferior vena cava after hepatectomy in anticipation of transplantation.

It has been demonstrated that, in patients with portal obstruction, there may be considerable shunting of blood from the portal to the pulmonary veins via the communications about the diaphragm and esophagus, with the azygos and bronchial veins acting as intermediaries (Schoenmackers and Vieten, 1954; Blackburn, 1956).

Edwards (1951) emphasized that connections of moderate size (2 or 3 mm. in diameter) may normally exist between the splenic and inferior mesenteric veins, and the left renal vein or its tributaries. He showed an example of a large connection (1.2 cm. in diameter) between the splenic and left ovarian veins, in a patient with cirrhosis. The hemodynamic effectiveness of such large spontaneous connections has been documented by Price and his colleagues (1963).

SURGICAL PORTASYSTEMIC SHUNTS

Three portasystemic shunts are commonly used surgically: the portacaval, superior mesenteric–caval, and the splenorenal (McDermott, 1974).

Exposure for *portacaval shunt* is obtained through an abdominal or a right thoracoabdominal incision. The peritoneum is opened over the cava behind the epiploic foramen, and the dissection is extended around the bend of the duodenum to allow elevation of the duodenum and the head of the pancreas, exposing the cava from the liver to the right renal vein (see Fig. 101). This segment of the vena cava seldom receives lumbar veins, which here usually course to the ascending lumbar or azygos system. Mobilization of the cava may require division of some small hepatic veins anteriorly. Occasionally the tip of a large caudate lobe must be amputated to gain exposure of the cava or the portal vein.

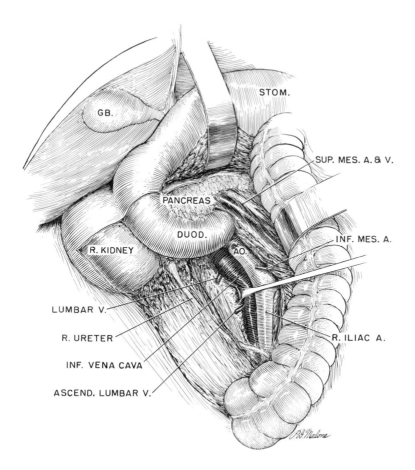

STOM.

GB.

SUP. MES. A. & V.

PANCREAS

DUOD.

INF. MES. A.

R. KIDNEY

AO.

LUMBAR V.

R. URETER

R. ILIAC A.

INF. VENA CAVA

ASCEND. LUMBAR V.

FIG. 118
Exposure for superior mesenteric–caval anastomosis. (After Rousselot, 1971.)

Mobilization of the portal vein may entail division of small tributaries above the head of the pancreas (Fig. 115).

A *superior mesenteric–caval anastomosis* can be done via medial retraction of the right colon and hepatic flexure (Fig. 118). A graft may be placed between the two vessels, or the cava can be divided above the iliac confluence and turned up for the anastomosis below the duodenum. In children adequate length of the cava may require using some of one common iliac vein as well.

For *splenorenal anastomosis* access is gained as for the pancreas, by incising the gastrocolic ligament or the transverse mesocolon, or by a paracolic incision mobilizing the splenic flexure of the colon to the right (Fig. 119). The splenic artery may be ligated above the tail of the pancreas to gain exposure or to decrease portal venous inflow. Splenectomy is not obligatory since there is adequate collateral arterial supply. Figure 119 demonstrates the

creation of the shunt with splenectomy. The dissection of
the splenic vein from its groove in the pancreas entails division of several fine pancreatic veins. Some surgeons ampu-
tate a portion of the tail of the pancreas. The renal vein and
its tributaries are exposed by incising the splenorenal ligament. The gonadal and adrenal veins are identified, and
divided if necessary. Blakemore and Voorhees (1964) displaced the adrenal gland medially from the kidney to establish a groove in which the splenic vein could lie above the
anastomosis, the tail of the pancreas falling back anterior
to the vein. Others bring the splenic vein down over the front
of the pancreas.

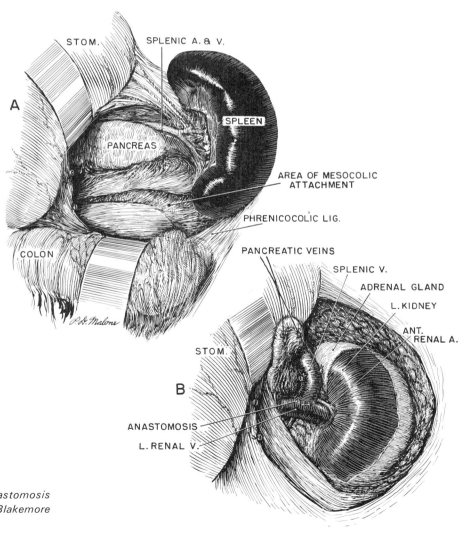

FIG. 119
*Splenorenal venous anastomosis
with splenectomy. (After Blakemore
and Voorhees, 1964.)*

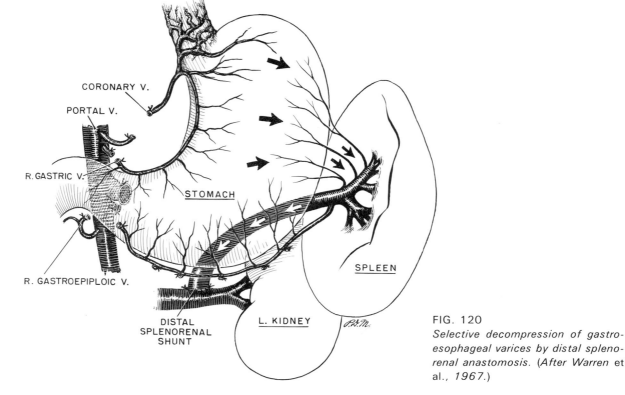

CORONARY V.

PORTAL V.

R. GASTRIC V.

R. GASTROEPIPLOIC V.

STOMACH

SPLEEN

DISTAL
SPLENORENAL
SHUNT

L. KIDNEY

FIG. 120
Selective decompression of gastro-esophageal varices by distal spleno-renal anastomosis. (After Warren et al., 1967.)

SELECTIVE DECOMPRESSION OF GASTROESOPHAGEAL VARICES BY DISTAL SPLENORENAL SHUNT

This operation (Fig. 120) was proposed by Warren and his colleagues in 1967. The spleen is not removed, and the splenic artery is left intact to promote more active spleno-renal flow to discourage anastomotic thrombosis. The splenic vein is divided near its right extremity, and the distal segment is anastomosed to the renal vein. The coronary, right gastric, and right gastroepiploic veins are divided. The rationale is to decompress the area critical for control of hemorrhage, while maintaining a high-pressure intestinal venous system and preserving portal flow to the liver.

UMBILICAL-PORTAL VENOUS CATHETERIZATION

The connections of the umbilical vein with the portal vein and with the vena cava are shown in Figure 121. It is widely recognized that the umbilical arteries and the vein can be

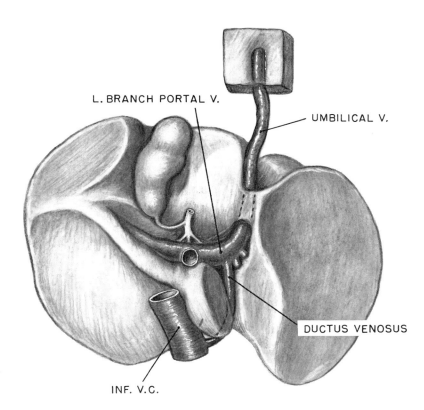

L. BRANCH PORTAL V.

UMBILICAL V.

DUCTUS VENOSUS

INF. V.C.

FIG. 121
Termination of the umbilical vein in the newborn. (After Testut and Jacob, 1914.)

easily catheterized in the neonate. Dangers of this procedure are emphasized by Egan and Eitzman (1971).

Wertheimer (1886) found that a vestigial lumen is usually present in the ligamentum teres. Butler (1954) observed that the lumen was narrowed by contraction and tissue proliferation, not by thrombosis. A persistent lumen was more constant in the hepatic end of the ligamentum teres than in its initial part. In the dissecting room we have commonly seen lumens in the ligamentum teres up to 2 or 3 mm. in diameter, with or without evident liver disease. Braastad and his co-workers (1967) found that an average of 8 cm. of the ligamentum teres could be mobilized in the extraperitoneal tissues above the umbilicus, beyond which it bent at an angle of about 40 degrees to descend in the free border of the falciform ligament. A lumen was grossly present in some part of its subaponeurotic course in 34 of 40 dissections. The vestigial umbilical lumen was separated from that of the portal vein by ''a small bit of fibrocollagenous tissue,'' with longitudinal elements of the walls of the two veins continuous in an end-to-end fashion. Thus, with the passage of progressively larger probes, one can penetrate the closure at the left branch of the portal vein, and catheterize the portal system (Gonzalez Carbalhaes, 1959; Bayly and Gonzalez Carbalhaes, 1964).

Initially this was done to perform portography and manometry, but the technique has been applied to emergency portasaphenous shunting (Christophersen and Jackson, 1967), and to filtration of schistosomes from the portal bed (Lima *et al.*, 1967; Kessler *et al.*, 1970).

The ligamentum teres can be exposed extraperitoneally by a midline incision above the umbilicus. If a distinct ligament with a central channel is not immediately encountered, dissection is continued into the cellular tissue of the falciform ligament, where the ligamentum teres may be more easily identified. The ligament is sectioned at progressively higher levels until a lumen is found. The passage of a Bakes dilator through the umbilical portal junction gives a sensation similar to that in passing the choledochal sphincter. Christophersen and Jackson open the peritoneum and identify the ligamentum teres in the free edge of the falciform ligament. They have been able to establish a lumen, when none was seen, by pushing a grooved director through the comparatively soft center of the ligamentum teres.

Asuncion and Silva (1971) found that the ligamentum venosum had no residual endothelium-lined channel, but could be opened by probing to its termination in the left hepatic vein close to the vena cava. They concluded, however, that it was impractical to attempt to form an umbilical-caval shunt by catheterization of the ligamentum teres continuing through the ligamentum venosum.

REfERENCES

Asuncion, Z. G., and Silva, Y. J.: Surgical significance of the ductus venosus Arantii. Amer. J. Surg. 122:109–111, 1971.

Bayly, J. H., and Gonzalez Carbalhaes, O.: The umbilical vein in the adult. Diagnosis, treatment, research. Amer. Surg. 30:56–60, 1964.

Blackburn, C. R. B.: Acquired portal-pulmonary venous anastomosis complicating partial oesophago-gastrectomy in a patient with portal hypertension. Thorax 11:30–35, 1956.

Blakemore, A. H., and Voorhees, A. B., Jr.: Splenectomy and End-to-Side Splenorenal Shunts. *In* Atlas of Technics in Surgery, Madden, J. L., Ed. 2nd ed. Vol. 2. Thoracic and Cardiovascular. New York, Appleton-Century-Crofts, 1964.

Bower, R. J., and Ternberg, J. L.: Preduodenal portal vein. J. Pediat. Surg. 7:579–584, 1972.

Braastad, F. W., Condon, R. E., and Gyorkey, F.: The umbilical vein. Surgical anatomy in the normal adult. Arch. Surg. 95:948–955, 1967.

Butler, H.: Post-natal changes in the intra-abdominal umbilical vein. Arch. Dis. Child. 29:427–435, 1954.

Christophersen, E. B., and Jackson, F. C.: A technique of transumbilical portal vein catheterization in adults. Arch. Surg. 95:960–963, 1967.

Douglass, B. F., Baggenstoss, A. H., and Hollinshead, W. H.: The anatomy of the portal vein and its tributaries. Surg. Gynec. Obstet. 91:562–576, 1950.

Edwards, E. A.: Functional anatomy of the porta-systemic communications. Arch. Intern. Med. 88:137–154, 1951.

Edwards, J. E.: Congenital Malformations of the Heart and Great Vessels. Chapter 9 *in* Pathology of the Heart and Blood Vessels, Gould, S. E., Ed., 3rd ed. Vol. I. Springfield, Charles C Thomas, 1968.

Egan, E. A., II, and Eitzman, D. V.: Umbilical vessel catheterization. Am. J. Dis. Child. 121:213–218, 1971.

Falconer, C. W. A., and Griffiths, E.: The anatomy of the blood-vessels in the region of the pancreas. Brit. J. Surg. 37:334–344, 1950.

Gonzalez Carbalhaes, O.: Portography. A preliminary report of a new technique via the umbilical vein. Clin. Proc. Child. Hosp. (Washington) 15:120–122, 1959.

Kessler, R. E., Amadeo, J. H., Tice, D. A., and Zimmon, D. S.: Filtration of schistosomes in unanesthetized man. J.A.M.A. 214:519–524, 1970.

Knight, H. O.: An anomalous portal vein with its surgical dangers. Ann. Surg. 74:697–699, 1921.

Lima, M. B. C., Caboclo, J. L. F., and Ribeiro, S. A.: Nova técnica de filtração do sangue portal na esquistossomose mansônica através de cateterismo da veia umbilical. Arq. Brasil. Med. 54:283–287, 1967.

McDermott, W. V., Jr.: Surgery of the Liver and Portal Circulation. Philadelphia, Lea & Febiger, 1974.

Marks, C.: Developmental basis of the portal venous system. Amer. J. Surg. 117:671–681, 1969.

Mayo, W. J.: The contributions of surgery to a better understanding of gastric and duodenal ulcer. Ann. Surg. 45:810–817, 1907.

Petrén, T.: Die Arterien und Venen des Duodenums und des Pankreaskopfes beim Menschen. Z. Anat. 90:234–277, 1929.

Price, J. B., Jr., Voorhees, A. B., Jr., and Blakemore, A. H.: Spontaneous hemodynamically effective portasystemic shunts. Ann. Surg. 158:189–194, 1963.

Rousselot, L. M.: Portal Hypertension with Bleeding Esophagogastric Varices. Chapter 65 *in* The Craft of Surgery, Cooper, P., Ed., 2nd ed. Vol. 2. Boston, Little, Brown, 1971.

Schoenmackers, J., and Vieten, H.: Atlas postmortaler Angiogramme. Stuttgart, Georg Thieme, 1954.

Testut, J. L., and Jacob, O.: Traité d'anatomie topographique avec applications medico-chirurgicales. Vol. IV. Paris, Doin, 1914.

Walsham, W. J.: Observations on the coronary veins of the stomach. J. Anat. 14:399–404, 1880.

Warren, W. D., Zeppa, R., and Fomon, J. J.: Selective transsplenic decompression of gastroesophageal varices by distal splenorenal shunt. Ann. Surg. 166:437–455, 1967.

Wertheimer, E.: Recherches sur la veine ombilicale. J. Anat. Phys. (Paris) 22:1–17, 1886.

Wilkie, D. P. D.: On the presence of valves in the veins of the portal system. Brit. Med. J. 2:602–604, 1911.

Woodwark, G. M., Vince, D. J., and Ashmore, P. G.: Total anomalous pulmonary venous return to the portal vein. J. Thor. Cardiovasc. Surg. 45:662–666, 1963.

SECTION 5
The Bowel

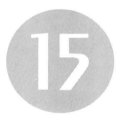

congenital anomalies
of the intestine
and mesentery

In this Chapter we will consider anomalies of rotation and malformations of the bowel, except those of the anorectum, which are presented in Chapter 17.

EMBRYOLOGY OF INTESTINAL ROTATION AND FIXATION

The description to be given is based largely on Huntington (1903), who clarified the embryology by extensive reference to comparative anatomy; Patten (1968), who presented a succinct account; and Dott (1923), who explained the embryologic basis for the spectrum of anomalies encountered clinically. In the embryo of four to seven weeks the gastrointestinal tract lies in the midline (Fig. 122; and see Fig. 55), some of the gut extending out of the abdomen through the umbilicus.

The definitive subdivisions of the gut are recognizable, as are the primordia of liver, pancreas, and spleen. The gut is suspended from the body wall by the mesentery, through

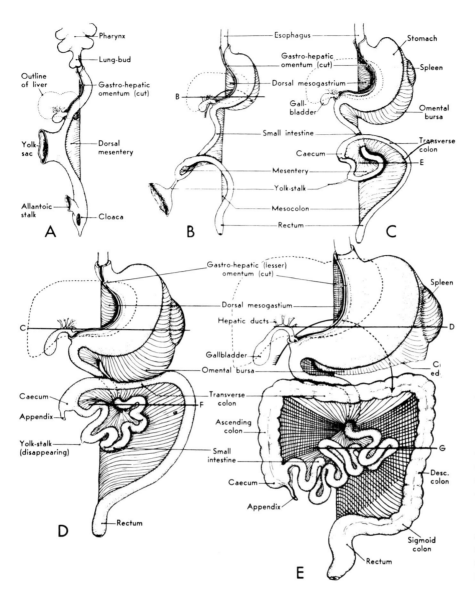

FIG. 122

Stages in development of position of the gut and relations of the mesenteries. Crosshatched areas in E indicate areas of mesenteries of duodenum and colon which become fused to the body wall. Arrow in E is within omental bursa. The heavy lines B to G refer to levels of cross sections not shown here. (From Patten, B. M.: Human Embryology, 3rd ed. Copyright 1968, McGraw-Hill Book Company, New York. Used with permission of McGraw-Hill Book Company.)

which pass the three gastrointestinal arterial trunks. That part of the alimentary tract supplied by the celiac artery is termed the foregut, and that supplied by the inferior mesenteric artery, the hindgut; the intervening portion, supplied by the superior mesenteric artery, is the midgut. The umbilical loop of the intestine protruding from the primitive celomic cavity is centered on the superior mesenteric artery. At the apex of the umbilical loop lies the omphalomesenteric, or vitelline, duct. Its connection with the yolk sac is generally lost by the fourth week; rarely it persists as some form of Meckel's diverticulum, or omphalomesenteric fistula (see

Fig. 129). That segment of the midgut proximal to the apex of the umbilical loop and the axis of the superior mesenteric artery is called the pre-arterial, or cephalic; the distal segment, the post-arterial, or caudal. Further growth of the intestine is accompanied by a return of the umbilical loop to the enlarging cavity of the abdomen, simultaneously with its rotation about the superior mesenteric artery.

Prior to rotation of the midgut, the stomach and duodenum have undergone their own rotation and repositioning, leaving the proximal duodenum fixed to the right of the aorta. At the same time, a retention band of mesenchyma has anchored the left colic angle (splenic flexure) high in the left upper quadrant. The superior mesenteric artery descends in the duodenocolic isthmus thus formed (see Fig. 123) to the midgut, which shows a general direction from right to left. These relations are maintained if the umbilical loop returns to the abdominal cavity in the state of non-rotation.

Normal rotation is initiated by a deviation of the proximal cephalic part of the umbilical loop to the left behind the superior mesenteric artery. Rotation of the remainder of the umbilical loop continues in a counterclockwise direction, when the embryo is viewed from the front. The rotation carries the region of the cecum from its pre-rotational position in the left lower quadrant upward, then to the right anterior to the superior mesenteric artery. The entire intestine normally rotated has generally been returned to the abdomen by the tenth or eleventh week.

Fixation of the mesentery, and of other parts destined to have a bare retroperitoneal surface, takes place about the twelfth week. Fixation is accomplished by fusion of the parietal and visceral mesothelium of the primitive peritoneum with transformation of these cells to a fusion fascia (Fig. 122 E). Arterial connections across these bare areas are insignificant except after extensive and long-standing occlusions of the visceral arteries when branches of parietal vessels can compensate for loss of even several of the gastrointestinal and renal trunks (Chiene, 1869; Rob, 1970). The viscera may thus be mobilized extensively in these zones in such operative maneuvers as pancreatectomy or colectomy. Portasystemic venous connections, however, are most significant in these places (see Fig. 117). Franke (1910) showed communications between parietal lymphatics and those of the cecum, appendix, and ascending colon, across the posterior fixation of these organs. Aside from this, the crossing of the fusion fascia by lymphatics has been described only in patients with cancer, where contiguous invasion of the parietes may be suspected. The passage of nerves across the fusion fascia has not been demonstrated.

MALROTATION

The midgut is often involved in major errors in location or attachment; such errors involving the foregut or hindgut are exceedingly rare. Such anomalies include non-rotation, incomplete rotation, and reversed rotation. Non-rotation, the commonest, may be an isolated anomaly (Fig. 123). It is also a feature of omphalocele and postero-lateral diaphragmatic hernia, and may be associated with duodenal atresia or other anomalies (Bill and Grauman, 1966). In incomplete rotation, the initial deviation of the duodenum and proximal jejunum has occurred, with these parts behind the superior mesenteric artery, but with the cecum arrested somewhere

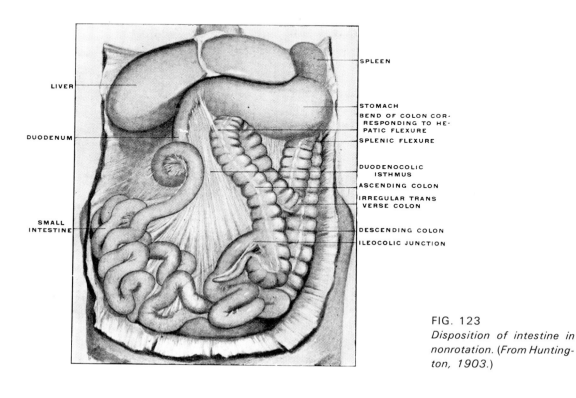

FIG. 123
Disposition of intestine in nonrotation. (From Huntington, 1903.)

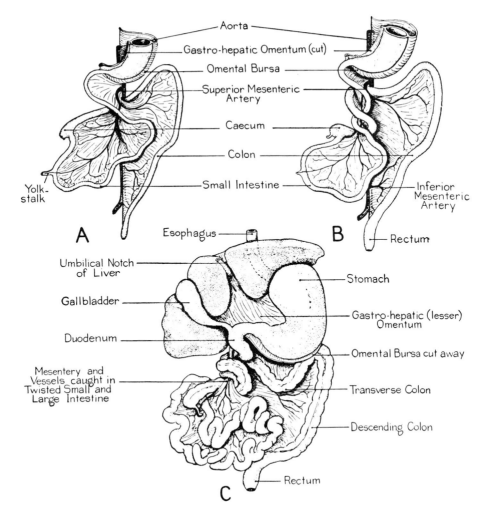

FIG. 124
Reversed intestinal rotation. A. Scheme of initiation of the rotation. In reverse of the normal (see Fig. 122), the small intestine passes anterior, and the large intestine posterior, to the superior mesenteric artery. B. Lack of fixation allows twisting of the gut. C. The resultant volvulus as seen in a newborn. (From Patten, B. M.: Human Embryology, 3rd ed. Copyright 1968, McGraw-Hill Book Company, New York. Used with permission of McGraw-Hill Book Company.)

in its counterclockwise course, most commonly just below the liver.

In the rare reversed rotation (Fig. 124) it is the caudal, rather than the cephalic, part of the umbilical loop that deviates behind the superior mesenteric artery, but toward the right. The cephalic part of the loop is thrown across the front of the artery, and the loop undergoes a clockwise rotation as viewed from the front. In individual cases, observers have not always been able to ascertain that this has indeed been the mechanism involved.

Hyper-rotation has been described, characterized by an excess of counterclockwise rotation, placing the cecum near the descending colon, to which it may be adherent.

The features of surgical significance in malrotation include (1) the unusual positioning of parts of the bowel, most

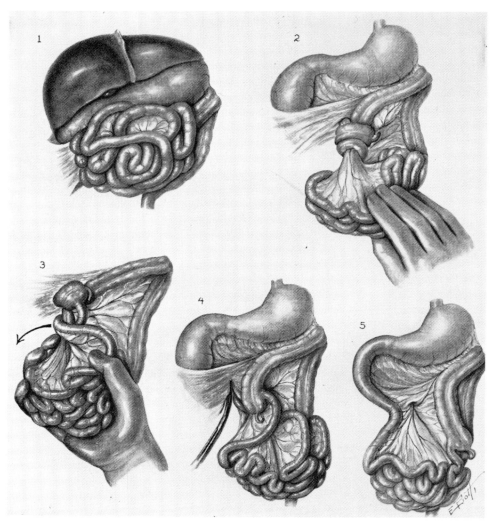

FIG. 125

Operative correction of intestinal obstruction with nonrotation and deficient fixation ('incomplete rotation'—Gross). 1. Appearance on opening abdomen. 2. Demonstration of the volvulus. 3. Untwisting the volvulus. 4. Dividing the peritoneal fold obstructing the duodenum ('Ladd's procedure'). 5. Condition at completion of operation. (From Gross, 1953.)

commonly the cecum, appendix, and ascending and transverse colon; (2) inadequate fixation of the mesenteries and viscera posteriorly, or of the omentum to the colon, with large peritoneal fossae predisposing to internal hernia (see Fig. 126) and excessive mobility of the bowel predisposing to volvulus; and (3) the presence of obstructing peritoneal bands, especially across the duodenum (Fig. 125).

The major steps to relieve the volvulus and the duodenal obstruction are shown in Figure 125. The proximity of the superior mesenteric artery should be kept in mind when dividing the peritoneal bands in the duodenocolic isthmus, as in step 4 of that Figure. Bill and Grauman advise concluding the operation by suturing the duodenum to the right parietal peritoneum and the cecum to the left.

CONGENITAL INTERNAL AND VENTRAL HERNIAS

The extent of fusion of the primitive peritoneum is variable, even in the presence of normal bowel rotation. This leads to variations in the size of peritoneal fossae, especially those about the cecum, duodenojejunal junction (Fig. 126), and sigmoid colon (Fig. 127). A deficiency in fixation predisposes to volvulus (most marked in malrotation) and to internal hernia. According to Jones (1964), the commonest type of internal hernia with a congenital basis is paraduodenal, both left and right (Fig. 128 1, 2). Hernia through the epiploic foramen is next in frequency. Excessive roominess of the intersigmoid fossa allows the formation of the rare sigmoid hernia. Defects within the various mesenteries, rather than inadequate fusion, form the basis for other hernias, as in the mesenteries of the jejunum or ileum, cecum or ascending colon, in the omentum, or in the broad ligament of the uterus.

Three varieties of ventral hernia are related either to in-

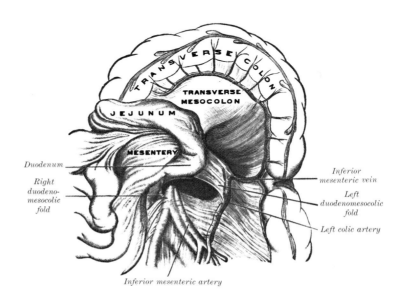

FIG. 126
Large paraduodenal fossa. (From Goss, 1973.)

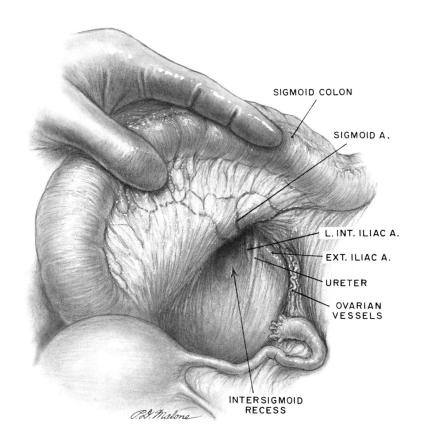

SIGMOID COLON

SIGMOID A.

L. INT. ILIAC A.

EXT. ILIAC A.

URETER

OVARIAN
VESSELS

INTERSIGMOID
RECESS

P.D. Malone

FIG. 127
The intersigmoid recess.

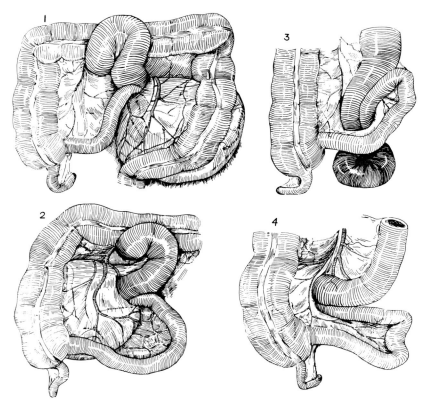

1

3

2

4

FIG. 128
*Forms of some intraperitoneal
hernias. 1. Left paraduodenal
(mesentericoparietal) hernia.
The left colic artery and inferior
mesenteric vein course in the
neck of the sac anteriorly,
the inferior mesenteric artery proper appears below.
2. Right paraduodenal (mesentericoparietal) hernia. The superior mesenteric artery and
vein lie in the neck of the sac
anteriorly, the inferior mesenteric vein lies more remotely
posterior and to the left. Forms
1 and 2 are related to inadequate embryonic parietal
fixation of mesenteries.
3. Hernia through defect in
ileal mesentery. 4. Hernia
through defect in ascending
mesocolon. (From Gross,
1953.)*

complete return of the embryonic bowel to the abdominal cavity or to failure of normal closure of the abdominal wall, or to both. The commonest form is congenital umbilical hernia. Here the bowel has returned to the abdominal cavity but a defect persists at the umbilicus, allowing protrusion of the bowel or omentum. The sac consists of peritoneum, subcutaneous fat, and skin. The spontaneous closure of such hernias, when small, is described in Chapter 2. In the second form, omphalocele, herniation occurs through the umbilicus and into the umbilical cord. The hernia is large, containing the entire umbilical loop of the gut, not returned to the abdominal cavity, and non-rotated. Other viscera—stomach, spleen, and liver—may also be present in the sac. The sac is translucent, consisting of peritoneum internally, and amniotic membrane externally (Gross, 1970). Swenson (1969) notes that extended postoperative observation in these patients reveals an otherwise sound abdominal wall. In the third variety, gastroschisis, the herniation is parumbilical, and usually right sided. The defect in the abdominal wall averages only about 2 cm., according to Bill (1969). The hernia is, however, very large, containing non-rotated or malrotated intestine, and other organs, as in omphalocele. Bill states that the small intestine is short, and occasionally is the seat of stenosis or duplication. The sac is of amniotic membrane alone, the peritoneum lacking here. Other bodily defects may be associated with either omphalocele or gastroschisis. Good reviews are given by Hutchin (1965) and by Wesselhoeft and his colleagues (1972).

DIVERTICULA, DUPLICATIONS, AND STENOSES

Meckel's diverticulum (diverticulum ilei), located on the antimesenteric border of the ileum proximal to the ileocecal junction, is an unobliterated remnant of the vitelline duct at the apex of the umbilical loop of intestine (Fig. 129). Jay and his colleagues (1950) found that, although the location on the ileum is usually between 90 and 100 cm. from the ileocecal junction, the distance may vary between 15 cm. and 167 cm. The incidence is generally given as 2 per cent. Rarely, the tip of the diverticulum may extend to the um-

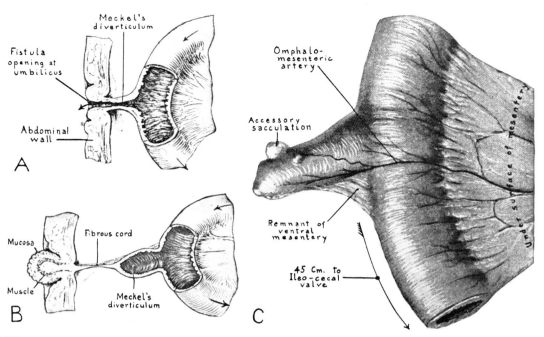

FIG. 129

*Forms of Meckel's diverticulum. A. With open fistula. B. With mucosa at umbilicus, and fibrous cord interven-
ing. C. With no connection at umbilicus, the commonest form. The distance from the ileocecal valve in this instance is shorter than the average. (From Patten, B. M.: Human Embryology, 3rd ed. Copyright 1968, McGraw-
Hill Book Company, New York. Used with permission of McGraw-Hill Book Company.)*

bilicus as a fibrous cord or, even more rarely, as a fistula.
Intestinal obstruction is a recognized complication of
Meckel's diverticulum. It may be caused by volvulus around
the vitello-umbilical cord extending from the diverticulum to
the umbilicus (Fig. 129 B), by herniation beneath a fibrous
vestige of the omphalomesenteric artery, or by intussusception (Rutherford and Akers, 1966). Bleeding may occur due
to the presence of gastric epithelium within the diverticulum.
Pancreatic or other epithelium may also be present (Gross,
1953).

Diverticula and duplications of the alimentary canal may
occur at any level from oropharynx to anus, but are most
common along the small intestine (Gross, 1953). They are
of disputed origin (Gray and Skandalakis, 1972). Duplications found in the thorax may be of the esophagus, or of
the stomach or intestine, with or without connection with
the parent organ. Gross (1970) emphasizes that the mucosa
of duplications often corresponds to that of some part of the
alimentary canal other than that to which the duplication is

attached. In 80 per cent there is a communication of the lumens of the normal tract and the duplication. The muscle of the two tubes, normal and abnormal, may be firmly united, rendering removal of the duplication hazardous. Treatment usually consists of excision, or of the creation of an anastomotic window between the two lumens.

Duplication of the appendix is rare, only 48 cases having been reported by 1945 (Menten and Denny). The two appendices may occur with or without duplication of the ileocolic segment. Waugh (1941) divided cases of double appendix into three types: (1) Double-barreled, where the two appendices share a common muscular coat, and often show a common lumen for part of their extent. (2) Symmetrically placed on the cecum, with one on either side of the ileocecal valve. (3) Tenia coli type, with one appendix at the usual site, and a smaller one at a tenia more proximally.

Atresia of the intestine is said to be present when the lumen is interrupted at one or more sites, stenosis when the lumen is narrowed. Either anomaly may be encountered from the duodenum distally, most often in the ileum (Gross, 1953). Several mechanisms for the production of these lesions have been postulated and are discussed by Gray and Skandalakis. These authors emphasize the frequency of Down's syndrome accompanying atresia or stenosis. Jimenez and Reiner (1961) found a high incidence of associated celiac and superior mesenteric artery anomalies. Parenthetically, a congenital diaphragm of the gastric antrum (antral web) has also been recorded (Hait *et al.*, 1972). The technical management of diverticula and stenoses is well described by Gross (1953, 1970), Shackelford (1955), and Madden (1964).

REFERENCES

Bill, A. H., Jr.: Gastroschisis. *In* Pediatric Surgery, Mustard, W. T., Ravitch, M. M., Snyder, W. H., Jr., Welch, K. J., and Benson, C. D., Eds., 2nd ed. Vol. I, pp. 685–689. Chicago, Year Book Medical Publishers, 1969.

Bill, A. H., Jr., and Grauman, D.: Rationale and technic for stabilization of the mesentery in cases of nonrotation of the midgut. J. Pediat. Surg. 1:127–136, 1966.

Chiene, J.: Complete obliteration of the coeliac and mesenteric arteries: the viscera receiving their blood-supply through the extra-peritoneal system of vessels. J. Anat. Phys. 3:65–72, 1869.

Cullen, T. S.: Embryology, Anatomy, and Diseases of the Umbilicus. Together with Diseases of the Urachus. Philadelphia, W. B. Saunders, 1916.

Dott, N. M.: Anomalies of intestinal rotation. Their embryology and surgical aspects, with report of five cases. Brit. J. Surg. 11:251–286, 1923.

Franke, K.: Über die Lymphgefässe des Dickdarmes. Arch. Anat. Physiol., Anat. Abt., pp. 191–213, 1910.

Goss, C. M.: Anatomy of the Human Body, by Henry Gray, 29th American ed. Philadelphia, Lea & Febiger, 1973.

Gray, S. W., and Skandalakis, J. E.: Embryology for Surgeons. The Embryological Basis for the Treatment of Congenital Defects. Philadelphia, W. B. Saunders, 1972.

Gross, R. E.: The Surgery of Infancy and Childhood. Its Principles and Techniques. Philadelphia, W. B. Saunders, 1953.

Gross, R. E.: An Atlas of Children's Surgery. Philadelphia, W. B. Saunders, 1970.

Hait, G., Esselstyn, C. B., and Rankin, G. B.: Prepyloric mucosal diaphragm (antral web). Arch. Surg. 105:486–490, 1972.

Huntington, G. S.: The Anatomy of the Human Peritoneum and Abdominal Cavity. Philadelphia, Lea Brothers, 1903.

Hutchin, P.: Somatic anomalies of the umbilicus and anterior abdominal wall. Surg. Gynec. Obstet. 120:1075–1090, 1965.

Jay, G. D., III, Margulis, R. R., McGraw, A. B., and Northrip, R. R.: Meckel's diverticulum. A survey of one hundred and three cases. Arch. Surg. 61:158–169, 1950.

Jimenez, F. A., and Reiner, L.: Arteriographic findings in congenital anomalies of the mesentery and intestines. Surg. Gynec. Obstet. 113:346–352, 1961.

Jones, T. W.: Paraduodenal Hernia and Hernias of the Foramen of Winslow. Chapter 37 in Hernia, Nyhus, L. M., and Harkins, H. N., Eds. Philadelphia, J. B. Lippincott, 1964.

Madden, J. L.: Atlas of Technics in Surgery, 2nd ed. Vol. I. General and Abdominal. New York, Appleton-Century-Crofts, 1964.

Menten, M. L., and Denny, H. E.: Duplication of the vermiform appendix, the large intestine and the urinary bladder. Arch. Path. 40:345–350, 1945.

Patten, B. M.: Human Embryology, 3rd ed. New York, McGraw-Hill, 1968.

Rob, C.: Vascular Diseases of the Intestine. Chapter 12 in Vol. 4 of Modern Trends in Gastro-enterology, Card, W. I., and Creamer, B., Eds. London, Butterworths, 1970.

Rutherford, R. B., and Akers, D. R.: Meckel's diverticulum: A review of 148 pediatric patients, with special reference to the pattern of bleeding and to mesodiverticular vascular bands. Surgery 59:618–626, 1966.

Shackelford, R. T.: Bickham-Callander Surgery of the Alimentary Tract. Philadelphia, W. B. Saunders, 1955.

Swenson, O.: Umbilical Anomalies. Chapter 32 in Pediatric Surgery, Swenson, O., Ed., 3rd ed. New York, Appleton-Century-Crofts, 1969.

Waugh, T. R.: Appendix vermiformis duplex. Arch. Surg. 42:311–320, 1941.

Wesselhoeft, C. W., Jr., Porter, A., and DeLuca, F. G.: Treatment of omphalocele and gastroschisis. Amer. J. Surg. 123:369–373, 1972.

16

topography, dimensions, arteries of the bowel

ARRANGEMENT OF SMALL INTESTINE
WITHIN THE PERITONEAL CAVITY

Relationships of the duodenum are considered in Section 3. Barring the presence of situs inversus (see page 28) or abnormalities of rotation (see Chapter 15), the jejuno-ileum will be found attached to the mesentery of the small intestine, within the perimeter of the large intestine. The parietal mesenteric attachment is 15 to 20 cm. (6 to 8 inches) long, starting on the left of the 2nd lumbar vertebra, and running down to the right iliac fossa overlying the right sacroiliac joint. The length of the mesentery from its parietal attachment to the bowel averages 20 cm. (8 inches). It is about 25 cm. (10 inches) for the distal jejunum and the ileum, allowing this part of the bowel to hang down into the pelvis. An approximation to the location of the segment of small intestine within the abdomen may be obtained by reference to the topography of the posterior line of mesenteric attachment (Fig. 130). The proximal third of the jejuno-ileum will generally be located within the upper left hypochondrium, the middle third from the right hypochondrium to the left iliac fossa, and the distal third in the right iliac fossa and the pelvis.

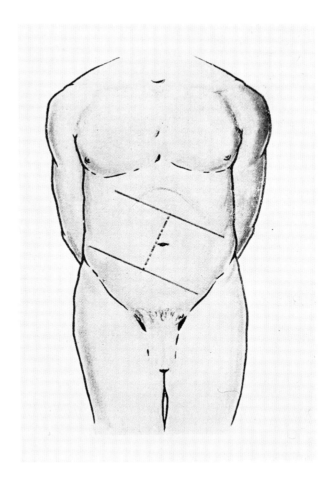

FIG. 130

Localization of small intestine within the peritoneal cavity. The (dotted) line of posterior attachment of the mesentery extends obliquely to the right of the umbilicus. Two lines drawn perpendicular to this line demarcate three zones. The upper third of the small intestine lies in the upper left zone, the middle third in the middle, and the lower third in the lowest right zone. (From Monks, 1903.)

To determine the direction taken by a loop of intestine, an assistant pulls the loop to render the mesentery taut. When the mesentery, held in the axis of the posterior attachment, is ascertained to be free of a twist one may infer that the end of the loop lying upward and to the left is indeed the proximal end. On occasion it is difficult to be certain that the mesentery is not twisted, and it is reassuring to identify both the part of the intestine and its direction by following it to one end at either the duodenojejunal or the ileocecal junction.

CHARACTERISTICS OF INTESTINAL SEGMENTS; COLONOSCOPIC VIEWS

The large intestine possesses teniae, haustra, and appendices epiploicae, which distinguish it from the small intestine. The three teniae are named libera, mesocolica, and omentalis, from their position on the transverse colon. The tenia libera lies inferior on the transverse colon, but anterior (and is often named anterior) on the cecum and the ascending and descending colon (see Fig. 133). On the cecum, the mesocolic tenia lies posteromedial, the omental tenia posterolateral. All of the teniae lead to the appendix, and they meet in its base. The teniae widen and become progressively less prominent on the rectum, where haustration is also lacking. The diameter of the large bowel diminishes from the cecum (about 7.5 cm.) to the sigmoid colon (about 2.5 cm.), and is then further widened in the ampulla of the rectum.

Several characteristics help to determine the proximodistal position of a piece of small intestine, granted there is a gradual transition of jejunum to ileum. The first is the appearance of its mesentery. In its proximal reaches, the mesentery is thin and its blood vessels show clearly. The mesenteric fat increases distally, progressively obscuring the vessels, especially in obese subjects. Toward the terminal ileum little tabs of fat project freely or onto the intestine. The anastomotic arcades between adjacent jejunal arteries are arranged in one or two tiers proximally. The number of arcades increases distally, until four or five tiers may be counted at the terminal ileum, arranged in a more haphazard pattern and at least partly obscured by fat. The vasa recta are long and straight on the upper small bowel, and rarely give off branches to the mesentery. On the lower ileum the vasa recta are shorter, smaller, and less regular, and give off frequent branches to the mesentery.

The diameter and thickness of the small bowel and the prominence of the valvulae conniventes diminish from above downward. In the average healthy bowel, the jejunum is about 4 cm. in diameter, the ileum about 3 cm. The jejunum is thicker and more vascular than the ileum; its valvulae conniventes are better developed and more evident by palpation or by inspection against the light. Peyer's patches may also thus be seen in the ileum. The consistency of the contents of the bowel increases toward the lower ileum.

The colonoscope, a flexible fiber-optic endoscope, can be introduced via the anus and advanced through the large bowel and into the terminal ileum. The instrument is passed with the patient on his back, or on his side. Photographs of the views obtained at several levels are shown in Figure 131. Guidance for the passing of the instrument is available from the light transmitted through the abdominal wall, and is afforded as well by certain gross landmarks visible within the bowel. The transmitted light is first seen in the left lower quadrant, as the tip of the colonoscope enters the mid sigmoid; it then disappears as the junction of the sigmoid and descending colon is traversed. It reappears in the left flank and becomes bright below the 11th and 12th ribs as the tip moves up the descending colon. The light moves up and down with respiration when the splenic flexure is entered. It travels across the abdomen at the level of the umbilicus during passage of the tip through the transverse colon, then disappears behind the liver to reappear at McBurney's point when the cecum is entered.

The first major internal landmark is the obstruction to easy advance encountered at the junction of the sigmoid and descending colon. Slight retraction and counterclockwise rotation of the instrument ('alpha maneuver'), with the patient in right lateral decubitus position, opens the bowel ahead and allows a relaxed 'slide-by' into the descending colon. At the splenic flexure one sees motion imparted by the heart beat, and here respiratory excursions are first noted. Both cardiac and respiratory movements are lost as the instrument enters the hepatic flexure. The transverse colon and cecum are close enough to the abdominal wall to allow an easy appreciation of localized pressure applied externally.

LENGTH OF THE INTESTINE

The total length of the intestine determined by postmortem measurement is generally given as 800 to 900 cm. (26 to 29 feet), but careful measurements made during life by means of a weighted tube passed through the nose show these figures to be excessive, the error being attributed to postmortem loss of tone in the intestine. Table 7, based on the work of Hirsch and his colleagues (1956), gives an average length during life for the entire intestine of close to 400 cm., or 13 feet. The length of the alimentary canal was related to body height. They emphasized that

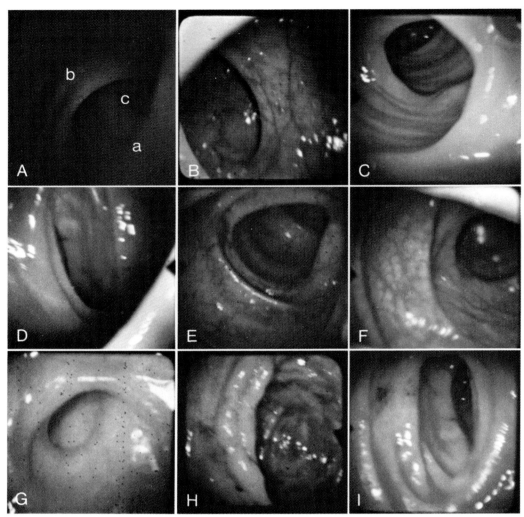

FIG. 131

Colonoscopy.

I. Interior of bowel as viewed through the colonoscope. These photographs are oriented as though the patient were lying on his back. Each segment is viewed from below. A. The rectum. The smooth-walled cavity is partially divided by the transverse rectal folds (valves of Houston). They are more prominent in the young, and may not be discernible in the old, especially when the rectum is distended with air. The inferior fold, a, lies on the patient's left and posterior, the middle fold, b, lies right and anterior, the superior fold, c, left and posterior. B. The rectosigmoid shows a prominent venous pattern. C. The sigmoid colon, characterized by low mucosal folds, tubular lumen, forceful peristaltic waves, and acute angulations. D. The descending colon, showing an open straight lumen compared with that of the sigmoid. A transition from mucosal folds randomly crossing the lumen to definite haustration is noted; the lumen may become somewhat triangular here. E. The transverse colon, characterized by a triangular lumen, with prominent repetitive drapery-like mucosal folds. Deep pockets, the haustra, separate segments with a triangular lumen. F. The upper ascending colon with capacious lumen, circular in outline; the folds between haustra are deep and widely separated. Here, as in the cecum, the wall is thin, with a prominent vascular pattern running across the long axis of the bowel. G. The cecum and the appendicular orifice, here widely patent. The orifice may be a mere dimple if the lumen of the appendix is scarred, or a shallow diverticulum if previous appendectomy has been done. H. The ileocecal valve, shown here in tight contraction, is often recognized by a fleck of ileal contents within it. I. The terminal ileum. Here the friable mucosa is arranged in closely spaced folds extending 180 to 270 degrees around the circumference of the oval lumen. Peristalsis is continuous and makes further advancement of the colonoscope difficult. (Courtesy of Dr. Paul H. Sugarbaker, Department of Surgery, Peter Bent Brigham Hospital, Boston.)

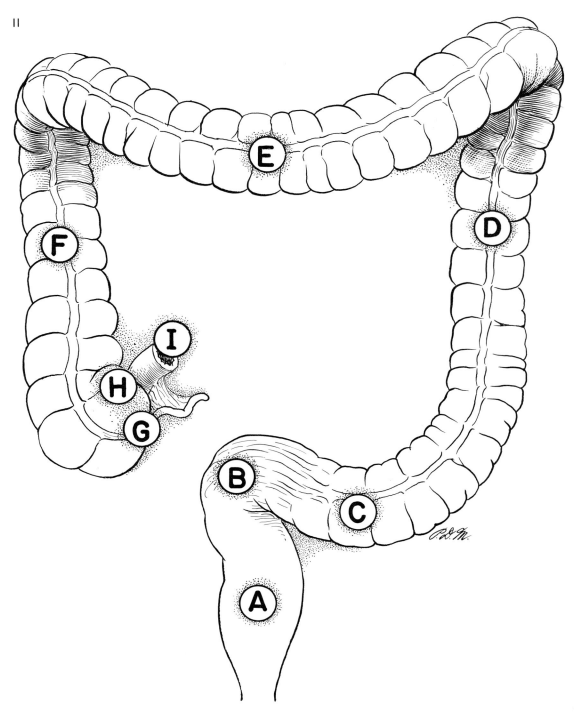

FIG. 131
Colonoscopy (continued).
   II. Sites in the bowel at which the colonoscopic views in I were obtained.

TABLE 7
Average Length of Alimentary Canal in
*Living Adult, Measured by Nasal Tube.**

Total Nose to Anus Length	453 cm. (15 feet)
Duodenum	21 cm. (8 inches)
Jejuno-ileum	261 cm. (8 feet, 8 inches)
Large Intestine	109 cm. (3 feet, 7 inches)

Total length of Alimentary Canal is 2.5 to 3 x Standing Body Height
Length of Jejuno-ileum is 1.6 x Standing Body Height

*Based on Hirsch *et al.* (1956).

the gut can shorten considerably upon a nasointestinal tube, that it is longer with solid than with a liquid diet, and that it is subject to changes in length with an increase or diminution in tone. The length of the intestine at birth is reported to be half that in the adult—300 to 350 cm. for the small intestine (apparently measured in the cadaver), with an increase of about 50 cm. in the first year of life, and doubling by puberty, at which time its length approximates that in the adult (Watson and Lowrey, 1962).

The length of bowel that can be resected safely varies with the level of resection. Total colectomy may result in loose and frequent movements, but does not appreciably alter the nutritional state. Loss of small intestine is more serious. There are reports of survival with the small intestine shortened to only a few feet, and occasionally even a few inches, but as Wright and Tilson (1971) sum it up "the nutritional consequences of loss of more than 80 per cent of the gut will be profound." Loss of the ileum is more serious than loss of the jejunum. Thus diarrhea, a particularly disabling feature of loss of the small bowel, may be avoided even after 70 per cent resection, provided the terminal ileum and the ileocecal valve are preserved. Weismann (1973) and Payne and his co-workers (1973) report their experiences with planned small bowel resection in many patients. Wright and Tilson state that the newborn can survive the removal of all but 10 per cent [30 cm., or 12 inches] of intestine, provided the ileocecal valve is intact. The gut in infancy shows some compensatory growth after resection.

SOURCE AND DISTRIBUTION OF THE
INTESTINAL ARTERIES

The superior mesenteric artery gives off the inferior pancreaticoduodenal, the middle colic, and the initial jejunal arteries, under cover of the neck of the pancreas (see Fig. 76). Additional jejunal and ileal arteries derive from the left side of the superior mesenteric, for a distance of 10 to 16 inches. Their arcade formation has been noted above.

Details of the blood supply to the large intestine are shown in Figures 132 and 133. Three arteries to the large intestine are given off from the right side of the superior

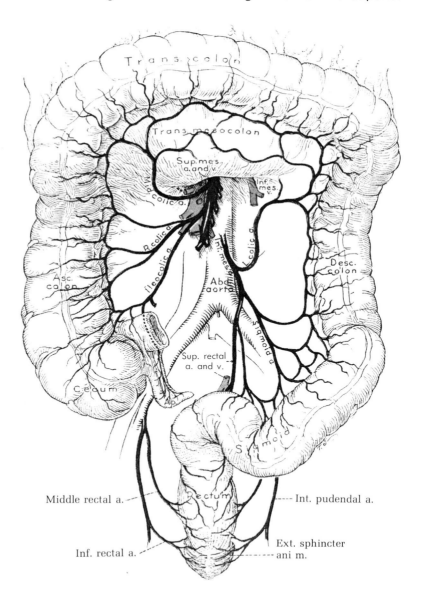

FIG. 132
Arteries of the large intestine. (From Jones and Shepard, 1945.)

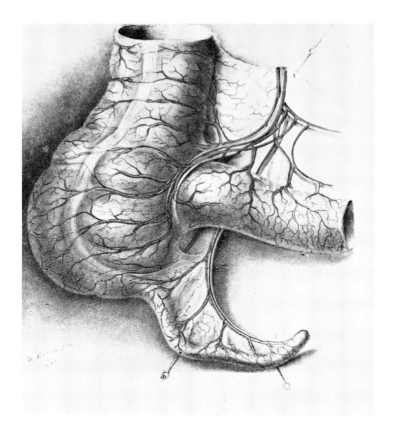

FIG. 133
Blood vessels and other features of the ileocecal region. Four branches of the ileocecal artery are shown: The anterior cecal in front of the ileocolic junction; the posterior cecal behind, its origin obscure; the appendicular in the mesoappendix behind the ileum; and an ileal branch. A thin termination of the ileocolic artery (the 'recurrent ileal') courses to the left where it will join the distal part of the superior mesenteric trunk. (This fourth branch was absent in over half of the specimens of Michels et al., 1963.) A narrow ileocecal fold (bloodless fold of Treves) extends from the antimesenteric border of the ileum to the cecum. The anterior tenia (tenia libera) extends down the anterior cecum to the base of the appendix. (From Kelly, 1909.)

mesenteric, usually quite proximally. These are the middle colic, the right colic, and the ileocolic. The initial branch of the inferior mesenteric is the left colic artery, which ascends sharply to supply the descending colon and often the splenic flexure. Next come the sigmoid arteries, generally three in number, the upper of which may be combined with the left colic. The inferior mesenteric continues downward as the superior rectal artery (Fig. 132). All the colic and the sigmoidal arteries bifurcate proximal to the bowel. The anastomoses between the bifurcations form a composite vessel, termed the marginal artery. A few secondary arcades may also be formed. The marginal artery lies 1 to 8 cm. from the bowel (Steward and Rankin, 1933).

The extent of the colon supplied by the various colic arteries is variable. In general, the ileocolic and right colic are distributed to the cecum and ascending colon; the middle colic is distributed to the transverse colon. The left colic artery ascends to reach the splenic flexure in 86 per cent, according to Michels and his colleagues (1965). Kahn and Abrams (1964) found by arteriography that the left colic extended even proximal to the flexure in 13 per cent. The replacement of one of the colic arteries by an adjacent vessel may be so complete as to justify the statement that the right, middle, or, rarely, the left colic artery is absent. Contrariwise, two vessels may represent one of these usually single arteries. The right colic artery originates from a common trunk with the middle colic in close to half of all subjects, and from the ileocolic less frequently. The middle colic in its initial course is vulnerable to injury in the performance of pancreatectomy, since it passes around the lower border of the gland, or through it (see Figs. 65 and 76). Its avoidance during gastrectomy has been mentioned (p. 117). The middle colic can originate from the celiac artery or from one of the three branches of that vessel passing behind the pancreas. Michels (1955) found the dorsal pancreatic artery occasionally giving rise to the middle colic or to an accessory left colic artery. Michels emphasized that frequent communications exist behind the pancreas between branches of the celiac and branches of the superior mesenteric, especially the middle colic and accessory left colic arteries. The communicating vessels are generally small, but may reach 2 mm. in diameter.

The 'arc of Riolan,' an accessory left colic artery, springs from the proximal superior mesenteric or the middle colic artery, and joins the left colic artery in the mesocolon close to the duodenojejunal junction. Its incidence is generally given as 10 per cent, but Adachi (1928) found it in 20 per cent. When present, the accessory left colic artery forms a large anastomosis between the superior and inferior mesenteric arteries parallel to the marginal artery, but closer to the base of the mesentery. It is likely that the 'meandering mesenteric artery,' seen after mesenteric artery obstruction, is made up of an accessory left colic artery plus portions of the colic and marginal arteries (Moskowitz *et al.,* 1964; Gonzalez and Jaffe, 1966).

The anorectum is supplied from three sources: the superior rectal, from the inferior mesenteric artery; the middle rectal, from the internal iliac; and the inferior rectal, from the internal pudendal artery (Fig. 132). The superior rectal artery bifurcates, or sometimes trifurcates unevenly, on the posterior aspect of the rectum, where, with the pararectal lymph nodes, it descends deep to the rectal fascia a few centimeters above the pelvic floor (see Fig. 150 II). The middle rectal is the most variable. Angiography shows the rectum receives many small arteries from the lateral and median sacral and adjacent visceral arteries (see Figs. 35 and 175). Incidence of the presence of a predominant large middle rectal artery extending from the internal iliac or one of its branches is variously given from 66 to 98 per cent (see page 66, and Boxall *et al.,* 1963). The middle rectal arteries course downward and medially beneath the peritoneal reflection, and traverse the rectal fascia anterolaterally to reach the rectum, usually less than 2 cm. above the levator ani muscles.

The arterial supply to the anorectum gains importance because of its role in determining the viability of the distal stump or segment after resection above it. Individual variation is great, and the surgeon is obliged to examine the distal segment after compressing or dividing the arteries to see whether the arterial supply is adequate. If it is not the bowel must be cut back to a well-vascularized level. In general, a rectal stump between 8 and 15 cm. above the peritoneal reflection will survive. Whether its vascularity depends on the inferior rectal or small remaining middle rectal vessels is debatable. Such small vessels may remain lying on or close to the levators. Boxall and his co-workers (1963) emphasize that a large middle rectal artery usually does not pass through the lateral rectal ligament but rather runs anterolaterally and may escape division when the bowel is mobilized.

The terminal arteries to the bowel are called the vasa recta. They derive from the para-intestinal artery composed of the arcades of the jejunal and ileal arteries, and, for the large intestine, the vessel called the marginal artery. The duodenojejunal junction is twisted prior to embryonic fusion, so that the relationships of the para-intestinal vessel and the vasa recta to the bowel are sharply divergent on either side of the junction of the duodenum and jejunum. Figure 76 shows the inferior pancreaticoduodenal arteries and their branches to the duodenum, comparable to the vasa recta, lying on the superior aspect of the duodenum; the first jejunal artery crosses the front of the jejunum to reach the mesentery to communicate with the second jejunal artery. From there down the intestinal arteries enter the bowel on

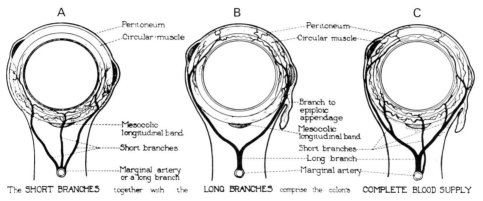

FIG. 134

Short and long vasa recta of the large intestine. A. Short vasa recta are distributed mainly to the depth of the bowel wall near the mesentery. B. Long vasa recta, fewer in number, pass closer to the serosa, then deep to the tenia on each side (where they are vulnerable to injudicious clamping) to supply the antimesenteric border. Here there are anastomoses between these branches but only of arteriolar caliber. C. The relations of the two sets of vasa recta. (From Steward and Rankin, Arch. Surg. 26:843–891, 1933. Copyright 1933, American Medical Association.)

the mesenteric border or fairly near it (Michels *et al.,* 1963). The vasa recta derived from the first jejunal artery course mainly anterior to the jejunum. A few vasa recta course posterior. Beyond the first jejunal artery the vasa recta pass to one side or the other of the small bowel in a haphazard fashion (Noer, 1943). Noer also noted that the vasa recta may give off some branches to the bowel before reaching that structure, but entered into no anastomoses. Mesenteric branches of the vasa have been mentioned above (p. 228). Steward and Rankin described long and short vasa recta for the large intestine (Fig. 134).

The vasa recta carry out the principle already noted for the small arteries to the duodenum (Chapter 7), namely, they are, in effect, end-arteries, and the bowel is subject to necrosis if they are injured. Thus, tearing of the mesentery close to the bowel for 1 or 2 cm. may result in necrosis. For the same reason, the bowel may be cut diagonally in resection to remove somewhat less bowel at the mesenteric than at the antimesenteric border.

COLLATERALS BETWEEN INTESTINAL BRANCHES; THE ROUX LOOP

The collateral system produced by the arcade formation in the small intestine is, in the main, good enough to allow the division of one or more arteries contributing to the arcades without producing bowel necrosis. As regards the marginal artery, its contributors may or may not be dispensable. Thus bowel necrosis may follow division of the middle colic artery. The anastomotic system of any part of the bowel may be ineffective because of variations in the size of the major intestinal branches and in their anastomoses, or because of the presence of arterial stenosis or thrombosis.

The proximal superior mesenteric artery forms a link between the inferior pancreaticoduodenal and the first jejunal artery, there often being no arch between the two vessels. Individual jejunal and ileal arteries vary considerably in size. Barlow (1956) found a break in the convexity of the arcades of the small intestine in 5.7 per cent of individuals, and a 'weakness' in 15.7 per cent.

Discontinuity or probable inadequacy of the marginal artery is likely to occur in three locations, with a frequency found in extensive studies by Michels and his colleagues (1963 and 1965) as follows: (1) Between the ileocolic and right colic arteries, 10 per cent. (2) Between the ascending and descending branches of the left colic artery (Griffith's point, Griffiths, 1956), 39 per cent, although a secondary proximal arcade between these two branches often compensates for the inadequacy of the marginal artery. (3) Between the last sigmoid and the superior rectal artery (Sudeck's critical angle, Sudeck, 1907), 84 per cent. Basmajian (1954) added a fourth location, the junction of the right and middle colic arteries, incidence 5 per cent.

Sudeck was commenting on the gangrene of the large bowel that followed operations for cancer as they were done early in this century, in which the inferior mesenteric artery or its branches were divided to allow a perineal 'pull-through' to be performed. He suggested that the last portion of the inferior mesenteric artery should remain intact at the point where it bifurcated into the last sigmoid and superior rectal artery. Thus blood from the marginal artery reaching the last sigmoid could continue into the superior rectal artery (Fig. 132). Even today operations are sometimes done in which the inferior mesenteric artery is divided and the rectosigmoid saved. In such instances the question of communication between the last sigmoid and the superior rectal artery remains pertinent. Because the collateral supply to any part of the bowel is subject to variation, one should temporarily occlude the relevant artery and note the effect on the bowel, before dividing the artery.

The presence of a para-intestinal artery in both the small and the large intestine allows one to mobilize a pedicled segment of bowel (the Roux loop) (Fig. 135), which may be transposed to re-establish the continuity of the alimentary tract, as in esophagojejunostomy, or to establish a conduit in other systems, as in creating a ureterocutaneous fistula ('ileal conduit'). Roux (1897) first fashioned such a jejunal loop 'en Y,' for gastrojejunostomy. Later he bypassed the esophagus by laying a similar Y loop subcutaneously from the stomach to a premanubrial stoma (Roux, 1907). The length of the loop to be fashioned and the adequacy of its arterial and venous pedicle become especially significant when the loop must be transposed some distance, as in esophageal replacement. The first and second jejunal arteries are short, and their arcades small. A more mobile jejunal loop may be prepared from the jejunum 30 to 40 cm. beyond the duodenojejunal junction (Rienhoff, 1946; Allison and DaSilva, 1953). Thomas and Merendino (1958) emphasized the importance of saving the intestinal veins, which may or may not lie adjacent to the arteries. Allison and

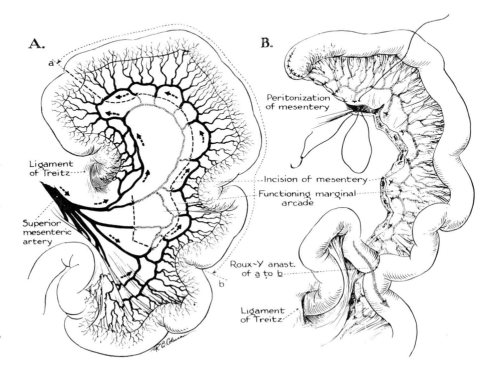

FIG. 135
The formation of a Roux Y loop of jejunum. A. The lines of the section of the bowel and of the jejunal arteries. Arrows indicate direction that anastomotic flow will take through the jejunal arterial arches. B. The completed loop with continuity restored and the pedicled loop of jejunum ready for anastomosis elsewhere. (From Reynolds and Young, 1948.)

DaSilva described details of technique, such as division of jejunal artery branches to mesenteric lymph nodes to improve mobility of the loop. Some length of the mobilized bowel may need to be removed if its circulation appears inadequate.

Either the terminal ileum with the cecum, ascending colon, and right half of the transverse colon pedicled on the middle colic artery (Petrov, 1964), or the left colon from the mid transverse part to the sigmoid below the first and second sigmoid arteries may be used to establish a very long intestinal graft when the vascular arcades of the jejunum are limiting. In an anatomic study Beck and Baronofsky (1960) found that such a 'left colon' centered on the middle colic was more satisfactory than the right. The frequent narrowing of the marginal artery near the splenic flexure (Griffith's point) could be overcome by preserving the often-present secondary arcade of the bifurcation of the left colic artery. Variations in the middle colic artery may reduce the adequacy of the pedicle of either the right or the left half of the colon.

Free grafts of jejunum or of the colon have been transposed to the neck or thorax to replace the esophagus, with the intestinal artery and vein anastomosed to the blood vessels of these regions (Longmire, 1947; Jurkiewicz, 1965).

REfERENCES

Adachi, B.: Das Arteriensystem der Japaner. Vol. II. Tokyo, Kenkyusha, 1928.

Allison, P. R., and DaSilva, L. T.: The Roux loop. Brit. J. Surg. 41:173–180, 1953.

Barlow, T. E.: Variations in the blood-supply of the upper jejunum. Brit. J. Surg. 43:473–475, 1956.

Basmajian, J. V.: The marginal anastomoses of the arteries to the large intestine. Surg. Gynec. Obstet. 99:614–616, 1954.

Beck, A. R., and Baronofsky, I. D.: A study of the left colon as a replacement for the resected esophagus. Surgery 48:499–509, 1960.

Boxall, T. A., Smart, P. J. G., and Griffiths, J. D.: The blood-supply of the distal segment of the rectum in anterior resection. Brit. J. Surg. 50:399–404, 1963.

Gonzalez, L. L., and Jaffe, M. S.: Mesenteric arterial insufficiency following abdominal aortic resection. Arch. Surg. 93:10–20, 1966.

Griffiths, J. D.: Surgical anatomy of the blood supply of the distal colon. Ann. Roy. Coll. Surg. Engl. 19:241–256, 1956.

Hirsch, J., Ahrens, E. H., Jr., and Blankenhorn, D. H.: Measurement of the human intestinal length *in vivo* and some causes of variation. Gastroenterology 31:274–284, 1956.

Jones, T., and Shepard, W. C.: A Manual of Surgical Anatomy. Philadelphia, W. B. Saunders, 1945.

Jurkiewicz, M. J.: Vascularized intestinal graft for reconstruction of the cervical esophagus and pharynx. Plast. Reconstr. Surg. 36:509–517, 1965.

Kahn, P., and Abrams, H. L.: Inferior mesenteric arterial patterns. An angiographic study. Radiology 82:429–441, 1964.

Kelly, H. A.: Appendicitis and Other Diseases of the Vermiform Appendix. Philadelphia, J. B. Lippincott, 1909.

Longmire, W. P., Jr.: A modification of the Roux technique for antethoracic esophageal reconstruction. Anastomosis of the mesenteric and internal mammary blood vessels. Surgery 22:94–100, 1947.

Michels, N. A.: Blood Supply and Anatomy of the Upper Abdominal Organs. Philadelphia, J. B. Lippincott, 1955.

Michels, N. A., Siddharth, P., Kornblith, P. L., and Parke, W. W.: The variant blood supply to the small and large intestines: Its import in regional resections. A new anatomic study based on four hundred dissections, with a complete review of the literature. J. Int. Coll. Surg. 39:127–170, 1963.

Michels, N. A., Siddharth, P., Kornblith, P. L., and Parke, W. W.: The variant blood supply to the descending colon, rectosigmoid and rectum based on 400 dissections. Its importance in regional dissections: A review of medical literature. Dis. Colon Rectum 8:251–278, 1965.

Monks, G. H.: Intestinal localization. A study on the cadaver for the purpose of determining to what extent the various parts of the small intestine may be identified through an abdominal wound. Trans. Amer. Surg. Assn. 21:405–424, 1903.

Moskowitz, M., Zimmerman, H., and Felson, B.: The meandering mesenteric artery of the colon. Amer. J. Roentgen. 92:1088–1099, 1964.

Noer, R. J.: The blood vessels of the jejunum and ileum: A comparative study of man and certain laboratory animals. Amer. J. Anat. 73:293–334, 1943.

Payne, J. H., DeWind, L., Schwab, C. E., and Kern, W. H.: Surgical treatment of morbid obesity. Sixteen years of experience. Arch. Surg. 106:432–437, 1973.

Petrov, B. A.: Retrosternal artificial esophagus created from colon. 100 operations. Surgery 55:520–523, 1964.

Reynolds, J. T., and Young, J. P., Jr.: The use of the Roux Y in extending the operability of carcinoma of the stomach and of the lower end of the esophagus. Surgery 24:246–263, 1948.

Rienhoff, W. J., Jr.: Intrathoracic esophagojejunostomy for lesions of the upper third of the esophagus, Southern Med. J. 39:928–940, 1946.

Roux, C.: De la gastro-entérostomie. Rev. gynécol. chir. abdom. 1:67–122, 1897.

Roux, C.: L'oesophago-jéjuno-gastrostomose, nouvelle opération pour rétrécissement infranchissable de l'oesophage. Sem. med. 27:37–40, 1907.

Steward, J. A., and Rankin, F. W.: Blood supply of the large intestine. Its surgical considerations. Arch. Surg. 26:843–891, 1933.

Sudeck, P.: Ueber die Gefässversorgung des Mastdarmes in Hinsicht auf die operative Gangrän. Munch. med. Wschr. 54:1314–1317, 1907.

Thomas, G. I., and Merendino, K. A.: Jejunal interposition operation—analysis of thirty-three clinical cases. J.A.M.A. 168:1759–1766, 1958.

Watson, E. H., and Lowrey, G. H.: Growth and Development of Children, 4th ed. Chicago, Year Book Publishers, 1962.

Weismann, R. E.: Surgical palliation of massive and severe obesity. Amer. J. Surg. 125:437–446, 1973.

Wright, H. K., and Tilson, M. D.: The short gut syndrome. Pathophysiology and treatment. Curr. Prob. Surg. June, 1971.

THE ANORECTUM

TOPOGRAPHY

Anatomists define the anal canal in terms of its muscle relationships. It is somewhat longer than 3 cm., extending from the anal orifice to the perineal flexure, where the puborectalis muscles (the medial fibers of the two levator ani muscles) produce an angulation, above which the rectum widens abruptly. The angulation of this 'puborectalis sling' can be palpated posteriorly (see Fig. 144). In frontal section the lower portion of the anal canal is seen surrounded by the external sphincter; the upper part contains the internal sphincter, and levator ani muscle bundles are interspersed between the two sphincters and through the external sphincter (Fig. 136).

Certain landmarks of the anorectum and the sigmoid colon may be observed endoscopically. The pectinate line lies at the bases of the anal papillae. This level is somewhat inferior to the perineal flexure of the anorectum. Proctologists sometimes indicate the pectinate line as the upper limit of the anal canal (as in Fig. 137); by this definition the segment is less than 3 cm. long. The line approximates the mucocutaneous junction, although stratified epithelium may be found somewhat above it. The pectinate line marks the upper limit of acute pain sensitivity, and the boundary between lymphatic drainage to the inguinal nodes and drain-

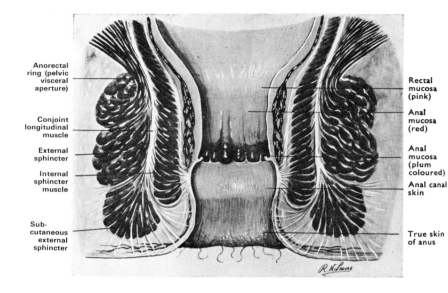

Anorectal ring (pelvic visceral aperture)

Conjoint longitudinal muscle

External sphincter

Internal sphincter muscle

Sub-cutaneous external sphincter

Rectal mucosa (pink)

Anal mucosa (red)

Anal mucosa (plum coloured)

Anal canal skin

True skin of anus

FIG. 136
The anal canal in frontal section to show the structure of the wall. The conjoint longitudinal muscle extends the fibers of the levator ani, of which the puborectalis ('anorectal ring') is a part, and the longitudinal smooth muscle of the bowel through the external sphincter to the skin. (From Morgan and Thompson, 1956.)

age to the iliac nodes. Internal hemorrhoids form by dilation of the submucous veins at the pectinate line; with progression the hemorrhoidal masses prolapse to a lower position.

Within the rectum the crescentic rectal folds (plicae transversales, or valves of Houston) project part way into the

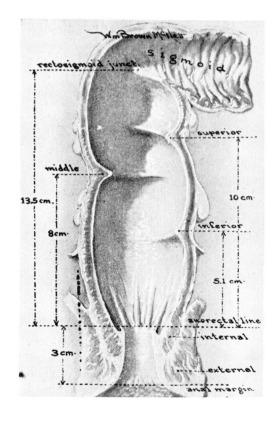

FIG. 137
Distances from the anus of the various features of the anorectum seen in frontal section. The distances shown represent the average of 161 determinations. The specimen is viewed from in front, the middle rectal valve being seen on the subject's right, the superior and inferior valves on his left (see Figs. 131, 147.) (From Bacon, 1949.)

lumen from the concavities of the rectal flexures (Figs. 131, 137, 147). There usually are three, but there may be two or four. The upper and lower are seen within, projecting from the left side of the rectum, the lower somewhat posterior; the middle projects from the right anterior side. The middle fold (the fold of Kohlrausch) is fairly constant. It lies about 8 cm. above the pectinate line, or 11 cm. above the anal orifice. The middle fold indicates the line of attachment of the peritoneum to the anterior rectum (see Fig. 140) and the lower limit of primary lymphatic drainage to the inferior mesenteric nodes. Thus a carcinoma lying above the middle rectal fold is usually amenable to anterior resection of the rectum. One lying below the fold may require other means (see Chapter 18). The bottom of the rectovesical pouch of peritoneum lies lower, between 7.5 and 9.0 cm. above the anal orifice, at lower levels in the female than in the male.

FECAL CONTINENCE

Fecal continence depends on the presence of a fecal reservoir—the rectum—maintained by the puborectalis muscles and anal sphincters that have adequate resting muscle tone and that can additionally respond to increases in intraluminal pressure. Pertinent to continence after anorectal operation are the structure of these muscles, their innervation, and the source of afferent stimulation for reflex contraction. Excellent reviews of the elements bearing on fecal continence are given by Denny-Brown and Robertson (1935) and by Stephens (1953), Scharli and Kiesewetter (1970), and Duthie (1971).

The puborectalis sling angulates the anorectal junction, indenting it sharply posteriorly, maintaining the rectal reservoir as a major factor in gross continence. The fibers of the external sphincter are mainly ringlike about the anus, but some are also attached to the coccyx posteriorly and to the central tendon of the perineum anteriorly. The deep part of the external sphincter blends with the puborectalis muscles on the posterior aspect of the anorectal junction. The structure of the external sphincter was carefully studied by Fowler (1957). He found that it could be divided into superficial and deep parts, but concluded that the existence of a subcutaneous part or of a corrugator cutis muscle was a myth. Fowler, as well as Wilde (1949) before him, concluded that corrugation of the anal skin was produced by the longitudinal muscle of the rectum and levator ani fibers which fan out into fibroelastic cords that extend through the external sphincter to the anal skin (Fig. 136). By palpation one can feel within the anal canal the slight groove marking the lower limit of the thickened circular non-striated muscle of the gut, termed the internal sphincter. Outside of the median fibers of the levator ani which constitute the puborectalis muscle, the levator itself sends bundles of its fibers down the long axis of the bowel. Here they mingle with the longitudinal non-striated muscle of the rectum. Morgan and Thompson (1956) point out that anesthesia alone, with or without traction on the anal mucous membrane, allows the internal sphincter to descend to a superficial position. The internal sphincter, although contributing less to sphincteric control than the striated components, is nevertheless of some importance. Bennett and Duthie (1964) found that after the internal sphincter was divided for anal fissure anal tone was measurably lessened both at rest and in response to experimental rectal distention. Moreover, Denny-Brown and Robertson (1935) observed that some anal tone and contractility remained after external sphincter paralysis caused by cauda equina lesions. They attributed this residual sphincteric action to the involuntary muscle found in the internal sphincter as well as that distributed throughout the pelvic floor.

The third and fourth sacral nerves innervate the levator ani and external sphincter muscles. The levator muscle is supplied by branches of their anterior rami that descend on the pelvic floor within the inferior hypogastric plexus. The external sphincter is innervated mainly by the inferior rectal branch of the pudendal nerve, supplemented by the anal branch of the perineal nerve (see Figs. 198, 212). The small perineal branch of the fourth sacral nerve perforates the posteromedial part of the ischiorectal fossa, but its significance is uncertain. The internal sphincter, as part of the pelvic intestinal musculature, is supplied by the inferior hypogastric plexus, probably only through its parasympathetic component (Denny-Brown and Robertson, 1935).

The resting tone and active contraction of the sphincters

depend on the presence of afferent stimulation. The source of these impulses may be deduced from observations after resection of varying lengths of the anorectum or removal of the anorectal mucous membrane. The sensation of rectal fullness appears to be mediated from propioceptive endings in the musculature of the rectal wall. Some of these endings are located in the perirectal tissues, including the levator muscles, since some of the sensation may persist when dissection of the rectum is done close to its wall, with anastomosis of colon to the anal canal. The discrimination of solid from liquid or gaseous content depends on sensory stimulation of the anorectal mucosa. Goligher and Hughes (1951) emphasized that the inferior hypogastric plexus carries the sensory nerves of the reflex arc serving sphincteric function and that it must be preserved. This precaution can easily be observed in rectal resection for benign disease; it preserves the innervation for proper vesical and genital function as well.

It appears that the puborectalis sling is all-important in maintaining resting rectal continence, aided by the resting tone of the external and internal sphincters. Gross resting continence can be maintained in the absence of external sphincter function provided the puborectalis muscles are intact. Relaxation of the internal sphincter occurs in response to waves of propulsion in the upper rectum, allowing the rectal contents to impinge on the mucous membrane of the anorectum, where sensory stimulation leads to the discrimination of the nature of the contents. The relaxation is probably the result of an intramural reflex, since it is not totally abolished by spinal anesthesia; it may or may not persist after resection of the rectum above the level of the internal sphincter (Scharli and Kiesewetter, 1970). The stimulation of sensory endings in the mucous membrane produces reflex contraction of the two voluntary sphincters to maintain continence, or to their inhibition if defecation is to proceed. External sphincter competence is undoubtedly important in the sharp termination of defecation and the maintenance of a clean perineum.

The minimal length of the anorectal stump which will allow *perfect* fecal continence after rectal resection is generally considered to be 6 cm. measured from the anus, in the adult. Segments shorter than this will be more or less deficient in continence, partly because of loss of sensation and partly because of loss of muscle function. Shortening to less than 4 cm. gives little hope of continence, mainly because of interference with the puborectalis muscles, with some effect from the loss of some of the internal sphincter. Loss of the mucous membrane, in operations which remove the anorectum to this depth, results in little impairment in continence although there is loss of fine discrimination of the nature of the bowel content. Even if the removal includes the internal sphincter, gross continence may still be maintained.

IMPERFORATE ANUS; CONGENITAL AGANGLIONIC MEGACOLON

The expression 'imperforate anus' includes the great variety of stenoses or atresias involving the anorectum. Gross (1953) created a simple classification of these anomalies (Table 8); a division into finer categories was presented by Stephens and Smith (1971). The commonest of these variations involves the lack of development of the anal canal, usually with fistulous connection to the bladder, vagina, urethra, or perineum. The surgeon's concern is to create not only an anal opening but one with a sphincteric mechanism. The internal sphincter is absent in those cases with anal atresia; external sphincter elements usually exist, but the muscle may function poorly after the bowel is brought

TABLE 8
*Types of Imperforate Anus Found in 507 Cases.**

	Frequency	Associated Fistula
Type I Stenosis of anus or rectum	6%	14%
Type II Membranous obstruction of anus	3%	14%
Type III High termination of rectum: atresia lower anorectum	87%	80%
Type IV High termination of rectum: normal lower anorectum	4%	None

*After Gross (1953).

through it. It remains for the puborectalis to supply the major sphincter control and proprioceptive sensation, as first pointed out by Stephens in 1953. The lower end of the rectum is most apt to terminate above the levator ani muscle in the male, whereas it usually, but not always, extends through the levator muscle to a lower position in the female (Fig. 138). The puborectalis sling therefore surrounds the urethra below a rectourethral fistula in the male, and surrounds the vagina when there is a high rectovaginal fistula in the female (Swenson and Donnellan, 1967).

The sacrococcygeal and perineal approach to imperforate anus with supralevator termination was proposed by Stephens (1953). Further descriptions are given by Stephens and Smith (1971) and Miller and Izant (1971). The blind end of the rectum is approached extra-peritoneally by an incision in the sacrococcygeal region. The cartilaginous coccyx is cut in the midline, and the rectum and its anterior fistula are exposed by blunt dissection. Dissection is facilitated by placing a sound within the urethra or vagina. The puborectalis muscles are not visualized, but a passage for the rectum is made within the muscle sling by dissecting bluntly in the midline behind the urethra or vagina, to a second perineal incision in the position of the anus. An N or Z incision is made at the site of the proposed anus, but Gross (1953) cautions that the deeper tissues, which contain the sphincter muscle, must be cut strictly in the midline. The rectum is then pulled through the perineal incision, opened, and sutured to the skin of the created anus. Swenson and Donnellan (Fig. 139) perform an abdominoperineal

FIG. 138
Relationship of the rectum to the puborectalis muscles in the commonest form of imperforate anus (I) in the male, and (II) in the female There is atresia of the lower anorectum in both, with a rectourethral fistula in the male, and a rectovaginal fistula in the female. The rectum has ended above the puborectalis muscles in the male, but terminates lower in the female, having already passed through the puborectalis muscles. (From Swenson and Donnellan, 1967.)

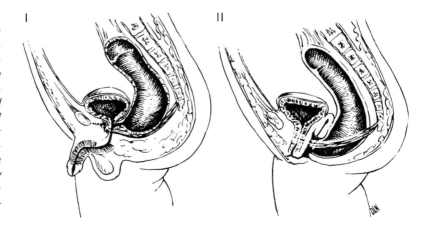

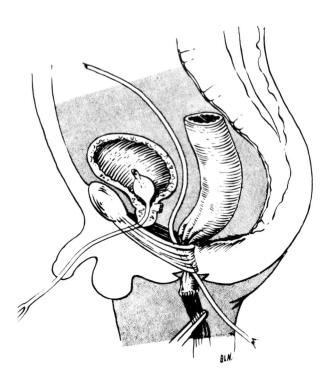

FIG. 139
Correction of imperforate anus in the male. The rectourethral fistula has been divided. A tape has been used to guide the dilation of the puborectalis muscles. The opened rectum is drawn through the muscles and the perineum. (From Swenson and Donnellan, 1967.)

operation, freeing up the rectosigmoid. They make no attempt to pass the rectum through the external sphincter, aiming at continence through the action of the puborectalis muscles alone. They bring these muscles down to a low position on the newly created anorectum by suturing them to the perineal skin and the rectum. Scharli and Kiesewetter found that the rectum after such procedures slowly regained the sensory and motor functions relating to continence.

Congenital aganglionic megacolon (Hirschsprung's disease) has been shown to be based on the absence of the intramural ganglion cells of the myenteric plexus (Swenson et al., 1949). The lack of propulsion in the aganglionic bowel constitutes a physiologic obstruction with secondary enlargement of the proximal colon. The aganglionic segment varies in length, but it extends to the internal sphincter in all cases, and usually involves the entire rectum. Faulty innervation of the bladder and other defects may accompany the rectal lesion (Gray and Skandalakis, 1972).

Treatment consists of resection of the aganglionic bowel with anastomosis of the proximal segment of divided colon to the anal canal. Swenson (1964) excises the bowel from a provisional level fairly high on the rectum, to a level demonstrating ganglionic cells, dividing the sigmoid and rectal branches of the inferior mesenteric artery, but saving the vein. The colon is mobilized, cutting close to the bowel wall. The rectal stump is then dissected, again very close to the bowel, avoiding the perirectal tissues to spare the inferior hypogastric nerve branches, until the rectum can be everted and the junction of anal mucosa and skin easily demonstrated. In the infant, Swenson advises transecting the anorectum obliquely about 2 cm. above the mucocutaneous junction anteriorly, and 1 cm. posteriorly. This ensures that at least part of the circumference of the remaining anorectum is not aganglionic. In addition, some of the internal sphincter (and probably some of the puborectalis sling) is divided, a maneuver which guards against postoperative sphincter spasm. The cut end of the colon, well mobilized and adequately vascularized, is pulled through the anus and anastomosed to the cut end of the anal canal, much as in Figure 145. The Duhamel (1960) procedure avoids much of the lateral pelvic dissection. The rectum is cut across and closed. After the proximal resection of bowel, the end of the colon is brought down through an incision in the posterior anorectum above the pectinate line. Subsequent application of crushing clamps to the adjacent walls of the rectum and colon creates a side-to-side enterostomy between the two segments (Pilling and Cresson, 1969). In the Soave (1964) procedure the anorectal stump is not mobilized, but its mucous membrane is removed and the proximal healthy colon is pulled through and anastomosed to the circumference of the anus.

PARARECTAL ABSCESS; ANAL FISSURE AND FISTULA

Abscesses in proximity to the anorectum may be located above or below the pelvic diaphragm (Fig. 140). Excluding intraperitoneal pelvic infection a supralevator abscess lies beneath the peritoneum, and is termed pelvirectal when it lies to the right or left, retrorectal when it lies behind the rectum. An infradiaphragmatic abscess is termed ischiorectal, since it occupies that fossa. Drainage of an ischiorectal abscess is from below, traversing the fat of the space bluntly

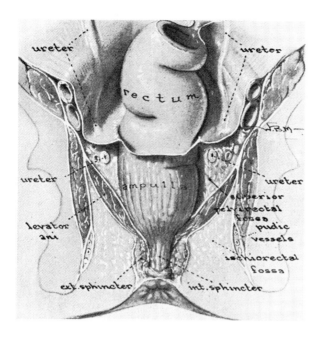

FIG. 140
Relationship of the rectum to the pelvic diaphragm and the peritoneum. Note that the right concavity of the rectal flexure, which indicates the position of the middle rectal fold, approximates the level of the peritoneal reflection. (From Bacon, 1949.)

to avoid injury to the inferior rectal nerve. Most surgeons also drain supralevator abscesses through the ischiorectal space, but Parks (1971) warns this should be done only if the supralevator abscess was formed by upward extension of an ischiorectal abscess. If the abscess originated above the levator he advises high drainage through the rectum, otherwise a total extrasphincteric pelvirectal fistula and incontinence will be produced. A retrorectal abscess is drained by incision between anus and coccyx. The coccyx may be removed for better drainage.

An anal fissure occupies the anal 'mucous membrane' most frequently in the posterior midline. Various operations proposed have in common the division or paralysis of the internal sphincter, with or without excision of the fissure and the sentinel pile (Notaras, 1971) (Fig. 141).

Fistula *in ano* of the usual variety represents a burrowing from an abscess in a rectal crypt, with a varying relationship to the sphincters and thence to the external opening (Fig. 142). The internal opening will quite invariably be at the pectinate line. The relationship between the location of the two openings usually follows 'Goodsall's rule,' as follows: If the external opening lies behind a line passing transversely across the anus, the internal opening is in the midline posteriorly, with the tract of the fistula curved. If the external

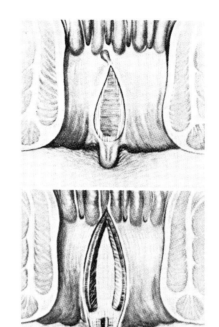

FIG. 141
Excision of fissure in ano *and internal sphincterotomy.* *1. Posterior fissure* in ano (*oval outline*) *with incidental polyp proximally and skin tag* (*sentinel pile*) *externally. Some fibers of the internal sphincter are bare.* *2. Fissure with skin tag and polyp excised; internal sphincter divided, slight partial division of subcutaneous external sphincter.* (*From Morgan and Thompson, 1956.*)

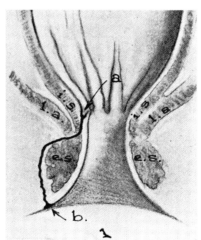

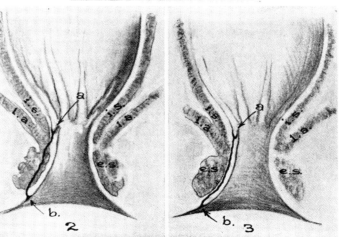

FIG. 142
Variable tract of complete anorectal fistula. *1. Tract a-b extending between external sphincter* (e.s.) *and internal sphincter* (i.s.). *l.a., the levator ani muscle.* *2. Tract extending through the superficial fibers of the external sphincter muscle.* *3. Tract beneath lining mucous membrane only. Lettering is the same in all the figures.* (*From Bacon, 1949.*)

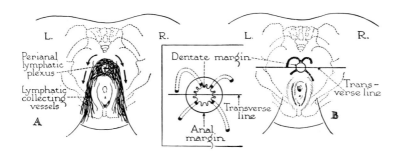

FIG. 143
*Explanation of Goodsall's rule.
A. Direction of perianal lymphatics.
B. Application of the rule, showing
direction taken by two posterior and
two anterior fistulas paralleling the
lymphatics. Insert indicates that the
internal openings are above the pectinate ('dentate') line. (From Nesselrod, 1964.)*

opening lies anterior to that line the internal opening is immediately opposite to it and the tract is straight (Fig. 143). Nesselrod (1964) points out that the direction of the fistula parallels that of the anal lymphatics and is explainable on the basis of the role of the lymphatics in carrying the infection which caused the fistula. The operation for fistula *in ano* consists in opening the fistula between the two ends and throughout any branching, dividing as much of the sphincters as lies within the tract (Fig. 142). Better sphincter function is said to return if the muscle fibers are divided at a right angle, rather than obliquely, but, in general, continence is maintained if the puborectalis sling is preserved.

PROLAPSE OF THE RECTUM

Prolapse of the rectum denotes a protrusion of this organ through the anus. It is called partial if only the mucous membrane descends, complete if all coats of the rectum protrude. Small protrusions may involve only the extraperitoneal part of the anorectum, but in the majority of cases of complete prolapse a regular feature is the presence of a peritoneal sac derived from the pouch of Douglas within the anterior part of the protruding mass (see Fig. 145 I). Thus complete prolapse may be termed a sliding hernia. Small bowel may or may not be present within the sac.

Three anatomical factors in the etiology of these cases require the surgeon's attention. First, and remarkably constant, is the presence of an abnormally deep rectovesical or recto-uterine peritoneal pouch, as though the embryonic fusion of the lower pouch which is thought to form the rectovesical septum (of Denonvilliers) was defective (see Fig. 192). Second is the presence of a wider than usual aperture between the fibers of the levator ani muscles forming the puborectalis sling. Third, laxity of the external anal sphincter. A loosening of the normal fixation of the rectum to its sacral bed may be a fourth etiological factor, but Goligher (1964) considers it rather a consequence of prolapse. Goligher also notes that some cases of prolapse ('sigmoidorectal intussusception') result from downward traction on neoplasms of the distal colon.

The treatment of incomplete rectal prolapse may be by radial fulguration so as to produce longitudinal shortening through scar formation. The large number of operative maneuvers suggested for complete prolapse may be divided into the following five categories: (1) Narrowing of the anal outlet, as by a circumanal wire suture. (2) Closure of the

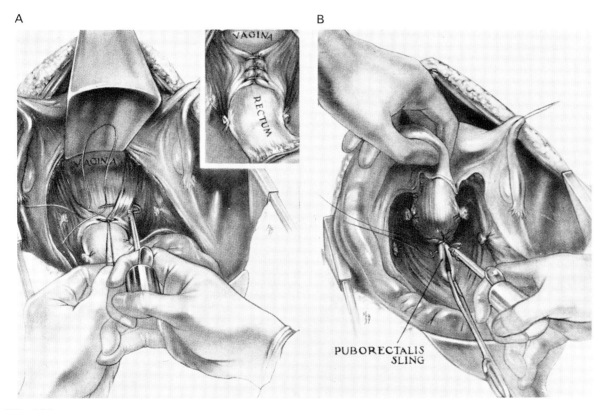

FIG. 144

Approximation of puborectalis muscles by abdominal approach for prolapse of the rectum. "Proper display [of the muscles] has demanded the fullest possible mobilization of the rectum down to the ano-rectal ring exactly as in the abdominal dissection of a Miles abdomino-perineal excision, except of course that the superior rectal vessels are not divided." It requires also that the mobilization remain close to the rectum and the superior rectal artery, leaving intact the hypogastric nerve plexuses. A. Method of suturing anterior to the rectum. The mobilization has been aided by division of the lateral ligaments of the rectum and their contained middle rectal vessels. These are shown ligated (insert). B. Alternative technique of posterior suture. The rectovesical pouch will be completely obliterated in the closure. (From Goligher, 1958.)

I

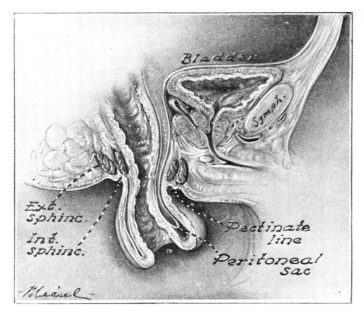

Ext.
sphinc.

Int.
sphinc.

Pectinate
line

Peritoneal
sac

Bladder

Symph.

—Maciel—

II

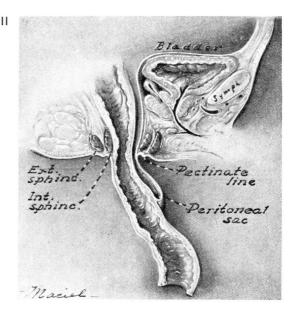

Bladder

Symph.

Ext.
sphinc.

Int.
sphinc.

Pectinate
line

Peritoneal
sac

—Maciel—

III

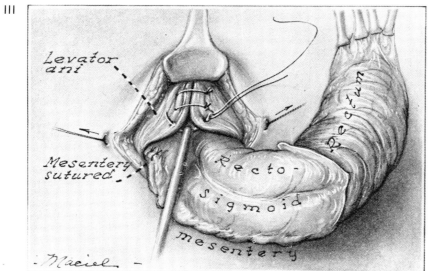

Levator
ani

Mesentery
sutured

Recto-
Sigmoid

mesentery

Rectum

—Maciel—

IV

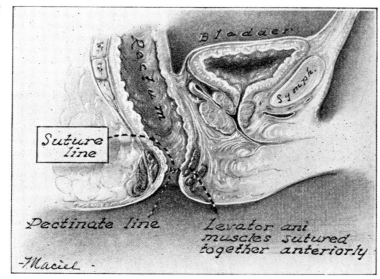

Bladder

Rectum

Symph.

Suture
line

Pectinate line

Levator ani
muscles sutured
together anteriorly

—Maciel—

FIG. 145

Perineal proctosigmoidectomy and levator ani approximation for rectal prolapse. I. Sagittal section demonstrating the presence of a peritoneal sac derived from the rectovesical pouch, lying between the outer and inner bowel anteriorly. When undisturbed the bowel lumen will point posteriorly because of the anterior sac. II. The prolapse converted to a single loop of bowel by circumferential incision of the outer bowel 3 cm. proximal to the pectinate line. III. The peritoneum has been sutured above the circumference of the rectosigmoid and the mesenteric vessels above the proposed line of resection of the inner bowel have been ligated. Now the levator ani muscles are brought together in the midline to strengthen the pelvic floor and snug up their medial or puborectalis portions. IV. The completed operation. The excess bowel has been amputated and its end anastomosed to the stump of the original outer layer of anorectum. (From Altemeier et al., 1955.)

pouch of Douglas, by suture or peritoneal elevation, sometimes on a bed of fascial grafts. An adequate closure of the pouch appears to require an abdominal approach. (3) Approximation of the levator ani muscles (puborectalis portions) in the midline. This is usually done anterior to the rectum, from an abdominal or perineal approach, but suturing behind the rectum has been tried and is satisfactory. Goligher (1958) makes an abdominal approach aiming at 'unequivocal' suture of the puborectalis muscles, and obliteration of the rectovesical pouch (Fig. 144). (4) Fixation of the rectum, from below or above, either to the sacrum or to neighboring muscle or fascia. (5) Shortening of the redundant bowel by plication or resection, either from below or above. Dunphy (1948) proposed a perineal proctosigmoidectomy, to which he added a closure of the peritoneal pouch through the abdomen. Altemeier and his associates (1955) amputated the bowel by a perineal approach and approximated the levator ani muscles anteriorly (Fig. 145). The range of these maneuvers and ways in which two or more may be combined within one procedure are discussed by Bacon (1949), Shackelford (1955), Goligher (1964), and Dunphy and Pikula (1969).

REFERENCES

Altemeier, W. A., Hoxworth, P. I., and Giuseffi, J.: Further experiences with the treatment of prolapse of the rectum. Surg. Clin. N. Amer. 35:1437–1447, 1955.

Bacon, H. E.: Anus, Rectum, Sigmoid Colon. Diagnosis and Treatment, 3rd ed. Philadelphia, J. B. Lippincott, 1949.

Bennett, R. C., and Duthie, H. L.: The functional importance of the internal anal sphincter. Brit. J. Surg. 51:355–357, 1964.

Denny-Brown, D., and Robertson, E. G.: An investigation of the nervous control of defaecation. Brain 58:256–310, 1935.

Duhamel, B.: A new operation for the treatment of Hirschsprung's disease. Arch. Dis. Child. 35:38–39, 1960.

Dunphy, J. E.: A combined perineal and abdominal operation for the repair of rectal prolapse. Surg. Gynec. Obstet. 86:493–498, 1948.

Dunphy, J. E., and Pikula, J. V.: Rectal Prolapse. Chapter 49 in Diseases of the Colon and Anorectum, Turell, R., Ed., 2nd ed., Vol. I. Philadelphia, W. B. Saunders, 1969.

Duthie, H. L.: Progress report. Anal continence. Gut 12:844–852, 1971.

Fowler, R., Jr.: Landmarks and legends of the anal canal. Aust. New Zeal. J. Surg. 27:1–18, 1957.

Goligher, J. C.: The treatment of complete prolapse of the rectum by the Roscoe Graham operation. Brit. J. Surg. 45:323–333, 1958.

Goligher, J. C.: Prolapse of the Rectum. Chapter 46 in Hernia, Nyhus, L. M., and Harkins, H. N., Eds. Philadelphia, J. B. Lippincott, 1964.

Goligher, J. C., and Hughes, E. S. R.: Sensibility of the rectum and colon. Its rôle in the mechanism of anal continence. Lancet 1:543–548, 1951.

Gray, S. W., and Skandalakis, J. E.: Embryology for Surgeons. The Embryological Basis for the Treatment of Congenital Defects. Philadelphia, W. B. Saunders, 1972.

Gross, R. E.: The Surgery of Infancy and Childhood. Its Principles and Techniques. Philadelphia, W. B. Saunders, 1953.

Miller, R. C., and Izant, R. J., Jr.: Sacrococcygeal perineal approach to imperforate anus. The Stephens procedure. Amer. J. Surg. 121:62–67, 1971.

Morgan, C. N., and Thompson, H. R.: Surgical anatomy of the anal canal. With special reference to the surgical importance of the internal sphincter and conjoint longitudinal muscle. Ann. Roy. Coll. Surg. Engl. 19:88–114, 1956.

Nesselrod, J. P.: Clinical Proctology, 3rd ed. Philadelphia, W. B. Saunders, 1964.

Notaras, M. J.: The treatment of anal fissure by lateral subcutaneous internal sphincterotomy—a technique and results. Brit. J. Surg. 58:96–100, 1971.

Parks, A. G.: Anorectal Surgery. Chapter 97 in The Craft of Surgery, Cooper, P., Ed., 2nd ed. Vol. II. Boston, Little, Brown, 1971.

Pilling, G. P., IV, and Cresson, S. L.: Hirschsprung's Disease. Chapter 59 in Pediatric Surgery, Mustard, W. T., Ravitch, M. M., Snyder, W. H., Jr., Welch, K. J., and Benson, C. D., Eds., 2nd ed., Vol. 2. Chicago, Year Book Medical Publishers, 1969.

Scharli, A. F., and Kiesewetter, W. B.: Defecation and continence: Some new concepts. Dis. Colon Rectum 13:81–107, 1970.

Shackelford, R. T.: Bickham-Callander Surgery of the Alimentary Tract. Vol. III. Philadelphia, W. B. Saunders, 1955.

Soave, F.: A new surgical technique for treatment of Hirschsprung's disease. Surgery 56:1007–1014, 1964.

Stephens, F. D.: Congenital imperforate rectum, recto-urethral and recto-vaginal fistulae. Aust. New Zeal. J. Surg. 22:161–172, 1953.

Stephens, F. D., and Smith, E. D.: Ano-Rectal Malformations in Children. Chicago, Year Book Medical Publishers, 1971.

Swenson, O.: Partial internal sphincterectomy in the treatment of Hirschsprung's disease. Ann. Surg. 160:540–550, 1964.

Swenson, O., and Donnellan, W. L.: Preservation of the puborectalis sling in imperforate anus repair. Surg. Clin. N. Amer. 47:173–193, 1967.

Swenson, O., Rheinlander, H. F., and Diamond, I.: Hirschsprung's disease: A new concept of the etiology. Operative results in thirty-four patients. New Eng. J. Med. 241:551–556, 1949.

Wilde, F. R.: The anal intermuscular septum. Brit. J. Surg. 36:279–285, 1949.

18

RESECTIONS of THE large intestine

LYMPHATIC DRAINAGE OF THE LARGE INTESTINE

The intramural lymphatics of the colon begin as a plexus in the muscularis mucosae, the collecting vessels communicating with submucosal, intramuscular, and subserosal networks in their centrifugal course. Some terminate in epicolic nodules along the antimesenteric teniae and in the base of appendices epiploicae, but most lymphatics collect along the mesentery to enter paracolic nodes lying near the marginal vessel.

The extramural lymphatics follow closely in distribution the segmental vascular arcades formed by the major named vessels of the colon (Fig. 146 VI). This applies unless the arcade is extremely narrow, as in the sigmoid colon; the tumor is located near the junction of two territories of arterial distribution; or the proximal lymphatic drainage of the segment is obstructed by tumor infiltration (Grinnell, 1966). The efferent lymphatics converge from the paracolic nodes to intermediate nodes located in the mesentery at major branchings of the colic vessels. When a major intestinal artery takes an anomalous origin, as is often the case with the middle colic artery (see page 235), the lymphatics follow that vessel to the corresponding proximal nodes. The larger lymphatic channels parallel the blood vessels to the principal nodes located on the superior and inferior mesenteric arteries at the base of the mesentery. The final lymphatic pathway from the superior mesenteric nodes is through the intestinal trunk to the cisterna chyli or the left lumbar trunk; from the inferior mesenteric distribution to aortic nodes and the left lumbar trunk, with some communication to superior mesenteric nodes (see Figs. 43, 44). An additional pathway from the splenic flexure and upper descending colon follows the inferior mesenteric vein to inferior pancreaticoduodenal lymphatics above the duodenojejunal junction, thence to the superior mesenteric nodes.

The anorectum possesses three lymphatic pedicles: a superior, along the superior rectal blood vessels; a middle, along the middle rectal vessels; and an inferior with two efferents—one along the inferior rectal and internal pudendal vessels, and a second to the superficial inguinal nodes (not shown in Fig. 146 VI). The mural lymphatic networks of the rectum collect to pass directly or through pararectal nodes (of Gerota) lying beneath the rectal fascia (see Fig. 150 II) to intermediate nodes at the junction of the superior rectal and last sigmoid vessels or, from the upper rectum, along the last sigmoid arcade. Injection studies have demonstrated a few direct communications to inferior mesenteric, left colic, and aortic nodes, and Slanetz and Herter (1972) have pointed out a few efferents passing parallel to the inferior mesenteric vein and terminating in medial inferior pancreaticoduodenal nodes. Inferior drainage at this level occurs only when there is obstruction along the superior route.

It is useful to consider three lymphatic territories of the anorectum, the upper lying above the middle transverse rectal fold and the peritoneum, the middle between that level and the pectinate line, and the lower below the pectinate line—the anal canal itself. From the middle territory primary drainage is still upward. Lateral drainage, particularly of lesions lying less than 2 cm. above the levators, occurs directly or through middle rectal nodes lying near the rectal wall in the pelvirectal space, to terminate in nodes of the middle rectal and internal and common iliac groups. Posteriorly spread may occur along the lateral and middle

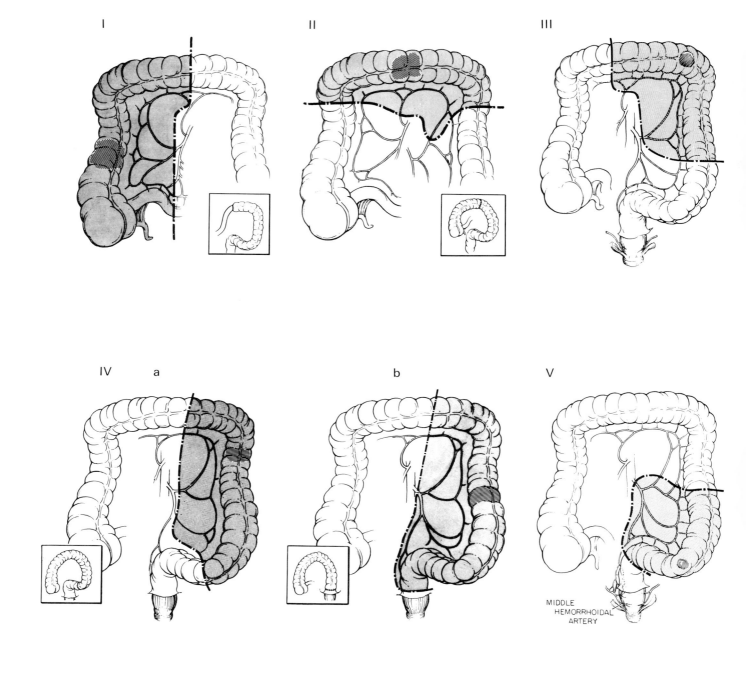

FIG. 146

Lymph and blood vessel determinants of resection for carcinoma of the large intestine.

I. Cecum and ascending colon. II. Mid-transverse colon. III. Splenic flexure. IV. Descending colon: a, of its upper part; b, of its lower. V. Sigmoid colon.

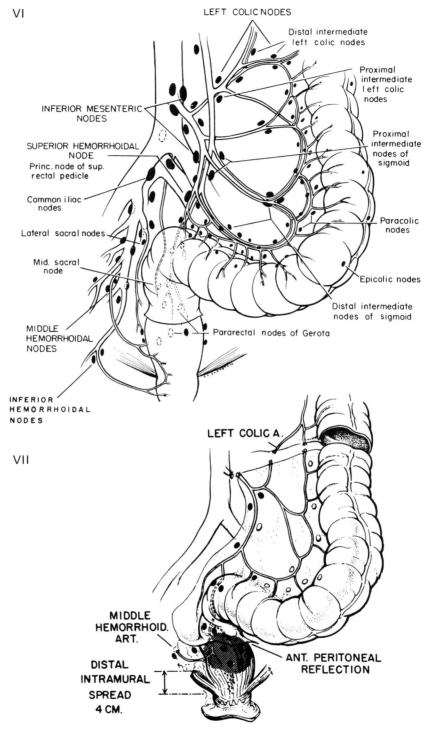

VI

LEFT COLIC NODES

Distal intermediate
left colic nodes

Proximal
intermediate
left colic
nodes

INFERIOR MESENTERIC
NODES

Proximal
intermediate
nodes of
sigmoid

SUPERIOR HEMORRHOIDAL
NODE

Princ. node of sup.
rectal pedicle

Common iliac
nodes

Paracolic
nodes

Lateral sacral nodes

Mid. sacral
node

Epicolic nodes

Distal intermediate
nodes of sigmoid

MIDDLE
HEMORRHOIDAL
NODES

Pararectal nodes of Gerota

INFERIOR
HEMORRHOIDAL
NODES

VII

LEFT COLIC A.

MIDDLE
HEMORRHOID.
ART.

DISTAL
INTRAMURAL
SPREAD
4 CM.

ANT. PERITONEAL
REFLECTION

FIG. 146
Lymph and blood vessel determinants of resection for carcinoma of the large intestine (continued).
   *VI. Lymphatic pathways for the sigmoid colon and anorectum.   VII. Lymphatic and intramural extension of
a carcinoma of the rectum. Abdominoperineal resection was chosen for this lesion below the anterior peritoneal
reflection. Lymph-node extension (solid outlines) occurred in the two directions expected for a lesion in this location.
(From Slanetz and Herter, 1972.)*

sacral vessels, penetrating the rectal fascia; anterior lymphatics penetrate the rectovesical (rectovaginal) septum (Denonvilliers' fascia) to terminate in internal iliac and para-aortic nodes.

The anal canal is supplied with a dense lymphatic plexus arranged longitudinally in the rectal columns to communicate weakly with the plexuses in the rectum (see Fig. 150 II) (Nesselrod, 1936). Primary drainage follows the blood vessels in the canal in the obturator fascia (of Alcock) to the internal pudendal and internal iliac nodes; and additionally, especially from the anus itself, across the anal verge and genitofemoral sulcus to the lower superficial inguinal nodes. Some of the drainage runs posteriorly via gluteal and lumbar lymphatics to reach the upper lateral superficial inguinal nodes (Nesselrod). Dye injected beneath the lining of the anal canal also spreads upward to the middle and superior rectal pedicles, staining in its passage the ischiorectal space, in the male the rectovesical septum, and in the female the posterior vaginal wall (Nesselrod; Hardy, 1971).

How cancer spreads in the bowel and its lymphatics, and the direction it can take are obviously important factors in planning resection for carcinoma. In spite of extensive intercommunications, and probably related to the presence of competent lymphatic valves, longitudinal intramural spread of malignancy seems limited to less than 5 cm., as demonstrated by tracer injection (Nesis and Sterns, 1973) and clinical study of tumors resected for cure (Grinnell, 1966). In their cases Slanetz and Herter (1972) found that intramural spread averaged 1.7 cm., and did not exceed 4 cm. (Fig. 146 VII). More extensive spread can be expected when the tumor is large and shows contiguous extension. In such instances the proximal lymphatic block gives rise to retrograde flow. The usually accepted mechanism of embolism for the transport of cancer cells from primary focus to lymph nodes seemed contradicted by the findings of Handley (1906) that cancer of the breast grows in continuity in the lymph trunk from primary focus to involved node ('permeation'). It was apparent from cleared specimen studies of carcinoma of the large bowel by Gilchrist and David (1948) and other data (Willis, 1952; Haagensen, 1972) that, although permeation can be seen, embolism is the more common mode of spread, at least in early cases; retrograde metastases are seen in instances of late and extensive growth (Grinnell).

The proximity of lymphatics and nodes to the mesenteries or corresponding peritoneum for each part of the colon requires that resections for carcinoma be done in continuity of the bowel, its lymphovascular pedicle, and the overlying peritoneum (as in Fig. 146). It is often feasible to remove the regional nodes off the anterior surface of the aorta and adjacent inferior vena cava (Stearns and Deddish, 1959), but currently resection of aortic or iliac nodes is generally not added since it appears that cure cannot be expected when cancer is found in these nodes. Coincidental injury to periaortic nerves is also likely to increase the incidence of postoperative bladder weakness (Slanetz and Herter, 1972).

RESECTIONS PROXIMAL TO THE RECTUM

Cecum and Ascending Colon (Fig. 146 I)

The lymphatic drainage of the portion of bowel supplied by the ileocolic artery is so interrelated to make impossible the separation of drainage from the various parts of this segment. In addition, direct communication from collecting lymphatics to intermediate or primary nodes is frequent. For example, trunks from the appendix have been demonstrated passing directly to central nodes at the origin of the ileocolic artery. The avascular space between ileal and ileocolic artery branches (see Fig. 133) precisely separates the lymphatic drainage of the colon and that of the ileum.

To encompass the pertinent vessels and lymphatic tissue, resection of the right colon should extend from the ileocolic vessels to the right branch of the middle colic artery (Fig. 146 I). The ileum is divided just distal to the last small bowel arcade (or 12 to 20 cm. proximal to the ileocecal valve) to ensure adequate vascularity of the proximal bowel. Because of the proximity of nodes to the superior mesenteric origin of the arteries involved, Goligher and his colleagues (1967) recommended extending the resection to include the middle colic artery at its source with anastomosis of the ileum to the distal transverse colon. This extension would also apply when the right colic artery is absent or originates from the middle colic, resulting in increased drainage by way of middle colic lymphatic pathways, or if the middle colic artery is absent, when arterial supply to the distal transverse colon may be compromised. As the location of the tumor approaches the hepatic flexure, the middle colic pedicle becomes increasingly important; the line of resection is moved to the splenic flexure and then includes the entire middle colic artery.

In thin patients preliminary division of the visible lymphovascular pedicles can be accomplished by incising the mesocolon close to their mesenteric origins (Turnbull *et al.,* 1967). The superior mesenteric vein, variably related to the artery (see page 199), should be protected. In the obese it is safer to divide the lateral peritoneal attachments, reflecting the colon to allow transillumination of the vessels and ligation at their origin. The right ureter, duodenum, inferior vena cava, and genital vessels are exposed in this dissection (see Fig. 36). An alternative technique is to mobilize the mesocolon from above downward along the middle colic vessels, identifying and ligating the structures of the vascular pedicle prior to lateral mobilization (Barnes, 1952).

Transverse Colon and Hepatic Flexure (*Fig. 146 II*)

Tumors of the transverse colon drain primarily to the middle colic system. Slanetz and Herter found drainage to nodes of left colic distribution in only 16 per cent. However, the central inferior mesenteric nodes were not involved in these specimens, allowing resection as pictured with proximal ligation of the middle colic lymphovascular pedicle and preservation of the inferior mesenteric artery. Tumors of the transverse colon occasionally spread along the gastrocolic omentum to omental and gastroepiploic nodes. For this reason resection should include the greater omentum. Absence of the middle colic artery, or its origin from the right colic artery, extends the lymphatic drainage to the ileocolic nodes and requires expansion of the resection to include the ileocolic lymphovascular pedicle.

For lesions of the hepatic flexure, the proximal line of resection is extended proximally to the same level as for lesions of the cecum and ascending colon, and distally onto the transverse colon to include the entire area of distribution of the middle colic artery.

Splenic Flexure (Fig. 146 III)

Lymphatic flow from this segment proceeds primarily to the middle colic nodes and to some less extent to the left colic nodes. Intermediate nodes along the left colic artery, particularly at its intersection with the left colic vein, effectively block direct lymphatic communication from the splenic flexure and proximal descending colon to central nodes. Resections should extend proximally to the middle colic artery at its origin, particularly if left colic arterial contribution is diminished (see Chapter 16). Tumor may spread retrograde to nodes in the greater omentum and the hilum of the spleen. The omentum is quite regularly included in the resection, but Slanetz and Herter advise against splenectomy since involvement of the splenic nodes indicates incurability. In the absence of the middle colic artery resection must extend to the right and should include the entire right colon with an ileal–descending colon anastomosis. Distally the resection extends to the origin of the left colic artery. When the first sigmoid artery arises from this vessel, the resection must include their common trunk and the part of the sigmoid supplied in order to ensure adequate lymphatic excision.

Descending Colon (Fig. 146 IV); Transverse Colostomy

A transverse colostomy may precede or accompany resection of the distal colon. It is best to choose a segment well to the right of the middle colic artery to avoid injury to this vessel, since it will be indispensable when the inferior mesenteric artery is sacrificed. The bowel is opened on its antimesenteric border to avoid cutting the stems of the vasa recta (see Fig. 134) or the marginal artery.

Lymphatic drainage from the upper descending colon is almost solely to the left colic nodes. For carcinoma in this location (Fig. 146 IV a) the colon and mesentery supplied by the entire left colic and first sigmoid arteries are removed. The inferior mesenteric vein is ligated just below the pancreas to the left of the duodenojejunal flexure. The left ureter and genital vessels are seen in the course of this dissection (see Figs. 36, 37).

When the left colic artery is absent (6 per cent) the highest sigmoid artery supplies the marginal arcade to the splenic flexure, and lymphatic flow is directed to the central inferior mesenteric nodes. In such cases, the resection must resemble that done for lesions of the lower descending colon (b). The proximal level of the bowel resection is then in the transverse colon, the lower limit is in the rectum, close to the peritoneal reflection. The inferior mesenteric artery is divided at the aorta.

Sigmoid Colon (Fig. 146 V)

The lymphatic drainage of the sigmoid is mainly to the nodes about the sigmoid vessels, but cleared specimens show that metastases do occur to the principal inferior mesenteric nodes as well. This has prompted extension of resection to include the origin of the inferior mesenteric artery. Goligher and his colleagues (1967) recommend total left colectomy for all left colic lesions with ligation of the inferior mesenteric artery on the aorta, and of the inferior mesenteric vein beneath the pancreas. Such a resection would be essential in cases previously mentioned where the left colic artery arises with the first sigmoid branch. If, as in Figure 146 V, the proximal descending colon is to be saved, the left colic artery is divided where it crosses the inferior mesenteric vein to allow adequate removal of the central inferior mesenteric nodes. Thus the bifurcation of its ascending branch remains to compensate for any inadequacy of the marginal artery at the splenic flexure.

The inferior mesenteric vein is ligated below the pancreas, saving the termination of the left colic vein to preserve the venous drainage of the retained descending colon. Some remove the nodes from in front of the aorta and promontory of the sacrum in continuity with the specimen. Distally, the bowel should be divided at least 5 cm. beyond the carcinoma to ensure removal of intramural spread. The rectosigmoid stump will rely on the inferior and middle rectal arteries. One must observe adequate blood supply at its cut end; a segment between 8 and 15 cm. long above the pelvic floor will generally survive.

ABDOMINOPERINEAL AND ANTERIOR RESECTIONS FOR CARCINOMA OF THE ANORECTUM

A host of limited procedures for cancer of the anorectum, developed prior to performance of abdominoperineal resections, were swept into the category of palliative procedures, once that operation was shown to be curative in a substantial proportion of patients. Because abdominoperineal resection carries the need for a permanent colostomy, the spread of the tumor was intensely restudied in the 1930's and 1940's in the hope of delineating a category of patients in whom operation could be curative while the anal canal and sphincter were saved. Anterior resection, the alternative procedure developed, is currently the only sphincter-saving operation in wide use for carcinoma of the upper rectum. Abdominoperineal resection remains the only operation done for cure of carcinoma of the lower rectum and the anal canal.

Early resistance to the adoption of anterior resection rested on three anatomical considerations: (1) The dictum of Miles (1908) that cancer of the rectum spread upward, laterally, and downward. This was modified by the differences in lymphatic drainage shown for the upper and lower rectum, and the demonstration of limits of retrograde lymphatic and intramural spread (see above) (Fig. 146 VI). (2) The assumption that the rectal stump could not be adequately supplied by the middle and inferior rectal arteries, later shown to be erroneous (see Chapter 16). (3) Some uncertainty as to the length of retained anorectum required for fecal continence (see Chapter 17). Information on these points joined to the observed satisfactory clinical results has led to the wide adoption of anterior resection for lesions above the peritoneal reflection and middle transverse rectal fold, equivalent to a level 10 to 11 cm. above the anus as measured by the sigmoidoscope, or somewhat higher according to Bacon's measurements (Fig. 147, and see Fig. 137). It is crucial that the location of the tumor must allow 5 cm. (extended to 10 cm. by some writers) of normal bowel

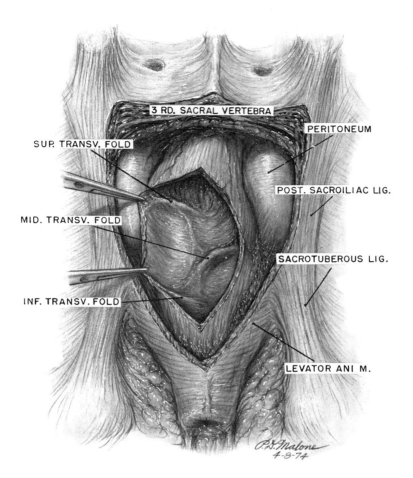

Labels on figure:
3 RD. SACRAL VERTEBRA
PERITONEUM
SUP. TRANSV. FOLD
POST. SACROILIAC LIG.
MID. TRANSV. FOLD
SACROTUBEROUS LIG.
INF. TRANSV. FOLD
LEVATOR ANI M.

P.S. Malone
4-8-74

FIG. 147
The transverse rectal folds. Note that the middle fold lies at the level of the peritoneal reflection. With the rectum distended in sigmoidoscopic examination, the folds appear thinner and much wider.

to be removed below the lesion, leaving enough of a stump to allow a technically good anastomosis.

Division of the superior and middle rectal pedicles and the intra-abdominal mobilization of the colon and rectal stump are carried out in the same manner for both anterior and abdominoperineal resections. Middle rectal branches, other than those in or near the lateral rectal ligament, may course close to the upper surface of the levators anteriorly and should be preserved in doing anterior resection (see page 236). The inferior mesenteric vessels are exposed and the bowel mobilized by incising the posterior peritoneum to the right of the vessels, and to the left of the sigmoid and rectum. Both ureters are visualized to their crossing by the vas deferens or the uterine vessels.

A thorough removal of pertinent lymph nodes is made possible by dividing the inferior mesenteric artery at its origin and by division of the vein where it disappears behind the pancreas (see Fig. 76). In obese or poor-risk patients the artery is often divided below the origin of the left colic or first sigmoid branches. As in resection of the sigmoid, the vein may be divided below its reception of the left colic vein, to avoid venous stasis of the upper descending colon. The remaining descending colon must be supplied by the marginal artery, aided by the arcade of the ascending branch of the left colic. If the vascularity of the bowel is considered inadequate, the bowel must be cut back to the splenic flexure or transverse colon. This upper end is used for the anastomosis if anterior resection is done, or for an end colostomy in the case of abdominoperineal resection.

Mobilization of the rectum is begun posteriorly where the superior pedicle is lifted off the bifurcation of the aorta, the common iliac veins, and sacral vessels. Anteriorly the peritoneum is lifted from the bladder base down to the rectovesical septum, which is dissected off the seminal vessels and base of the prostate, and left attached to the rectum. In the female the rectum is mobilized from the vagina. For lesions below the pelvic floor, particularly if anteriorly placed, the uterus, tubes, ovaries, and broad ligaments, along with the posterior part of the vaginal wall to a level well below that of the tumor, may be removed. Laterally, the lateral ligaments of the rectum are ligated and divided (Fig. 148). The rectum, thus freed down to the levators, is ready for division and anastomosis for anterior resection, or ready for perineal resection when the abdominoperineal operation is being done.

The perineal phase of abdominoperineal resection starts with an incision surrounding the anus; the coccyx may be divided or disarticulated (see Fig. 150 I). The incision is carried deeply to excise the ischiorectal fat, the inferior rectal vessels being sectioned laterally. The posterior part of the levators, and their upper and lower fascias are now cut well out laterally, exposing the rectum covered by its strong fascia propria. The circumferential attachment of this fascia to the posterior part of the parietal pelvic fascia is divided, giving access to the presacral retroperitoneal space, already entered from above. Anteriorly the dissection is deepened across the central perineal tendon, and in the male the recto-urethralis muscle and rectovesical septum (see Figs. 191, 192). The septum is dissected off the prostate and seminal vesicles. In the female the posterior part of the vagina may be resected with the rectum.

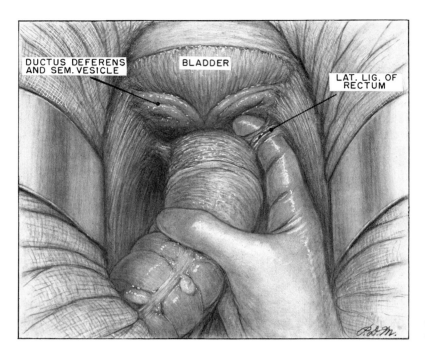

DUCTUS DEFERENS AND SEM. VESICLE

BLADDER

LAT. LIG. OF RECTUM

FIG. 148
Securing the lateral rectal ligaments in abdominoperineal resection.

Abdominoperineal resection for cancer is followed by impotence in many men—95 per cent according to Jones (1942). Vesical atony with incontinence is an uncommon sequel. It is attributed to interruption of the path of innervation of the bladder and urethra by branches of S-2,3,4 nerves. The pertinent branches emerge through the anterior sacral foramina, then pass through the parietal pelvic fascia to follow the blood vessels as the inferior hypogastric plexus at the sides of the pelvis and on the levators (see Chapter 6). The preservation of the sympathetic innervation in the male is necessary for ejaculation. It is possible that distortion of the bladder neck through loss of pelvic support (Bacon and McCrae, 1947), or malignant infiltration about the bladder neck in late cases (Ward and Nay, 1972) may play a part. Goligher and his colleagues (1967) warn against a presacral dissection behind the parietal pelvic fascia during which the sacral branches to the plexus would be endangered. It is noteworthy that such complications are rare following dissection of the rectum for benign disease, when carried out close to the bowel (Donovan and O'Hara, 1960).

SPHINCTER-SAVING RECTAL RESECTIONS

It is feasible to resect the rectum, while preserving sphincteric function, for a variety of benign conditions. Moreover, there are occasions when an anterior resection can be planned for cure of rectosigmoid carcinoma but the anastomosis from above is difficult or dangerous because of obesity or a narrow pelvis. In these instances, once the abdominal resection is completed, the colon may be brought down by one of the techniques to be described, and anastomosed below. Sphincter-saving operations are chosen by some for the cure of malignancy of the mid-rectum.

From the considerations of continence in Chapter 17, it is apparent that the expectation of normal or near normal postoperative continence will rest upon the preservation of an anal tube at least 4 cm. long in the adult, including the internal and external sphincters and the puborectalis sling, plus a relatively intact inferior hypogastric plexus. The puborectalis sling may or may not escape injury in operations in which some anal canal is preserved. It may be removed with much of the levators in operations for low-lying cancer (Fig. 149) and at least partially removed in others in which the anal canal is greatly shortened, as for aganglionic megacolon (see Chapter 17).

Sphincter-saving resections fall into one of three categories: (1) 'Pull-through' operations when the colon remaining after a prior resection or mobilization by the abdominal route, or a prolapsed rectum, is evaginated through the anal canal. (2) Anterior perineal rectal resections. (3) Transsacral (Kraske) resections.

The pull-through technique is exemplified by operations for congenital megacolon (Chapter 17) or the operation for prolapse of the rectum shown in Figure 145. When done for carcinoma of the middle rectum, the perineal approach begins with wide dilation of the anus, through which the anal wall just below the pectinate line is cut through circumferentially into the ischiorectal fossae to allow excision of the fat of the fossae and the levators (Fig. 149). Thus the dissection meets that done previously from above, in which the lymphovascular pedicle of the rectum has been divided as it would be in abdominoperineal resection. The rectosigmoid is pulled through the anus, excised at the desired level, and

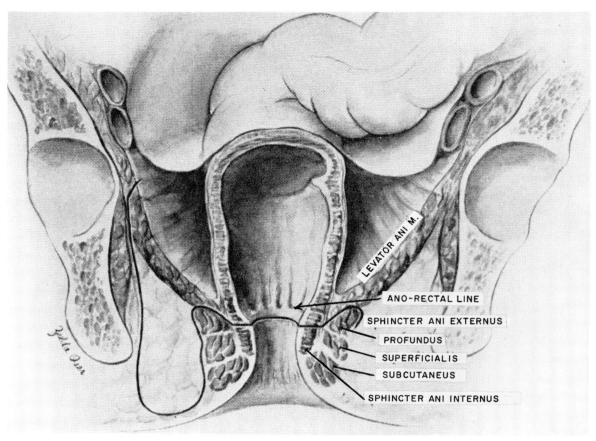

LEVATOR ANI M.

ANO-RECTAL LINE

SPHINCTER ANI EXTERNUS

PROFUNDUS

SUPERFICIALIS

SUBCUTANEUS

SPHINCTER ANI INTERNUS

FIG. 149

Lower line of resection for carcinoma of the rectum by the pull-through technique. (From Bacon, 1949.) Continence is likely to be quite imperfect with such extensive removal of the levator ani muscles.

the proximal end anastomosed to the everted stump of the anal canal (Bacon, 1949). The anal mucosa may be excised in this and other pull-through operations, but Bacon (1971) warns against removing too much lest it result in anal deformity and 'wet anus.' Techniques of various pull-through operations are described in Turell (1969).

The anterior perineal approach to exploration or resection of the rectum follows the same path as that used for perineal prostatectomy, that is, anterior to the rectovesical septum (see Figs. 191, 192). The attachment of the rectal fascia to the parietal fascia will be felt as strong lateral pelvirectal processes, extending backward to the sacrum below the fourth segment. The rectum is mobilized by cutting the rectal fascia around the bowel (Fig. 150 I). Griffith (1970) describes the anterior perineal as an excellent approach to the mid and distal rectum to be used for excisional biopsy in

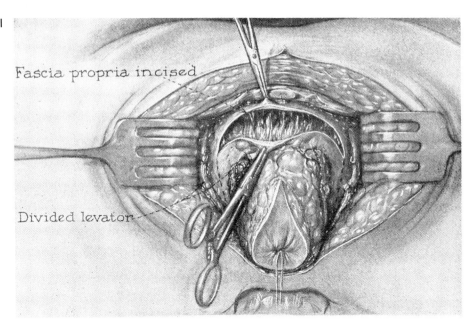

I

Fascia propria incised

Divided levator

FIG. 150
Posterior relationships of the rectum.

I. The rectal fascia (fascia propria) as seen in the perineal phase of abdominoperineal resection. The fascia is being divided around the rectum as it reflects from this structure onto the parietal fascia behind and above the levator ani muscles.

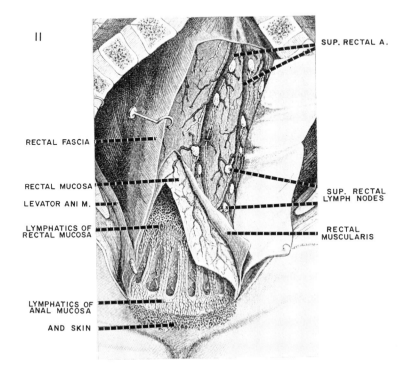

II

SUP. RECTAL A.

RECTAL FASCIA

RECTAL MUCOSA

LEVATOR ANI M.

LYMPHATICS OF
RECTAL MUCOSA

SUP. RECTAL
LYMPH NODES

RECTAL
MUSCULARIS

LYMPHATICS OF
ANAL MUCOSA

AND SKIN

FIG. 150
Posterior relationships of the rectum (continued).

II. Structures beneath the rectal fascia.

III

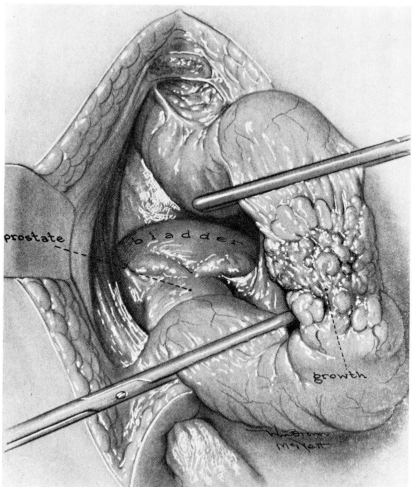

FIG. 150

Posterior relationships of the rectum (continued).

III. The anorectum as seen in transsacral palliative resection of carcinoma of the rectosigmoid. The bowel has been previously mobilized through the abdomen by division of the peritoneum on either side and section of the inferior mesenteric artery above the first sigmoid branch. The sigmoid was then pushed down below the restored peritoneal floor. The coccyx and fifth sacral segment have been removed. The median and lateral sacral arteries (not shown) usually require ligation. The posterior parts of both levator ani muscles have been divided. The left muscle is seen. A gauze pack lies against the peritoneum of the rectovesical pouch. The attachment of the rectal fascia to the presacral parietal pelvic fascia, the rectovesical septum, and the lateral ligaments of the rectum are not shown but have been divided to give this exposure. The bowel between the clamps will be excised and the ends anastomosed. (I. From David and Gilchrist. II. Modified from Gerota, 1895. III. From Bacon, 1949.)

tumors of doubtful malignancy or in the completion of an abdominoperineal operation with or without removal of the anal canal. If the canal is preserved, the colon-anal anastomosis is performed through this exposure.

The transsacral (Kraske) sphincter-saving operation can be done for carcinoma, either with a preliminary abdominal phase (Donaldson *et al.,* 1966; Localio and Baron, 1973) or by the lower dissection alone for villous tumors or large adenomatous polyps (Wilson and Gordon, 1969). Significant increase of exposure is gained by the resection of the coccyx and fifth sacral segment with division of the attached gluteus maximus fibers and sacral ligaments. Adjacent neural and vascular structures limit the extent of soft tissue division (see Fig. 14 I and II). Section of the fourth sacral segment may cause injury to the third sacral nerve, with possible loss of urinary and fecal continence (see page 21). Moreover, the dural-arachnoidal sac, which usually ends at the S-2 level, may on occasion be prolonged one segment lower. Figure 150 III shows the sacral resection of a high rectal carcinoma. In this instance a preliminary abdominal phase has been performed. A more limited excision for benign disease is possible through the sacral approach alone. The peritoneum can be opened from below once the attachment of the rectal to the parietal fascia has been divided (Fig. 147).

REFERENCES

Bacon, H. E.: Anus, Rectum, Sigmoid Colon. Diagnosis and Treatment, 3rd ed. Philadelphia, J. B. Lippincott, 1949.

Bacon, H. E.: Present status of the pull-through sphincter-preserving procedure. Cancer 28:196–203, 1971.

Bacon, H. E., and McCrea, L. E.: Abdominoperineal proctosigmoidectomy for rectal cancer. The management of associated vesical dysfunction. J.A.M.A. 134:523–526, 1947.

Barnes, J. P.: Physiologic resection of the right colon. Surg. Gynec. Obstet. 94:722–726, 1952.

David, V. C., and Gilchrist, R. K.: Surgery of the Rectum and Anus. Chapter VI in Nelson New Loose-Leaf Surgery. Whipple, A. O., Ed. Vol. V. Hagerstown, W. F. Prior.

Donaldson, G. A., Rodkey, G. V., and Behringer, G. E.: Resection of the rectum with anal preservation. Surg. Gynec. Obstet. 123:571–580, 1966.

Donovan, M. J., and O'Hara, E. T.: Sexual function following surgery for ulcerative colitis. New Eng. J. Med. 262:719–720, 1960.

Gerota, D.: Die Lymphgefässe des Rectums und des Anus. Arch. Anat. Physiol., Anat. Abt., pp. 240–256, 1895.

Gilchrist, R. K., and David, V. C.: Prognosis in carcinoma of the bowel. Surg. Gynec. Obstet. 86:359–371, 1948.

Goligher, J. C., Duthie, H. L., and Nixon, H. H.: Surgery of the Anus, Rectum and Colon, 2nd ed. London, Baillière, Tindall & Cassell, 1967.

Griffith, C. A.: Perineal exposure of the rectum. Amer. Surg. 36:652–655, 1970.

Grinnell, R. S.: Lymphatic block with atypical and retrograde lymphatic metastasis and spread in carcinoma of the colon and rectum. Ann. Surg. 163:272–280, 1966.

Haagensen, C. D.: The Spread of Cancer in the Lymphatic System. Chapter 4 in The Lymphatics in Cancer, Haagensen, C. D., Feind, C. R., Herter, F. P., Slanetz, C. A., Jr., and Weinberg, J. A. Philadelphia, W. B. Saunders, 1972.

Handley, W. S.: Cancer of the Breast and Its Operative Treatment. London, John Murray, 1906.

Hardy, K. J.: The lymphatic drainage of the anal margin. Austr. New Zeal. J. Surg. 40:367–369, 1971.

Jones, T. E.: Complications of one stage abdominoperineal resection of rectum. J.A.M.A. 120:104–107, 1942.

Localio, S. A., and Baron, B.: Abdomino-transsacral resection and anastomosis for mid-rectal cancer. Ann. Surg. 178:540–546, 1973.

Miles, W. E.: A method of performing abdomino-perineal excision for carcinoma of the rectum and of the terminal portion of the pelvic colon. Lancet 2:1812–1813, 1908.

Nesis, L., and Sterns, E. E.: Lymph flow from the colon under varying conditions. Ann. Surg. 177:422–427, 1973.

Nesselrod, J. P.: An anatomic restudy of the pelvic lymphatics. Ann. Surg. 104:905–916, 1936.

Slanetz, C. A., Jr., and Herter, F. P.: The Large Intestine. Chapter 11 *in* The Lymphatics in Cancer, Haagensen, C. D., Feind, C. R., Herter, F. P., Slanetz, C. A., Jr., and Weinberg, J. A. Philadelphia, W. B. Saunders, 1972.

Stearns, M. W., Jr., and Deddish, M. R.: Five-year results of abdominopelvic lymph node dissection for carcinoma of the rectum. Dis. Colon Rectum 2:169–172, 1959.

Turell, R., Ed.: Diseases of the Colon and Anorectum, 2nd ed. Philadelphia, W. B. Saunders, 1969.

Turnbull, R. B., Jr., Kyle, K., Watson, F. R., and Spratt, J.: Cancer of the colon. The influence of the *no-touch isolation* technic on survival rates. Ann. Surg. 166:420–427, 1967.

Ward, J. N., and Nay, H. R.: Immediate and delayed urologic complications associated with abdominoperineal resection. Amer. J. Surg. 123:642–648, 1972.

Willis, R. A.: The Spread of Tumours in the Human Body, 2nd ed. London, Butterworth, 1952.

Wilson, S. E., and Gordon, H. E.: Excision of rectal lesions by the Kraske approach. Amer. J. Surg. 118:213–217, 1969.

SECTION 6
Suprarenal Glands; Urinary and Male Genital Organs

19

ThE SUPRARENAL Glands

THE NEONATAL GLAND; DEVELOPMENTAL ANOMALIES

The suprarenal glands are large at birth (Fig. 151), with a disproportionate size of the cortex. About 50 per cent of the cortex is lost in the first two weeks of postnatal life, and the adult ratio of cortex to medulla is reached in the third year (Swinyard, 1943).

A good account of developmental anomalies of the suprarenal glands is given in Gray and Skandalakis (1972). The gland usually develops in its high position in cases of absence of a kidney, but is flattened in shape. However, in 10 per cent of agenesis of the kidney the suprarenal gland also fails to develop. Hypoplasia is also recognized, often associated with anencephalus. The commonest ectopic position of the gland is beneath the capsule of the upper pole of the kidney. In the rarer hepatic heterotopia the gland may be lodged beneath the capsule of the liver. Remarkably, three instances of intracranial heterotopia have also been reported. Fusion of the suprarenals has been seen, often accompanying fusion of the kidneys.

Appreciation of the presence of accessory suprarenal tissue is important when attempt is made to control malignancy of other organs by total adrenalectomy, or to locate tumors of the suprarenal gland (Falls, 1955). True accessory

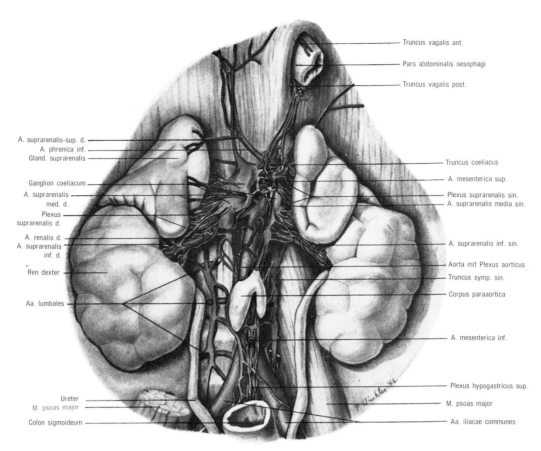

A. suprarenalis-sup. d.
A. phrenica inf.
Gland. suprarenalis

Ganglion coeliacum
A. suprarenalis
med. d.
Plexus
suprarenalis d.
A. renalis d.
A. suprarenalis
inf. d.
Ren dexter
Aa. lumbales
Ureter
M. psoas major
Colon sigmoideum

Truncus vagalis ant.
Pars abdominalis oesophagi
Truncus vagalis post.

Truncus coeliacus
A. mesenterica sup.
Plexus suprarenalis sin.
A. suprarenalis media sin.

A. suprarenalis inf. sin.
Aorta mit Plexus aorticus
Truncus symp. sin.
Corpus paraaortica

A. mesenterica inf.

Plexus hypogastricus sup.
M. psoas major
Aa. iliacae communes

FIG. 151
Suprarenal glands and adjacent structures in the newborn. (From Töndury, 1970.)

glands comprise both cortical and medullary tissue. Graham (1953) serially sectioned the tissues about the aorta and vena cava from above the celiac to just below the superior mesenteric arteries in 100 subjects at postmortem examination. He found accessory glands in 16 per cent. They were located in front of the aorta or to one side between the celiac and superior mesenteric arteries, eight to the left of the aorta, three to the right, three in the midline. In two instances the supernumerary glands were bilateral. In some contrast is the report of Schteingart and his associates (1972), who identified residual adrenal tissue after total adrenalectomy, all on the right side. This led them to conclude that such masses of adrenal tissue represent fragments of the usual right gland, consistent with the greater difficulty in dissection of the right gland than the left. Accessory suprarenal glands have also been observed in various parts of the retroperitoneum and along the kidneys, ureters, and the genital tract.

Accessory cortical tissue is much more common than accessory true glands, but both occur in about the same locations (Hollinshead, 1971). Thus Graham found 16 per cent of cortical masses in the celiac mesenteric area in addition to the 16 per cent of true glands, and a number of such masses have been identified at lower levels. A few isolated cases have been reported of recrudescence of Cushing's syndrome after total adrenalectomy, cured by the removal of an ectopic suprarenal gland at the inferior pole of the kidney (Chaffee et al., 1963) or by the removal of ectopic cortical tissue situated near the ovary (Strauch and Vinnick, 1972; Bennett et al., 1972).

Medullary ectopia is hard to define since, as Hollinshead (1971) says, chromaffin tissue characteristic of the adrenal medulla also normally occurs along the sympathetic ganglia and their plexuses (see also Page and Copeland, 1968). The largest of these, the para-aortic bodies (organs of Zuckerkandl) are prominent in the newborn (Fig. 151) but become grossly unrecognizable by puberty.

BLOOD VESSELS; LYMPHATICS; NERVES

The arteries to the suprarenal gland are termed inferior, middle, and superior. These are in reality sets of fine arteries totaling as many as 60, with an occasional predominant vessel, stemming, respectively, from the renal artery below, the aorta medially, and the inferior phrenic artery above (Solotuchin, 1929) (Fig. 152). Inferior suprarenal arteries may come off the superior polar renal artery or from other renal branches—the adipose, gonadal, or ureteric. Prior to entering the gland they ramify within the fat which separates the gland from the kidney. The middle suprarenal artery supplies the celiac ganglion as well as the suprarenal gland. Both structures usually receive additional twigs from the celiac. The celiac may give off the middle suprarenal or the inferior phrenic arteries.

On each side a single large vein leaves the gland at a small depression, in the lower anterior surface of the right, and from the lower medial border of the left. The left supra-

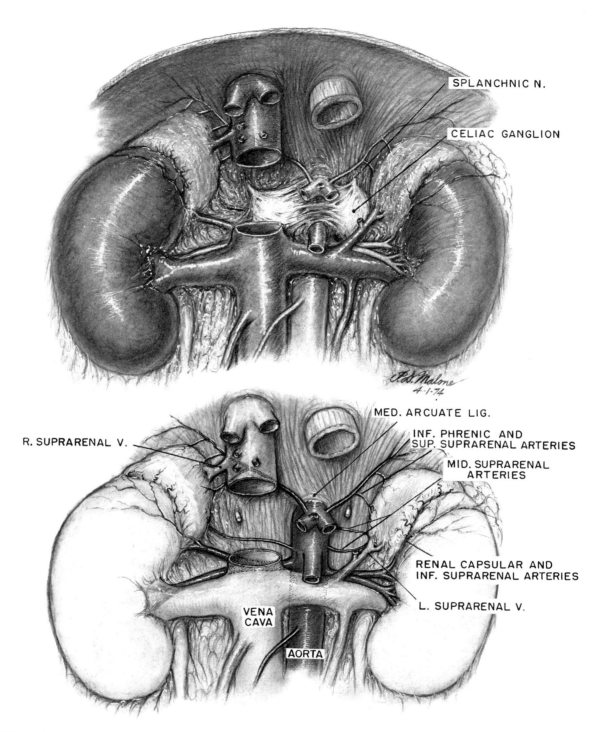

SPLANCHNIC N.

CELIAC GANGLION

MED. ARCUATE LIG.

R. SUPRARENAL V.

INF. PHRENIC AND
SUP. SUPRARENAL ARTERIES

MID. SUPRARENAL
ARTERIES

RENAL CAPSULAR AND
INF. SUPRARENAL ARTERIES

L. SUPRARENAL V.

VENA
CAVA

AORTA

FIG. 152
Arteries to the suprarenal glands and celiac ganglia.

renal vein is usually joined by the inferior phrenic, then enters the renal vein close to that part receiving the gonadal, occasionally joining that vessel. The right suprarenal vein is short, averaging 1 cm. It ends in the inferior vena cava close to the small posterior hepatic veins (see Fig. 101). Johnstone (1957) observed occasional doubling of the right suprarenal vein, with or without junction with a hepatic vein. Sudden interruption of the suprarenal vein may be damaging to the gland. Thus in animal experiments there was a better chance for survival, when the vena cava was ligated above the renal veins, if the ligature was placed distal to the entrance of the right suprarenal vein (Béjan and Cohn, 1911). Yet subtotal adrenalectomy usually includes removal of the major vein, the remaining portion of the gland being drained by the small veins accompanying the arteries from the inferior phrenic or renal arteries.

Lymph vessels are found only in the capsule of the gland. They pass medialward through a few small nodes at its medial edge, or directly to the cisterna chyli and the thoracic duct (Merklin, 1966).

The glands are well supplied with sympathetic nerve branches from the celiac plexus and from the splanchnic nerves and upper lumbar sympathetic ganglia. The fibers are preganglionic, ending directly upon the cells of the medulla.

EXPOSURES OF THE SUPRARENAL GLANDS

The suprarenal glands may be exposed: (1) Anteriorly— the abdominal approach. (2) Laterally—the flank approach. (3) Posteriorly—the lumbar approach. (4) By a thoracoabdominal incision.

The abdominal approach, while transperitoneal, allows one to operate on both glands at the same sitting, to gain good control of adjacent vessels, and to explore the abdomen for tumor metastases. For unilateral procedures, a long subcostal incision may be used; an upper rectus muscle—detaching incision (see Fig. 9) gives better access to one or both glands.

For exposure of the right suprarenal gland the liver is retracted upward. Incision of the peritoneum lateral to the duodenum allows displacement of the duodenum medially, and of the hepatic flexure of the colon downward. The view obtained is much like that shown in Figure 170. Mobilization and downward retraction of the kidney facilitates exposure of the suprarenal gland. The gland is a golden yellow compared with the perirenal fat. The dissection is begun by dividing the inferior suprarenal vessels. One can then bluntly separate the lateral border and the posterior surface of the gland from the right crus of the diaphragm. The vena cava is disclosed 5 or 10 mm. away, and the suprarenal vein is divided if adrenalectomy is to proceed. The gland is mobilized from its medial relationship to the celiac ganglion and its superior relationship to the inferior phrenic artery, and the middle and superior suprarenal arteries are divided.

An anterior view of the left suprarenal gland is usually gained by entering the omental bursa either through the gastrocolic ligament, through the gastrosplenic ligament, or through the transverse mesocolon. After the posterior peritoneum of the bursa is incised, the pancreas and splenic vessels are retracted downward (Fig. 153) (or upward if the bursa was entered through the transverse mesocolon). The left gland is semilunar in shape, and in contrast to the right is applied to much of the medial border of the kidney, where it may reach the renal vessels. Its medial border lies 1 or 2 cm. from the aorta, in intimate contact with the left celiac ganglion, with the left splanchnic nerve quite invariably posterior.

The lateral or flank approach in which the patient lies on his opposite side does not allow simultaneous exposure of both glands, but it has the advantage of being extraperitoneal and subpleural. The incision can resemble that of the posterolateral approach for nephrectomy or it may be transverse, below or across the 11th or 12th rib. One or both of these ribs are usually removed subperiosteally. Splitting the transversus abdominis muscle in the anterior part of the incision allows entry into the retroperitoneal fat; continuing in the same plane posteriorly one may push upward the costal attachment of the diaphragm and the pleura. The kidney is identified anterior to the quadratus lumborum muscle and is retracted downward. Blunt dissection exposes the vena cava on the right and the renal pedicle on the left, to allow recognition of some adjacent part of the suprarenal gland. Without this initial exposure one may proceed blindly

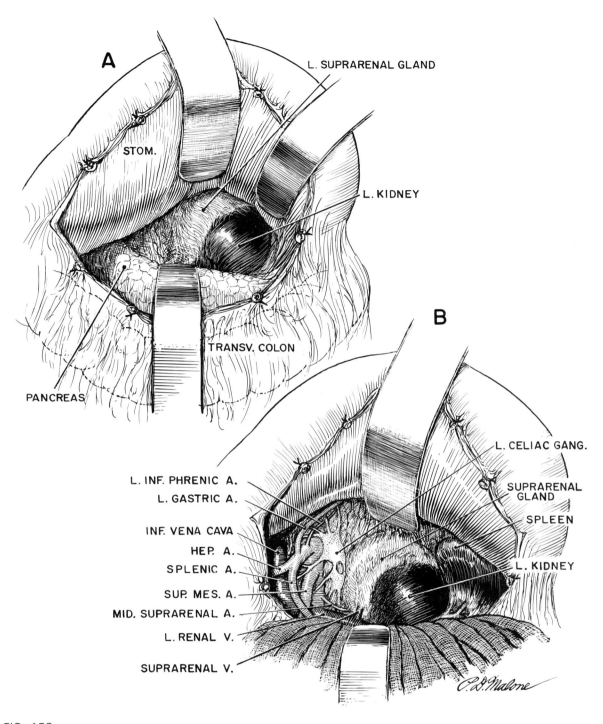

FIG. 153
Anterior approach to left suprarenal gland. A. Exposure on entering the omental bursa. B. Structures seen beneath the posterior peritoneum and on retracting the pancreas.

in the retroperitoneum, where on the left one may produce excessive mobilization of the tail of the pancreas and splenic artery.

The posterior approach, with the patient prone, is again extraperitoneal and subpleural and allows simultaneous exposure of both glands (Figs. 154, 155). The procedure resembles that of the flank approach with removal of the 11th or 12th rib.

The thoracoabdominal approach is particularly applicable

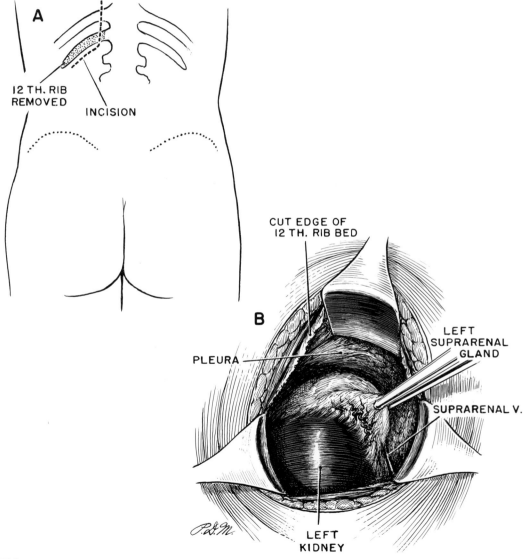

FIG. 154
Posterior approach to left suprarenal gland. A. The incision. B. Initial view of the gland, the inferior suprarenal vessels, and the suprarenal vein.

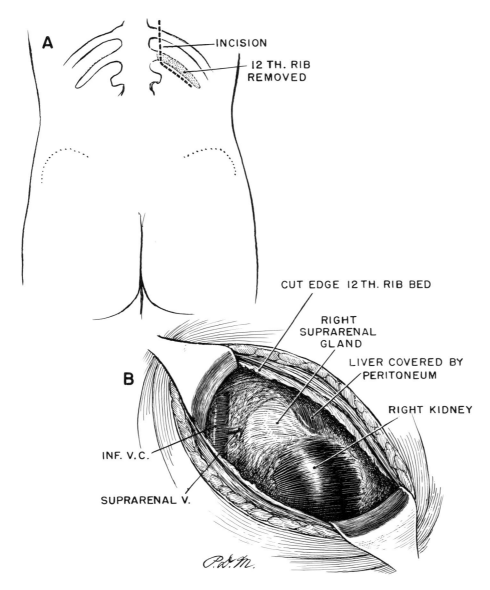

FIG. 155
Posterior approach to right suprarenal gland.   A. The incision.   B. Initial view of the gland.

for carcinoma of either suprarenal gland. It allows wider retraction of the liver and spleen than do other exposures. The incision resembles the thoracoabdominal approach to the kidney (see Fig. 170), passing through the pleura and diaphragm. Opening the peritoneum allows one to gain control of the blood supply early in the operation. Concomitant nephrectomy or splenectomy is often required and is accomplished through the same exposure (Bennett *et al.,* 1971).

REFERENCES

Béjan, J., and Cohn, M.: Sur la ligature de la veine cave inférieure. Étude expérimentale. Rev. Chir. 43:302–316, 1911.

Bennett, A. H., Cain, J. P., Dluhy, R. G., Tynes, W. V., Harrison, J. H., and Thorn, G. W.: Surgical treatment of adrenocortical hyperplasia: 20-year experience. Trans. Amer. Assn. Genito-Urinary Surg. 64:90–94, 1972.

Bennett, A. H., Harrison, J. H., and Thorn, G. W.: Neoplasms of the adrenal gland. J. Urol. 106:607–614, 1971.

Chaffee, W. R., Moses, A. M., Lloyd, C. W., and Rogers, L. S.: Cushing's syndrome with accessory adrenocortical tissue. J.A.M.A. 186:799–801, 1963.

Falls, J. L.: Accessory adrenal cortex in the broad ligament. Incidence and functional significance. Cancer 8:143–150, 1955.

Graham, L. S.: Celiac accessory adrenal glands. Cancer 6:149–152, 1953.

Gray, S. W., and Skandalakis, J. E.: Embryology for Surgeons. The Embryological Basis for the Treatment of Congenital Defects. Philadelphia, W. B. Saunders, 1972.

Hollinshead, W. H.: Anatomy for Surgeons, 2nd ed. Vol 2. The Thorax, Abdomen, and Pelvis. New York, Harper & Row, 1971.

Johnstone, F. R. C.: The suprarenal veins. Amer. J. Surg. 94:615–620, 1957.

Merklin, R. J.: Suprarenal gland lymphatic drainage. Amer. J. Anat. 119:359–374, 1966.

Page, L. B., and Copeland, R. B.: Pheochromocytoma. Disease-a-Month. January, 1968.

Schteingart, D. E., Conn, J. W., Lieberman, L. M., and Beierwaltes, W. H.: Persistent or recurrent Cushing's syndrome after "total" adrenalectomy. Adrenal photoscanning for residual tissue. Arch. Intern. Med. 130:384–387, 1972.

Solotuchin, A.: Über die Blutversorgung der Nebennieren. Z. Anat. 90:288–292, 1929.

Strauch, G. O., and Vinnick, L.: Persistent Cushing's syndrome apparently cured by ectopic adrenalectomy. J.A.M.A. 221:183–184, 1972.

Swinyard, C. A.: Growth of the human suprarenal glands. Anat. Rec. 87:141–150, 1943.

Töndury, G.: Angewandte und topographische Anatomie, 4th ed. Stuttgart, Georg Thieme, 1970.

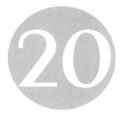

THe kidNEy ANd URETERS

ANOMALIES OF THE KIDNEYS AND URETERS

A succinct account of anomalies of the kidneys and ureters is given by Hollinshead (1971), with further detail given by Gross (1953), Lowsley and Kirwin (1956), and Gray and Skandalakis (1972). Anomalies of the kidney include those of number, size, position, and form. The incidence of such anomalies is variously reported as 3 to 9 per cent.

The most frequent anomaly is duplication of the kidney to the extent of a bifid collecting system, either complete or partial. A separate supernumerary kidney is exceedingly rare. The extra kidney is small and located inferior to the regular kidney, and their two ureters often are fused. When agenesis of both kidneys occurs, the infant is usually still-born. Unilateral agenesis occurs in about 1 per cent of otherwise normal individuals. The solitary kidney is usually in the normal position, but it may be ectopic in the pelvis or crossed with the ureter on the opposite side. The hazard of its being mistaken for a tumor and removed is stressed by Anderson and Harrison (1965).

Hypoplasia differs from agenesis in that a small rudimentary kidney is present along with a ureter, pelvis, and calices. The opposite kidney shows compensatory hypertrophy. Parenthetically, although discrepancy in size between two kidneys of normal form and location suggests atrophy from disease, such a discrepancy may exist without any demonstrable lesion.

An ectopic kidney is one arrested or deviated during its embryonic ascent. Sixty per cent of ectopic kidneys are pelvic in position; the remainder are lumbar, crossed, or, rarely, thoracic (Thompson and Pace, 1937). Abnormality of ascent is often associated with other renal and bodily abnormalities (Malek *et al.,* 1971). Thus 10 per cent of ectopic kidneys are said to be solitary (Gray and Skandalakis). Fusion of two ectopic kidneys is not unusual. Anomalous origin and multiplicity of the blood vessels are quite constant, as is a failure of rotation with retention of the ventral position of the kidney pelvis. A kidney of normal position may exhibit similar abnormal rotation.

Anomalies of form include lobulated kidney, multicystic and polycystic disease, and fused kidney. Lobulation is a regular feature in the kidney of the newborn (see Fig. 151) and traces may persist in the adult. Multicystic disease is usually unilateral, whereas polycystic disease is bilateral. The usual explanation for production of polycystic disease is a lack of communication between secreting and collecting elements of the kidney, but this explanation has been questioned. Other abnormalities are often associated with polycystic renal disease; these include skeletal deformity, cysts in other organs, and congenital 'berry' aneurysms of the cerebral arteries. The most common expression of fusion is the horseshoe kidney of symmetrical type (Fig. 156 A). The main portions lie in relatively normal position, their lower ends joined across the aorta and vena cava by an isthmus of varying thickness. In crossed ectopia with fusion, the kidneys join on one side to form an elongated structure (Fig. 156 F). Intermediate between these types are those in which the fused kidney overlies the midline to some degree (Fig. 156 B, C, D). Finally, the kidneys may fuse within the pelvis to form a discoid, or 'lump,' kidney (Fig. 156 E).

Common to all fused kidneys is the retention of the nonrotated position with an anteriorly placed pelvis and a multiplicity of renal vessels. The symmetrical horseshoe kidney may be supplied by a bifurcating single artery arising from the aorta (Fig. 156 A). Fused kidneys are predisposed to obstruction and infection, and division of the isthmus is

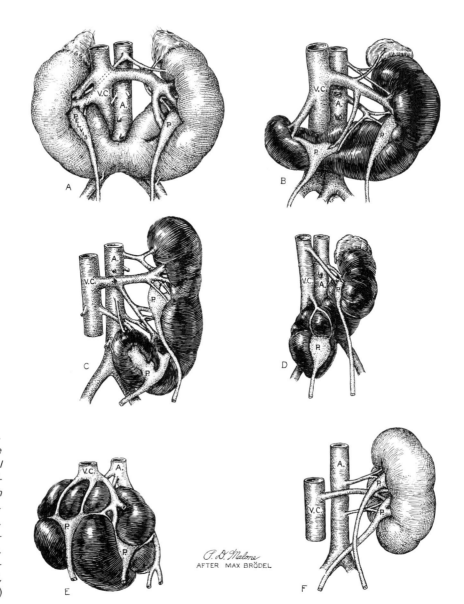

FIG. 156
*Types of fused kidneys.
A. Symmetrical horseshoe
kidney. B. Asymmetrical
horseshoe kidney. C. Uni-
lateral horseshoe kidney with
right ureter crossing to opposite side (crossed ectopia).
D. Sigmoid kidney. E. Discoid, or 'lump,' kidney.
F. Crossed ectopia with fusion. (From Everett, 1947,
after Kelly and Burnam, 1914.)*

AFTER MAX BRÖDEL

often indicated, with or without amputation pyeloplasty. The delineation of the internal anatomy requires pyelography and angiography. Although the arterial distribution is distorted, Graves (1969) found that the lack of communication between segmental arteries was maintained (see below).

Ureteral anomalies are clinically important because of the predisposition to obstruction and infection they cause, plus urinary incontinence in instances of ectopic termination. Duplication of the ureter is a frequent anomaly found more often in females than in males; it can exist as an incidental finding. The duplication may be associated with bifid pelvis and, very rarely, with duplication of the bladder. The two ureters may fuse, or may open separately in the bladder or ectopically below. Rarely multiplicity may exist to the extent of three or four ureters. A ureter may be anomalous in position; that is, it may be retrocaval (see Fig. 40). The course of a ureter behind an iliac artery is extremely rare. Ectopic termination of a ureter occurs three times as often in females as in males. The termination is in the lower urinary or genital tract (Fig. 157) (Stephens, 1963). Finally, there is a miscellany of lesions of functional importance. These include megaureter (Hendren, 1970), ureteropelvic intraluminal valves or external vascular compression (De Weerd, 1969), and obstruction or reflux at the ureterovesical junction (see Chapter 21).

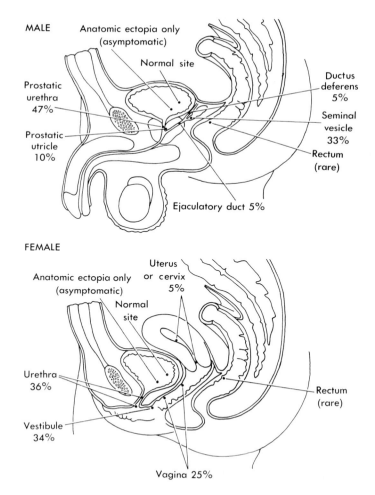

FIG. 157
Ectopic ureteral orifices and the relative frequency of their occurrence in men and women. (From Gray and Skandalakis, 1972.)

SEGMENTS OF THE KIDNEY;
THE RENAL PEDICLE

The division of the kidney into segments, determined by the mode of its arterial supply, is important in relation to the development of necrosis secondary to division of a branch of the renal artery or of a supernumerary artery, or of hypertension from localized ischemia, and to the possibility of resection of a diseased or injured segment. The lobed appearance of the kidney in the newborn suggests such localized territories. Externally, the adult kidney often shows some notching or incomplete fissures suggesting the persistence of fetal lobulation. Brödel (in Kelly and Burnam, 1914) suggested that small stellate veins on the surface of the kidney can sometimes indicate the location of such fissures. No explicit correlation has been made between these fetal lobes and the arterial segments of the adult kidney.

The presence of localized segments was indicated by the observations of Brödel (1901) and of older anatomists (see Merklin and Michels, 1958) of a lack of communication between branches of the renal artery except by capsular capillaries and arterioles. The actual segmentation was demonstrated by Graves (1954) and is generally accepted, although nomenclature varies (Fig. 158). The renal artery divides into anterior and posterior divisions. The branching of the anterior division is somewhat radial. The posterior division artery arches across the top of the kidney pelvis then descends in a short arc across the pelvis or the major calices (Fig. 159). This arch may sometimes be palpated beneath the posterior lip of the kidney sinus, or it may be embedded

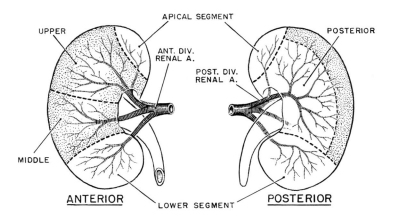

FIG. 158
Diagram of segmental arterial supply to the kidney. (After Graves, 1954.)

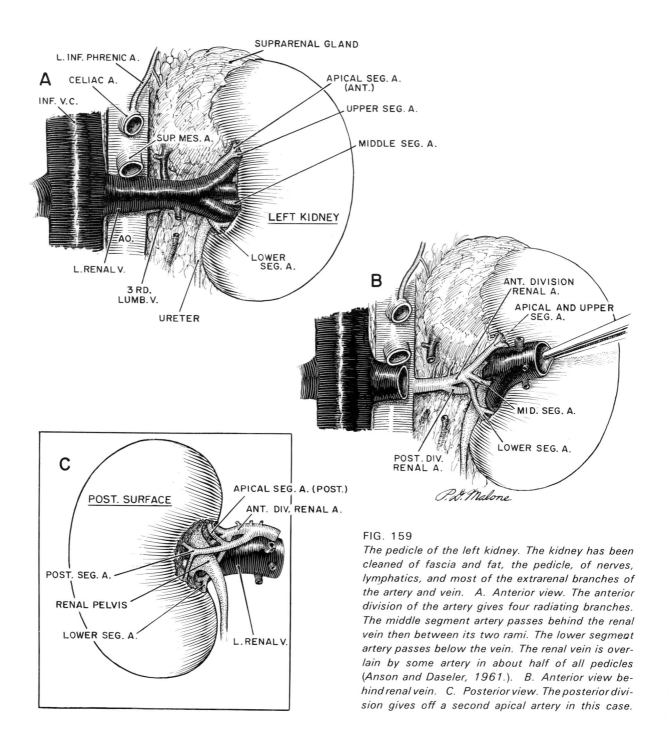

A

L. INF. PHRENIC A.

CELIAC A.

INF. V.C.

SUP. MES. A.

SUPRARENAL GLAND

APICAL SEG. A. (ANT.)

UPPER SEG. A.

MIDDLE SEG. A.

LEFT KIDNEY

LOWER SEG. A.

AO.

L. RENAL V.

3 RD. LUMB. V.

URETER

B

ANT. DIVISION RENAL A.

APICAL AND UPPER SEG. A.

MID. SEG. A.

LOWER SEG. A.

POST. DIV. RENAL A.

P. L. Malone

C

POST. SURFACE

APICAL SEG. A. (POST.)

ANT. DIV. RENAL A.

POST. SEG. A.

RENAL PELVIS

LOWER SEG. A.

L. RENAL V.

FIG. 159

The pedicle of the left kidney. The kidney has been cleaned of fascia and fat, the pedicle, of nerves, lymphatics, and most of the extrarenal branches of the artery and vein. A. Anterior view. The anterior division of the artery gives four radiating branches. The middle segment artery passes behind the renal vein then between its two rami. The lower segment artery passes below the vein. The renal vein is overlain by some artery in about half of all pedicles (Anson and Daseler, 1961.). B. Anterior view behind renal vein. C. Posterior view. The posterior division gives off a second apical artery in this case.

within the kidney substance. The anterior division is the larger, supplying the apical and lower segments and the upper and middle segments, the region between the poles anteriorly and along the convex border. The posterior division supplies the posterior segment.

Further arterial branching, as noted by Brödel for the poles, suggests the presence of subsegments; the 'interlobar' branches of the segmental arteries cannot be considered subsegmental since the interlobar arteries supply adjacent pyramids (Fig. 160). Löfgren's study (1949) suggests the possibility for a subdivision into subsegments. He found that the kidney medulla of the fetus consists of 14 major pyramids, 7 ventral and 7 dorsal. In the newborn, these are partially fused into a cranial part, comprising the first three ventral and dorsal pyramids (V1–3, D1–3), an intermediate (V4–5, D4–5), and a caudal (V6–7, D6–7). Boijsen (1959) has at least partially confirmed this subdivision angiographically.

The line of incision in partial nephrectomy will do least damage to the remaining parenchyma if it follows the boundaries of the segment to be resected. The surgeon can determine the segmental boundary by the blanching caused by tentative clamping of the pertinent artery, or by the intra-arterial injection of a dye.

Variations of the extrarenal portion of the renal arteries

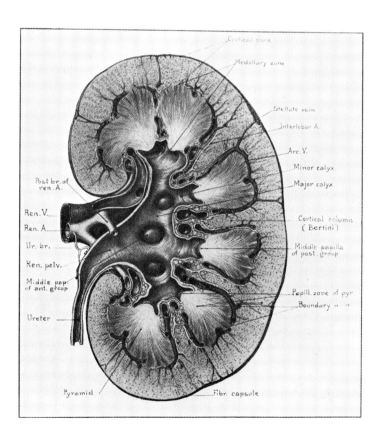

FIG. 160
Intrarenal branching of renal vessels seen in longitudinal section of the kidney. (From Kelly and Burnam, 1914.)

concern their number, source, and mode of branching. In the usual kidney Sykes (1963) found Graves' pattern of division in 59 of 71 specimens. In half of the remaining 12 kidneys the renal artery divided into three branches, each subdividing into anterior and posterior arteries. In the other six two renal arteries of equal size stemmed from the aorta ('dual renal arteries'). In five of these six kidneys the upper artery supplied the apical and posterior segments, the lower artery the upper, middle, and lower segments. In the sixth kidney, the upper artery went to the two polar segments, the lower to the anterior and posterior parts between.

Multiple renal arteries are present in over 20 per cent of all individuals (Adachi, 1928; Pick and Anson, 1940; Merklin and Michels, 1958; Olsson, 1971). In usual kidneys, multiple renal arteries occur mainly as the dual renal arteries mentioned above, or as supernumerary arteries (one or more) to either pole of the kidney, those to the lower pole being more frequent. Supernumerary polar arteries usually stem from the aorta, but a superior polar artery may come off the inferior phrenic artery. As in the liver, such an 'accessory' artery cannot act as a collateral for the other renal vessels, for its distribution is limited to some one segment or subsegment. Multiple arteries are the rule in the case of congenitally abnormal kidneys (see above). Brödel and Kelly and Burnam emphasized that an anomalous renal pelvis, including 'split' pelvis, is often associated with supernumerary arteries, and that an unusual complexity of internal branching is also to be expected. There is a wide source for the multiple arteries of renal anomalies, ranging from the sacral and internal, external, and common iliac arteries below—to the aorta, lumbar, inferior and superior mesenteric, hepatic, colic, and inferior phrenic above (Adachi). The height of location of the kidney determines the probable source in the individual case.

Collaterals for the renal artery come from the perimeter of the kidney and ureter, using the extrarenal branches of the renal artery to reach the kidney (Abrams and Cornell, 1965). The arterial collaterals are usually inadequate to prevent the production of ischemic hypertension.

The renal vein is formed by the union of two or three major rami, which usually leave the kidney anterior to the pelvis (Figs. 159, 161). Anson and Daseler (1961) found

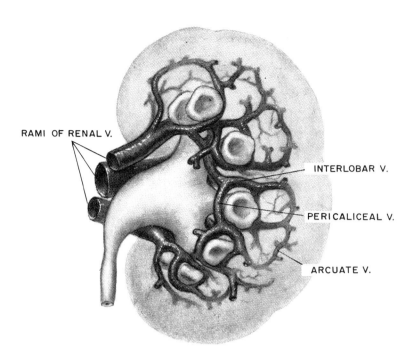

RAMI OF RENAL V.

INTERLOBAR V.

PERICALICEAL V.

ARCUATE V.

FIG. 161
The intrarenal veins.

a second renal vein behind the pelvis in about 14 per cent of kidneys, more often on the right (see Fig. 40). In about 6 per cent of their subjects the left renal vein either split to enclose the aorta ('renal collar') or ran behind the aorta as a single vessel. This is the same incidence reported by Reis and Esenther (1959).

Within the kidney major rami receive large interlobar veins which run between the pyramids. These are interconnected by a peripheral set of anastomoses—the arcuate veins which drain the cortex, and pericaliceal veins at the apices of the pyramids (Figs. 160, 161). The freedom of venous anastomosis between all parts of the kidney was pointed out by Brödel (1901) and has been confirmed by others (Kelly and Burnam, 1914; Graves, 1954; Smith, 1963; Poisel and Sirang, 1972). Thus, while a nephrotomy along Brödel's 'avascular line' cuts across several arcuate and pericaliceal veins, no interference with venous drainage ensues. Likewise, during kidney transplantation, only one of two renal veins requires anastomosis, as compared with the requirements regarding supernumerary arteries (Smith).

Occlusion of a renal vein seldom gives rise to hypertension or nephrosis, because of the rich anastomosis between the perinephric branches of the renal vein and adjacent veins of the body wall and of the portal system (Edwards, 1958). This is particularly true of the left renal vein (see page 60).

Of the other elements of the renal pedicle, the nerves are shown in Figure 48, and the renal lymphatics are indicated in Figure 44.

THE KIDNEY PELVIS; PYELOTOMY AND NEPHROTOMY

The form of the collecting system of the kidney was carefully described by Brödel (1901, and in Kelly and Burnam, 1914). In a kidney of regular form and location, the pelvis usually shows a division into two (sometimes three) major calices. The upper calix is the smaller, and becomes the upper pelvis in instances of bifid pelvis. The major calices typically receive 8 minor calices (Fig. 162), but the number may range from 4 to 18. Two or more papillae, as many as six near the poles, project into each minor calix (Fig. 160). The papillae, in turn, are the terminations of one or more pyramids.

The typical four calices pertaining to the anterior and posterior segments usually join the pelvis in two rows, at such angles that the posterior calices ''point to a line just

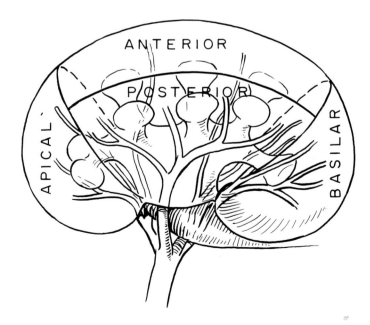

FIG. 162
Pelvic calices and segments. The 'anterior' segment includes the upper and middle segments of Graves. (From Boyce, 1969.)

a little posterior to the lateral convex border of the kidney, while the anterior calices are directed straight forward into the convex anterior region of the organ'' (Brödel, 1901). The pelvis may be completely hidden within a deep renal sinus (intrarenal pelvis); in such an instance the calices are short. The pelvis may be completely extrahilar, with major or even minor calices visible beyond the lips of the sinus. The pelvis of a fused kidney will usually be found in an anterior rather than a posterior position. The precise anatomy displayed by pyelography and arteriography has rendered somewhat superfluous the elaborate correlations between external form and intrarenal configuration presented by Kelly and Burnam.

In a kidney of regular form pyelotomy is best done from behind. Not only are fewer vascular structures related to its posterior surface, but the posterior lip of the renal sinus projects over the pelvis to a lesser extent than does the anterior. However, if the renal arteries are of the predominant variety (see page 295) the posterior division artery is consistent in its position, first crossing the superior border of the pelvis then curving downward posterior to the lateral part of the renal pelvis or to the calices, either beneath the posterior lip of the sinus or embedded within the parenchyma. As noted above, an element of the renal vein may also lie behind the pelvis, more often on the right. Removal of the posterior hilar fat, preserving as many of the fine blood vessels to the pelvis as possible, and retraction of the posterior lip of the sinus, exposes the entire posterior and medial aspects of the pelvis of the kidney. With a trap-door incision in the posterior aspect of the pelvis, and the posterior lip of the sinus and posterior segment artery well retracted, Gil-Vernet (1972) is able to extract most staghorn calculi. Boyce (1969) states that a circumferential incision is preferable to a longitudinal one because it gives more exposure of the interior and follows more closely the circulospiral arrangement of the muscle of the pelvis.

An additional reason for opening the renal pelvis from behind is that a nephrotomy, if indicated, is also best carried out with this approach. ''The only anatomically permissible extension of pyelotomy into the renal parenchyma is that which follows the line between the posterior and lower segments and opens into the lower [major] calyx'' (Boyce) (Fig. 163). It may be well to note the description (in Kelly and

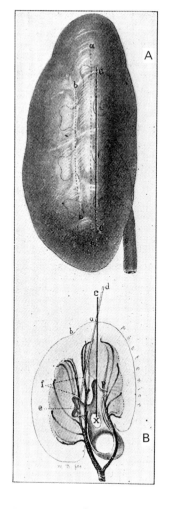

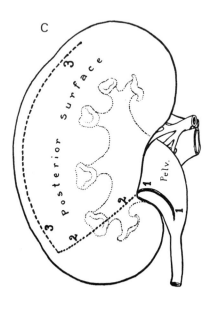

FIG. 163

Brödel's 'white line' and his favored nephrotomy incision. A right kidney is shown. A. External landmarks: a-a', convex border. b-b', "This is the so-called white line and should be avoided." c-c', the safe incision. B. Cross section of the kidney: c-x, the safe incision, passing through the plane of cleavage between the anterior and posterior divisions of the renal artery and entering the posterior calices. If deflected anteriorly, d-e, the incision cuts across the arteries. C. Brödel's pyelonephrotomy incision: 1. The pyelotomy. 2. Continuation of incision to open lower calices. 3. Continuation to open entire pelvis. (From Kelly and Burnam, 1914.)

Burnam, 1914) of Brödel's 'white line,' since it is so often mentioned as a landmark for nephrotomy. It is described as a longitudinal "whitish band to which the perirenal fat appears more intimately attached than elsewhere," located *anterior* to the convex border, and on the part of the kidney between the two polar regions. It lies within the anterior segments and marks the location of the longitudinal cortical column carrying anterior and posterior interlobar arteries of the anterior segments. A nephrotomy incision is advised, not through the white line, but entering the posterior calices through their concave distal ends. The incision is begun on the posterior surface of the kidney, medial to the convex border, and directed to the posterior calices so as to avoid the large vessels of the longitudinal cortical column (Fig. 163).

Some renal papillae are transected in such an incision.

To avoid this, Boyce advises a nephrotomy which enters the anterior aspect of the posterior calices—his 'posterior segment approach,' or one which enters the posterolateral margin of the renal pelvis between the two rows of calices—his 'intersegment approach.' Externally the incision is made according to Brödel's suggestion, dividing the cortex sharply. The deeper part of the incision is carried out bluntly, slanted according to which of the two objectives is to be gained, and keeping in mind the angulation of the calices with respect to the kidney referred to above. Preliminary roentgen study of the kidney, and intra-operative dye injection or temporary arterial occlusion helps delineate the individual vascular pattern. In the posterior segment nephrotomy the anterior surfaces of the posterior calices are opened transversely in the middle of their extent, well away from their fornices and the papillae. If both major calices are opened and their incisions joined, a relatively large pyelotomy is achieved. In the intersegment nephrotomy the deep dissection proceeds to the pelvis, somewhat closer to the posterior than to the anterior calices. The incision will pass through the large venous plexus between the two rows of calices, termed the 'median vein' (of Hauch, in Kelly and Burnam, and Poisel and Sirang, 1972). The pelvis is first opened between the calix of the middle segment and the lower of the two posterior calices, where the plexus is relatively small. To avoid arteries of the apical and basilar segments, these calices are opened on their lateral surfaces and in the frontal plane of the kidney; the anterior and posterior calices are opened on their opposing surfaces and in the transverse plane of the kidney. "It must be said, however, that the calices, in a few instances, form very complex cavities, minor calices giving rise again to secondary minor calices, so that even if the kidney be opened from pole to pole, an operator cannot always guarantee that all the pockets have been explored, and palpation of the two halves is by no means a satisfactory method of detecting a small-sized stone" (Kelly and Burnam).

When the renal pelvis is bifid, a separate nephrotomy is advised for each half, the upper nephrotomy joining neither the lower nephrotomy nor a pyelotomy, since large arteries and veins will be endangered in the bifurcation of the pelvis.

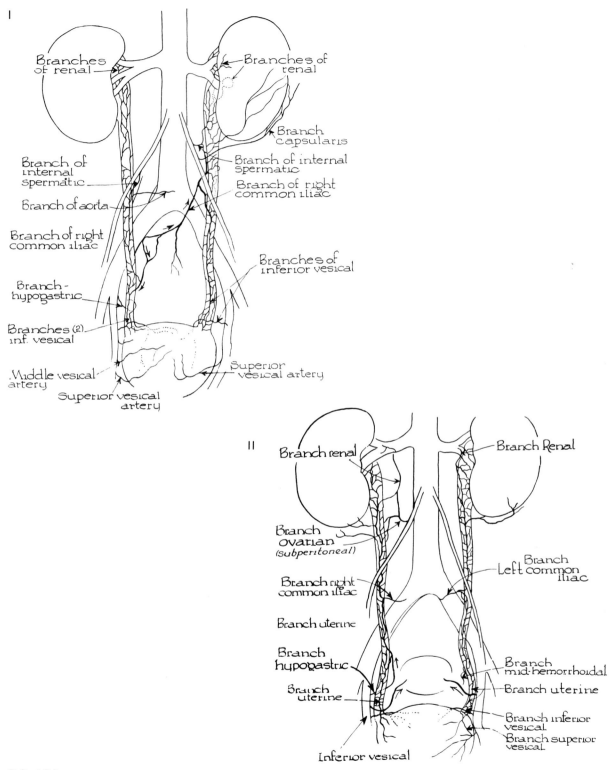

FIG. 164

Arterial supply of the ureter in the male (I) and female (II). (From Michaels, 1948. By permission of Surgery, Gynecology & Obstetrics.)

COURSE AND BLOOD SUPPLY
OF THE URETER

We may briefly emphasize that the ureter courses retroperitoneally at a variable distance lateral to the spine, crossing the brim of the pelvis over the iliac bifurcation then passing on the floor of the pelvis to its termination in the bladder. Three areas of narrowing are significant for the lodgment of calculi—the first at the origin of the ureter from the kidney pelvis, second as it crosses the brim of the pelvis, and the third just before it passes through the bladder wall.

The blood supply is given by a number of small arteries from adjacent vessels (Fig. 164). In spite of the arterial anastomoses, ischemic slough is a well-known complication of operations on the ureter, particularly in kidney transplantation and in pelvic lymphadenectomy, as for cancer of the cervix uteri. To prevent ischemia it is important to save as many of the arterial sources as possible, and it is also important not to clean too assiduously the spiderweb-like connective tissue clinging to the ureter, in which the fine arteries course and communicate (Fig. 165). When transplanting the ureter, as for urinary diversion, the peritoneum should be left in place where it is adherent to the ureter. One should avoid cleaning the end of a divided ureter of adhering tissue any more than necessary—never for a distance of more than 2.5 cm.

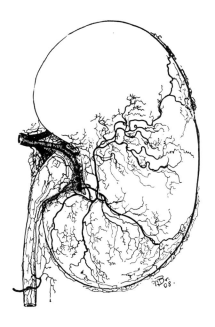

FIG. 165
Delicacy of the extrarenal branches of the renal artery. (From Kelly and Burnam, 1914.)

APPROACHES TO THE KIDNEY
AND URETER

Knowledge of the posterior surface topography of the kidney (Fig. 166) is helpful in planning a limited approach, such as a needle biopsy. For this procedure Muehrcke and his associates (1955) place the patient prone upon a sandbag to push the kidneys well backward. The needle is inserted below the 12th rib, lateral to the erector spinae muscle, but medial to the lateral border of the kidney as determined by roentgenography. The insertion of the needle into the kidney is signaled by marked movements of the needle's hub with respiration. One is certain to enter the pleura if the needle is inserted close to the rib when the lowest rib is actually the 11th. This is an added reason for consulting the x-ray films or ultrasound scan prior to doing the biopsy.

The most commonly used open approach to the kidney and upper ureter is the lumbar extraperitoneal (Fig. 167). The incision can be made more commodious posteriorly by

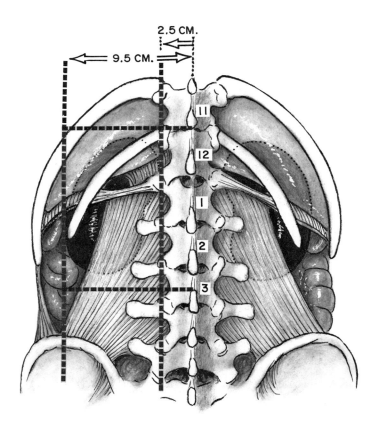

FIG. 166
Posterior surface relationships of kidneys. About one-third of the kidney lies above the inferior border of the 12th rib, the left being about 1 cm. higher than the right. The two vertical and two horizontal lines shown mark out a parallelogram which generally contains the kidney. Each kidney is tilted laterally below, so that the hilum lies 5 cm. from the spine of the first lumbar vertebra.

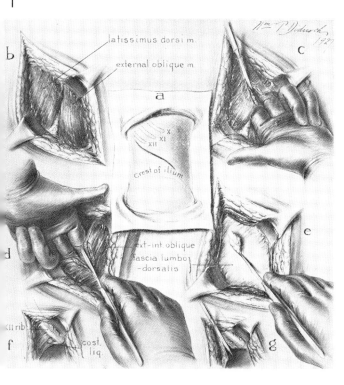

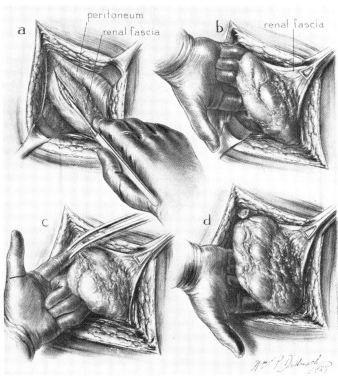

FIG. 167

Lumbar extraperitoneal approach to the kidney. I. Incision in abdominal wall: a. Line of incision. Its anterior part may be extended for ureterectomy. b, c, d. Exposure and division of muscles. The 12th intercostal (sub-costal), iliohypogastric, and ilioinguinal nerves should be spared if encountered. They lie outside the endoabdominal fascia posteriorly but gradually enter the abdominal wall to run between the tranversus and internal oblique muscles from about the anterior axillary line forward. e. Incision of the endoabdominal (lumbodorsal) fascia. f, g. Exposure and division of costovertebral ligament. II. Delivery of kidney. a. Incision of the renal fascia. b, c, d. Mobilization of the kidney by blunt and sharp dissection of perirenal tissues. Polar arteries must be preserved if the kidney is not to be removed. (From Lowsley and Kirwin, 1956.)

subperiosteal removal of the 12th rib, or the 11th if the 12th is short or absent. The posterior relationships of this approach, including those of the pleura, are described in Chapter 1. Anteriorly, the incision can be extended in the manner of a transverse abdominal, or rectus muscle–detaching incision, still staying extraperitoneally (O'Conor and Logan, 1966) (see Figs. 5, 6). Exposure of the ureter alone can be accomplished by using only the anterior part of this incision or an anterior extraperitoneal incision of some other variety (see Chapter 1).

An anterior abdominal approach (Figs. 168, 169) opens the peritoneum, but has the following advantages: (1) Early control of the pedicle, as when there is a tumor which extends into the renal vein and vena cava and which might otherwise embolize during the procedure, or when there is a highly vascular tumor. (2) Safeguarding the duodenum and colon when an *en bloc* removal of the kidney and peri-

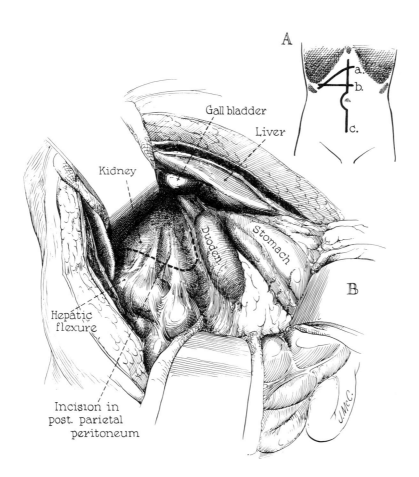

FIG. 168
Right abdominal transperitoneal nephrectomy.

A. Choice of incisions, line a being used here. B. Initial view of right kidney area. Line of incision of posterior peritoneum is indicated.

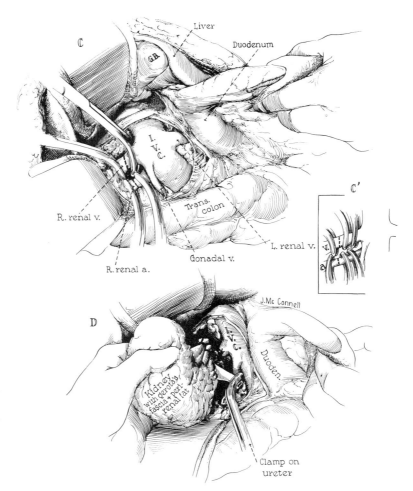

FIG. 168
*Right abdominal transperitoneal ne-
phrectomy* (continued).

*C. Duodenum is mobilized to the
left, exposing vena cava and right
renal vein and artery which are
clamped and, in C', transected.
D. Incision in peritoneum has been
extended and the hepatic flexure of
colon mobilized, allowing en bloc
removal of kidney and upper ureter
with renal fascia and perirenal fat.
Prior separation of the kidney from
the suprarenal gland is not shown.
(From Grayhack and Graham, 1969.)*

renal fat is to be done, or when adhesions are present between the kidney and those segments of the intestines. (3)
Better exposure of large tumors or tumors involving adjacent
organs. (4) Simultaneous lymph node removal. Two other
approaches are available to attain these same objectives.
These are the thoracoabdominal (Fig. 170), especially useful
for large tumors (Chute *et al.,* 1949), and the Nagamatsu
(see Fig. 13).

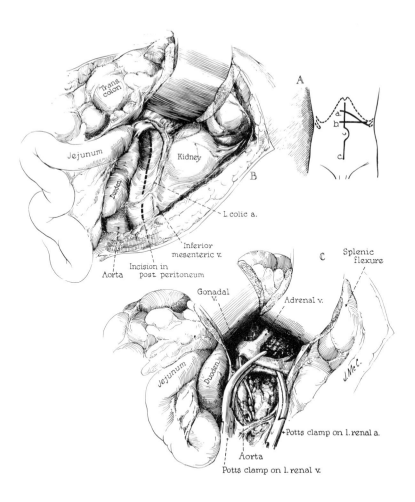

FIG. 169

Abdominal transperitoneal approach to left kidney. A. Choice of incisions. B. Initial view of left kidney area. C. The duodenum and splenic flexure of the colon have been displaced to expose the renal pedicle. A second incision into the posterior peritoneum lateral to the splenic flexure allows mobilization of the kidney with its fascia and fat. (From Grayhack and Graham, 1969.)

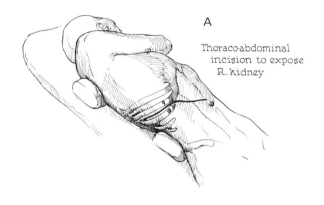

A

Thoraco-abdominal
incision to expose
R. kidney

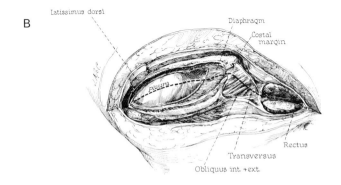

B

Latissimus dorsi

Diaphragm

Costal
margin

pleura

Rectus

Transversus

Obliquus int. + ext.

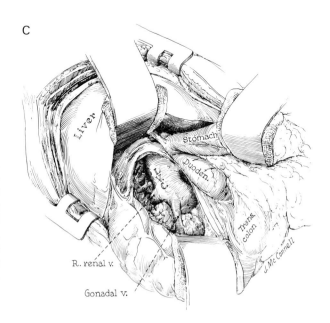

C

Liver

Stomach

Duoden.

I.V.C.

Trans.
colon

J. McConnell

R. renal v.

Gonadal v.

FIG. 170

Thoracoabdominal transpleural, transperitoneal exposure of right kidney. A. Line of incision. B. The muscles and costal arch have been divided. Line of incision in pleura and anterior peritoneum is indicated. C. The posterior peritoneum is opened over the renal pedicle, with further procedure as in Figure 168, C, D. (From Grayhack and Graham, 1969.)

REFERENCES

Abrams, H. L., and Cornell, S. H.: Patterns of collateral flow in renal ischemia. Radiology 84:1001–1012, 1965.

Adachi, B.: Das Arteriensystem der Japaner. 2 vols. Tokyo, Kenkyusha, 1928.

Anderson, E. E., and Harrison, J. H.: Surgical importance of the solitary kidney. New Eng. J. Med. 273:683–687, 1965.

Anson, B. J., and Daseler, E. H.: Common variations in renal anatomy, affecting blood supply, form, and topography. Surg. Gynec. Obstet. 112:439–449, 1961.

Boijsen, E.: Angiographic studies of the anatomy of single and multiple renal arteries. Acta Radiol., Suppl. 183, 1959.

Boyce, W. H.: Surgery of Renal Calculi. Chapter 3 *in* Glenn, J. F., and Boyce, W. H., *op. cit.*, 1969.

Brödel, M.: The intrinsic blood vessels of the kidney and their significance in nephrotomy. Bull. Johns Hopkins Hosp. 12:10–13, 1901.

Chute, R., Soutter, L., and Kerr, W. S., Jr.: The value of the thoracoabdominal incision in the removal of kidney tumors. New Eng. J. Med. 241:951–960, 1949.

De Weerd, J. H.: Surgery of the Renal Pelvis and Ureteropelvic Juncture. Chapter 4 *in* Glenn, J. F., and Boyce, W. H., *op. cit.*, 1969.

Edwards, E. A.: The anatomy of collateral circulation. Surg. Gynec. Obstet. 107:183–194, 1958.

Everett, H. S.: Gynecological and Obstetrical Urology, 2nd ed. Baltimore, Williams & Wilkins, 1947.

Gil-Vernet, J. Mª.: Extended Pyelolithotomy for Removal of Staghorn Calculus. Chapter 18, Essay 2 *in* Current Controversies in Urologic Management, Scott, R., Jr., Gordon, H. L., Scott, F. B., Carlton, C. E., and Beach, P. D., Eds. Philadelphia, W. B. Saunders, 1972.

Glenn, J. F., and Boyce, W. H., Eds.: Urologic Surgery. New York, Hoeber Medical Division, Harper & Row, 1969.

Graves, F. T.: The anatomy of the intrarenal arteries and its application to segmental resection of the kidney. Brit. J. Surg. 42:132–139, 1954.

Graves, F. T.: The arterial anatomy of the congenitally abnormal kidney. Brit. J. Surg. 56:533–541, 1969.

Gray, S. W., and Skandalakis, J. E.: Embryology for Surgeons. The Embryological Basis for the Treatment of Congenital Defects. Philadelphia, W. B. Saunders, 1972.

Grayhack, J. T., and Graham, J. B.: Surgery of the Kidney. Chapter 2 *in* Glenn and Boyce, *op. cit.*, 1969.

Gross, R. E.: The Surgery of Infancy and Childhood. Its Principles and Techniques. Philadelphia, W. B. Saunders, 1953.

Hendren, W. H.: Functional restoration of decompensated ureters in children. Amer. J. Surg. 119:477–482, 1970.

Hollinshead, W. H.: Anatomy for Surgeons, 2nd ed. Vol. 2. The Thorax, Abdomen, and Pelvis. New York, Harper & Row, 1971.

Kelly, H. A., and Burnam, C. F.: Diseases of the Kidneys, Ureters and Bladder, with Special Reference to the Diseases in Women. New York, Appleton, 1914.

Löfgren, F.: Das topographische System der Malpighischen Pyramiden der Menschenniere. Lund, Ohlsson, 1949.

Lowsley, O. S., and Kirwin, T. J.: Clinical Urology, 3rd ed. Baltimore, Williams & Wilkins, 1956.

Malek, R. S., Kelalis, P. P., and Burke, E. C.: Ectopic kidney in children and frequency of association with other malformations. Mayo Clin. Proc. 46:461–467, 1971.

Merklin, R. J., and Michels, N. A.: The variant renal and suprarenal blood supply with data on the inferior phrenic, ureteral and gonadal arteries. A statistical analysis based on 185 dissections and review of the literature. J. Int. Coll. Surg. 29:41–76, 1958.

Michaels, J. P.: Study of ureteral blood supply and its bearing on necrosis of the ureter following the Wertheim operation. Surg. Gynec. Obstet. 86:36–44, 1948.

Muehrcke, R. C., Kark, R. M., and Pirani, C. L.: Biopsy of the kidney in the diagnosis and management of renal disease. New Eng. J. Med. 253:537–546, 1955.

O'Conor, V. J., Jr., and Logan, D. J.: Nephroureterectomy. Surg. Gynec. Obstet. 122:601–603, 1966.

Olsson, O.: Variations in Renal Blood Supply. Chapter 48 *in* Angiography, Abrams, H. L., Ed., Vol. 2. Boston, Little, Brown & Co., 1971.

Olsson, O., and Wholey, M.: Vascular abnormalities in gross anomalies of kidneys. Acta Radiol. (Diagn.) 2:420–432, 1964.

Pick, J. W., and Anson, B. J.: The renal vascular pedicle: An anatomical study of 430 body-halves. J. Urol. 44:411–434, 1940.

Poisel, S., and Sirang, H.: Die Verästelungstypen der Vena renalis im Hinblick auf den venösen Blutabfluss aus dem Parenchym der Niere. Acta Anat. 83:149–160, 1972.

Reis, R. H., and Esenther, G.: Variations in the pattern of renal vessels and their relation to the type of posterior vena cava in man. Amer. J. Anat. 104:295–318, 1959.

Smith, G. T.: The renal vascular patterns in man. J. Urol. 89:275–288, 1963.

Stephens, F. D.: Congenital Malformations of the Rectum, Anus and Genito-Urinary Tracts. Edinburgh, Livingstone, 1963.

Sykes, D.: The arterial supply of the human kidney with special reference to accessory renal arteries. Brit. J. Surg. 50:368–374, 1963.

Thompson, G. J., and Pace, J. M.: Ectopic kidney. A review of 97 cases. Surg. Gynec. Obstet. 64:935–943, 1937.

THE bladder
and pelvic URETERS

EXSTROPHY AND OTHER CONGENITAL ABNORMALITIES

Exstrophy is by far the most serious congenital abnormality of the bladder. Its incidence is low—about 1 in 40,000 or 50,000 births, with a male-to-female ratio of about 5 to 1 (Lowsley and Kirwin, 1956). The lesion consists of a gap in the anterior abdominal wall in front of the bladder, with an open, everted bladder. There is complete incontinence. In the rare incomplete exstrophy the opening is small, with but little of the posterior bladder wall presenting to view. In the more common complete exstrophy all the mucous membrane is exposed and the trigone protrudes. The defect often continues into the urethra as an epispadias (see Fig. 184). The defect in the abdominal wall involves a wide separation of the pubic bones, with a lateral rotation of each half of the pelvis, and therefore a lateral rotation of the lower limbs. The rectus muscles are widely separated. There may be associated anomalies in other parts of the body, such as spina bifida, anal atresia, and cleft palate.

Operative treatment of exstrophy may consist of urinary diversion and simple cystectomy, or of reconstruction of the bladder and urethra. The proponents of urinary diversion base their choice on the fact that continence may not be achieved with the reconstruction. Recent improvements in the technique of ureterosigmoidostomy have made urinary diversion more popular than in former years (Bennett, 1973). Details of reconstruction are given by Smith and Lattimer (1966) and by Chisholm (1969). The edges of the bladder and urethra are freed from adjacent tissues so that they may be sutured to form an anterior wall. Chisholm notes that in freeing the urethra a firm band can be felt between the pubes, representing the epispadic external urethral sphincter. He frees this structure subperiosteally from the pubes and adds its suture anteriorly in the reconstruction. A preliminary osteotomy of the ilia is sometimes advised to allow the pubes to be brought together in front of the reconstruction and to correct the lateral rotation of the limbs (Chisholm; Campbell, 1970). It also aids in the approximation of the lateral edges of the bladder and urethra, as well as the medial borders of the rectus muscles. A preliminary iliac osteotomy is also advised when cystectomy is done (Scott and Carlton, 1969).

Agenesis or hypoplasia of the bladder is exceedingly rare and usually is associated with widespread severe malformations. The bladder may be duplicated to the extent of two separate urethras, or by the presence of a sagittal or frontal septum. Diverticulum of the bladder may be congenital, or secondary to outflow obstruction. Malformations at the vesicoureteral junction are considered below.

Urachal cysts and fistulas are rare, but of some interest. At birth, the epithelial-lined urachus extends from the apex of the bladder, but its upper end is already below the umbilicus. Above this it is ligamentous—the median umbilical ligament (Begg, 1930) (see Fig. 15). The urachus and the ligament possess a single artery derived from a superior vesical artery, usually the left, and a single vein. The ligament may hypertrophy in pregnancy (Begg) (see Fig. 224). The apex of the adult bladder shows a dimple at the urachal junction. Begg found a residual urachal lumen in one third of the adult bladders he examined. However, the lumen admitted only a bristle, and for a distance of 1 cm. or less. Congenital umbilical urinary fistula represents persistent patency of the urachus. Postnatal urachal cysts are based on the presence of nests of epithelium found along the original path of the urachus. Such cysts may or may not communicate with the bladder. Adenocarcinoma derived from the urachal lining may develop at the apex of the bladder.

EXTERNAL AND INTERNAL TOPOGRAPHY; THE VESICOURETERAL JUNCTION

The bladder is firmly attached at its base by the ureters and urethra and by the continuity of the vesical fascia with the fascia of the pelvic diaphragm, reinforced by the pubo-vesical ligaments, also called the puboprostatic in the male (see Fig. 178), and the pubocervical ligaments or pillars of the bladder in the female (see Fig. 206). From this basal attachment the fundus expands upward with distention within the loose tissue of the extraperitoneal space (of Retzius). Emptying it prior to laparotomy helps avoid injury to the bladder; filling it allows intentional cystotomy with less risk of entering the peritoneum.

The bladder of the young child, even when empty, lies partly above the symphysis. At birth its anterior surface is in contact with the abdominal wall for about two-thirds of the distance between the symphysis pubis and the umbilicus, and the internal urethral orifice lies behind the symphysis (Symington, 1887) (Fig. 171). By the age of four or five the bladder has descended to allow a pouch of peritoneum to separate the abdominal wall and the pubes from the empty bladder.

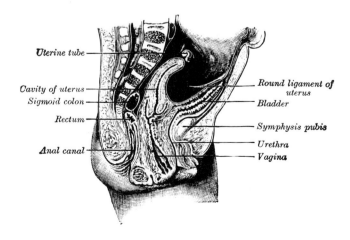

FIG. 171
The bladder in the newborn. (From Goss, 1973.)

The exterior of the bladder fundus can be recognized at operation by the coarsely lobulated dark-yellow fat and large, easily ruptured veins, lying beneath the thin vesical fascia (Fig. 172).

The interior of the bladder presents trabeculation which is low in profile in the normal, increasing in thickness with age, especially with outflow obstruction. The trigone shows the ureteral orifices at the two angles, connected by the interureteric ridge as its base, and the internal urethral orifice at its apex (Fig. 172). Above and behind the bladder neck, in the male, lies the median lobe of the prostate; on either side lie the lateral lobes. The bladder neck merges with the prostatic urethra.

Malformations or functional disorder of the vesicoureteral junction or of the ureters may occasion ureteral obstruction or ureteral reflux. The anatomy of the junction has been interpreted in a number of ways (see Paquin, 1969; Hutch and Amar, 1972). According to Woodburne (1968), bundles of the fundal (detrusor) musculature course prominently on the extravesical terminal ureter. As the ureter passes through the bladder wall, it lies within a space ('Waldeyer's separation'). It is firmly attached to the wall of the trigone by the junction of the ureteral and bladder mucosa, and the continuity of the ureteric muscle with that of the trigone, particularly at the interureteric ridge. Paquin states that the junction functions mainly as a valve, not as a sphincter. When the bladder is filled, the intramural ureter is compressed by the intravesical pressure within, against the supporting bladder wall behind. In this action the obliquity of the intravesical ureter, its relative softness, and the resistance of bladder wall exterior to it, are all significant factors. Paquin acknowledges that the competence of the junction is to some extent dependent on normal neuromuscular activity in two ways. First, normal tone of the ureteral muscle, including that of the fascicles extending from the detrusor muscle, helps keep the ureter closed between peristaltic waves. Second, stimulation of the trigone, as in voiding, pulls the intravesical ureter downward, lengthening its oblique intramural part, increasing the length of ureter to be compressed.

Conditions which produce reflux may be congenital or acquired. These conditions include (1) congenital malforma-

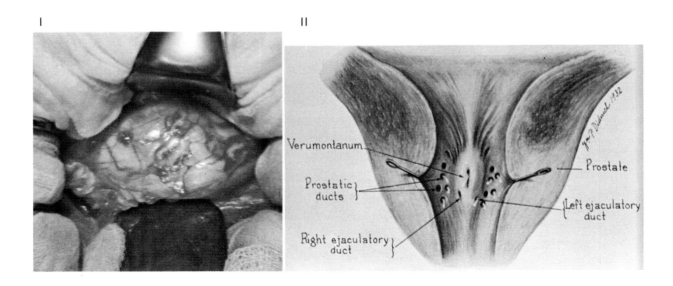

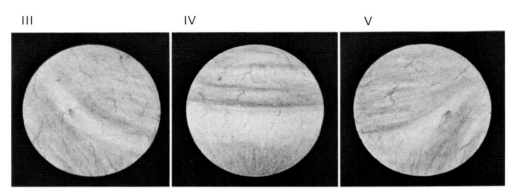

FIG. 172

Exterior and interior of the bladder and of the prostatic urethra. I. Exterior of dome of the bladder seen on suprapubic exposure. The coarsely lobulated and deep-colored fat and the large veins beneath the vesical fascia are characteristic. II. The prostatic urethra in prostatitis and seminal vesiculitis. III. Normal right ureteral orifice. IV. Interureteric fold. V. Left ureteral orifice. (I. Courtesy of Dr. J. Hartwell Harrison. II. Drawn from cystoscopic views, Didusch, 1952. III, IV, V. Drawn from cystoscopic views, Young and Davis, 1926.)

tions of the ureter, as paraureteral diverticulum, ureterocele, inadequate obliquity of the intravesical portion, or ectopic bladder termination; (2) inflammation of the bladder or ureter; (3) weakness of the bladder wall, congenital or acquired; and (4) increased intravesical pressure. Recounting his experiences in children, Hendren (1968) says: "A refluxing ureter usually has a patulous orifice, often too far lateral in the trigone, and a straight course through the bladder wall, with a short submucosal segment of ureter, in contrast to a normal ureter which passes obliquely through the bladder wall and has a tunnel 6 to 12 mm. long." Paquin, Hutch and Amar, and Hendren give details on the operative correction of reflux, which consists either of reimplantation of the ureter through the bladder wall, attempting to approximate the normal course, or of plastic procedures on the ureter in conditions such as megaureter.

MICTURITION AND INCONTINENCE

The structural basis for continence and micturition may be considered under three headings: the roles of (1) the bladder and bladder neck, (2) the urethra, and (3) the urethrovesical angulation. As Woodburne (1968) emphasized, the sacral nerves, through their sensory and motor fibers, control all the events of micturition, the sympathetic system playing no recognizable part. No anatomically defined sphincter muscle can be found in the vesical neck, yet this structure constitutes an effective sphincter. This is adequately confirmed by the presence of continence after the operation of Waterhouse and his associates (1973) for injury or stricture of the membranous urethra. In this procedure, the distal urethra (bulbar and penile) is implanted into the prostatic urethra, bypassing the external sphincter of the membranous urethra.

The descending fibers of the detrusor muscle extend the entire length of the urethra in the female, and into the prostatic urethra of the male. As the muscle fibers of the bladder contract, this extension draws the bladder neck and proximal urethra radially, accounting for the 'funneling' of the bladder seen in a voiding cystourethrogram. Concomitant relaxation of the levator ani and sphincter urethrae muscles contributes

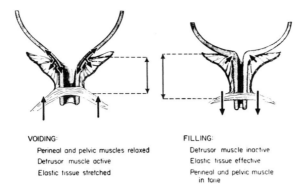

VOIDING:
 Perineal and pelvic muscles relaxed
 Detrusor muscle active
 Elastic tissue stretched

FILLING:
 Detrusor muscle inactive
 Elastic tissue effective
 Perineal and pelvic muscle
   in tone

FIG. 173
Schema of structural relations in voiding and filling of the bladder. (From Woodburne, 1961.)

to lessening the resistance in the urethra, not only by the removal of their resting sphincteric tone, but also by shortening the tube. Urine is now expressed by the increase in intravesical pressure produced by contraction both of the fundus and of the abdominal muscles (Fig. 173).

During filling of the bladder, the urethra regains its continence through the return of resting tone in the external sphincter and levator ani muscles, the relaxation of the detrusor muscle extension, the recoil of its elastic tissue (which Woodburne (1961) has shown to be abundant in the urethra), and by the regaining of its resting length, which Lapides and his colleagues (1960) have demonstrated to be a significant factor.

Muscle of the urethra which plays a part in continence consists of smooth muscle continuing here from the bladder, as well as the striated external sphincter of the membranous urethra. Through pressure determinations Lapides and his co-workers (1960) concluded that primary sphincter action resides in the distal prostatic and the membranous urethra of the male, and in the mid portion of the urethra of the female. Tanagho (1971) concluded, from pharmacological and other evidence, that the smooth muscle of the urethra can maintain continence at rest, although the striated muscle is needed to overcome increase in bladder pressure caused by sudden contractions of the abdominal wall.

It is apparent from observations on stress incontinence that continence is also considerably dependent on the maintenance of normal angulation between bladder and urethra by the pubococcygeus muscles. The angle normally formed by the junction of these two parts posteriorly is 90 to 100 degrees (see Fig. 202). This angle is widened in the funneling of micturition and in stress incontinence simply with the patient in the erect position. The responsibility for this widening of angulation lies in the relaxation of the pelvic floor, primarily posteriorly through loss of strength of the decussation of the pubococcygeus muscles and their fascia (see Chapter 23). Hutch (1965) proposed that the region of the base of the bladder which meets the urethra acts as a unit, sliding forward to pinch off the urethra in the non-voiding state. He called this part of the bladder, which extends somewhat beyond the trigone, the 'base plate.'

Stress incontinence is overwhelmingly a postpartum problem, and operations for its cure by restoration of the urethrovesical angle are discussed in Chapter 23. However, stress incontinence may occur in nulliparous women. Here it is explained by a congenital weakness (paralytic or non-paralytic) of the pelvic floor with a similar loss of support for the urethrovesical junction. For incontinence following prostatectomy, Kaufman (1973) has devised a procedure to augment closure of the urethra by implanting against it a sac containing silicone gel. Urinary incontinence after resection of the rectum for cancer apparently may also be based on loss of pelvic support, or on interference with the sacral nerve supply. Other causes of incontinence include congenital lesions of the bladder, urethra, or the spine (Stephens and Smith, 1971); paralysis caused by organic neurologic disease or induced by drugs (Talbot, 1958); distortion by urethral scarring, or distortion and paralysis through infiltration of the pelvic floor by malignancy (Muellner and Fleischner, 1949).

BLOOD VESSELS; LYMPHATICS; NERVES

On the basis of the arterial supply the bladder is divisible into three regions in both sexes (Figs. 174, 175, 176). The dome and apex are supplied by the branches from the umbilical artery termed superior vesical; the most posterior of these branches is sometimes called the middle vesical. In the male, the lower anterior region is supplied by the inferior vesical, and the lower posterior region by the deferential artery. The connective tissue about each artery, containing also veins, lymphatics, and nerves, is sometimes termed a

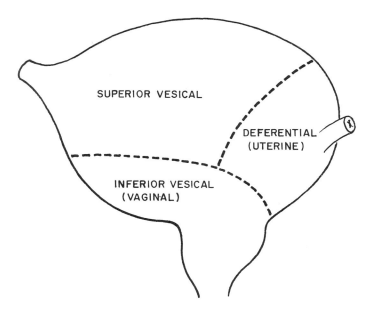

FIG. 174
Arterial territories of the bladder.
(After Braithwaite, 1952.)

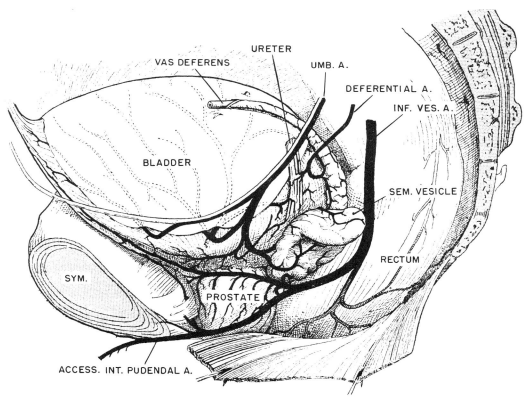

FIG. 175
Arteries to the male bladder and pelvic genital organs. (From Farabeuf, 1905.)

ligament of the bladder. This is a substantial structure about the inferior vesical artery, forming a pedicle called the posterior ligament of the bladder.

The inferior vesical artery (see Fig. 185) most often stems from the internal pudendal, or from a gluteopudendal trunk (see Chapter 4). The deferential, sometimes also called the middle vesical, arises from the umbilical artery (Braithwaite, 1952; Darget *et al.,* 1957), less often from the inferior vesical. It regularly supplies the seminal vesicles, as well as the vas, and plays a role in the blood supply of the testis (see Fig. 181). In the female the vaginal artery, when large, represents the inferior vesical, and a 'middle vesical' is the counterpart of the deferential (Fig. 176). The uterine artery gives a variable contribution to the bladder.

The veins of the bladder (Fig. 177) run into the capacious paired vesical or, in the male, prostatovesical plexuses. A particularly large vein in the vesical plexus was called by Farabeuf the collecting vein of the bladder, and another large vein along the prostate, the collecting vein of the prostate. The plexuses receive the deep dorsal vein of the penis, or clitoris anteriorly. On each side, the plexuses communicate with the internal pudendal veins, and quite freely with the veins of the prostate, or vagina and uterus, to empty posteriorly into the internal iliac veins. Further communications

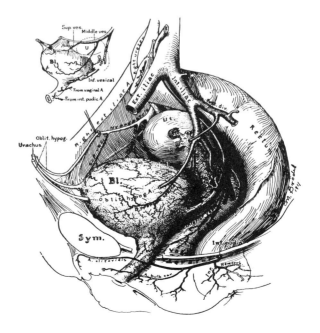

FIG. 176
Arteries to the female bladder and ureter. (From Kelly and Burnam, 1914.)

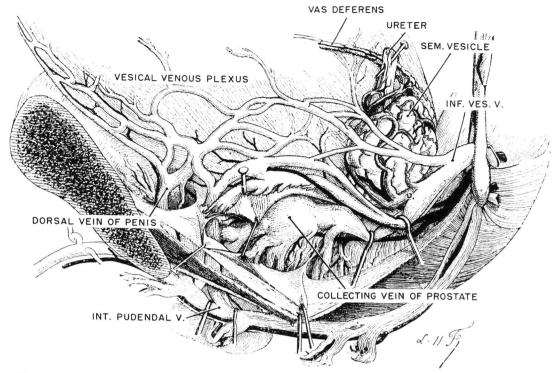

FIG. 177
Veins of the male bladder and pelvic genital organs. (From Farabeuf, 1905.)

with the vertebral system of veins is thought to facilitate distant hematogenous spread of cancer (Chapter 5).

The lymphatics of the anterior part of the bladder extend along the umbilical arteries to external iliac nodes. Those from the posterior part reach external, internal, and common iliac and sacral nodes. The lymphatics of the trigone, as well as those in the prostate and seminal vesicles, pass along the ureters partly through peri-ureteral nodes, thence to external iliac nodes. Some of the trigonal lymphatics pass between the superior and inferior vesical arteries to internal iliac nodes (Parker, 1936). In the female the lymphatics of the lower part of the bladder mingle with those from the cervix and upper vagina (see Chapter 26).

Both sensory and motor (parasympathetic) fibers reach the bladder and prostatic urethra from the second, third, and fourth sacral nerves, through the peri-arterial vesical subsidiaries of the inferior hypogastric plexus. Sympathetic fibers from the presacral nerves and sacral sympathetic chains also pass through these plexuses, but no definite function has been ascribed to them except for the mechanism of ejaculation (see Chapter 6). The role of sensory fibers traveling with the sympathetic nerves is discussed with presacral neurectomy (p. 374). Sensation of the membranous and penile urethra and function of the internal urethral sphincter are subserved by the pudendal nerves. The levator ani muscles, which play a part in continence (see above), receive special branches from the sacral nerves on their superior and from the pudendal nerves on their inferior aspect.

APPROACHES TO THE BLADDER; CYSTECTOMY

The simplest approach to drainage or exploration of the bladder is the suprapubic, staying below the level of peritoneal reflection. The incision in the abdominal wall may be vertical, or low transverse, often with rectus muscle detachment (see Fig. 6). A suprapubic cystotomy is employed, as in one method of prostatectomy for benign disease (see Fig. 188) or for exploration of the interior of the bladder. For procedures on the bladder wall, as for diverticulum or vesico-ureteral reflux, the initial exposure of the anterior wall of the bladder may continue in the extraperitoneal space around the bladder to its sides or base, and to the pelvic ureter. Division of the urachal ligament and some superior vesical arteries may be necessary. The dissection will produce less venous bleeding if one remains outside of the vesical fascia. The connections between the dorsal vein of the penis or clitoris with the vesical venous plexus must be avoided or controlled. Aberrant arterial and venous connections between the vesical and obturator vessels may exist here, and aberrant internal pudendal components from the inferior vesical or other arteries may extend forward in relation to the neck of the bladder (see Fig. 175).

An exposure of the neck of the bladder and of the membranous and posterior urethra may be obtained by excision of the bodies of the pubic bones and the symphysis pubis (Waterhouse et al., 1973), or by division of the upper and lower pubic rami at the medial edges of the obturator foramina (Pierce, 1962). The authors cited did not find it necessary to replace the bone.

Partial cystectomy and plastic repair of the bladder, as

for the removal of a diverticulum, can be readily done by suprapubic exposure. Removal of the bladder neck, either for primary tumor or for involvement by prostatic cancer, may be accomplished by the extension of either the retropubic or the perineal operation as for carcinoma of the prostate, described in Chapter 22.

Total cystectomy for benign disease, or for cancer if lymphadenectomy is not planned, can be performed through suprapubic exposure. Urinary diversion precedes the removal of the bladder. For benign disease in the male, the prostate and seminal vesicles, with their blood supply, are retained, and the vesicourethral junction is divided sufficiently proximal so as not to interfere with the ejaculatory ducts. In the female, the vagina is spared. For benign disease in both sexes, the vesical arteries are divided close to the bladder; this makes for less dissection and does least damage to the nerve plexuses of the pelvic organs. When cystectomy is performed for malignant disease, as much as possible of the cellular tissues about the vesical arteries is taken and the peritoneum on the posterior aspect of the bladder or of the entire pelvis is also removed if there is adjacent tumor.

The steps in cystectomy (Fig. 178) are well described by Leadbetter (1969). In simple cystectomy by the anterior approach, the peritoneum is separated from the bladder, or incised if it is to be removed. Laterally, the branches from the umbilical arteries are divided. In the male the vasa deferentia are divided and the stumps of the ureters are freed toward the bladder. The umbilical arteries are divided close to the internal iliac arteries. Further blunt dissection exposes the posterior ligaments of the bladder containing the inferior vesical neurovascular structures. Division of the ligaments leads to the plane of cleavage between the two layers of the rectovesical septum (see Fig. 191). The lateral extensions of the prostatic fascia to the pelvic fascia—the puboprostatic ligaments—and the dorsal vein of the penis are now all divided. This brings the membranous urethra into view, which, when cut across, frees the specimen. A preliminary perineal stage preceding the abdominal dissection is preferred by some. This resembles a perineal prostatectomy and has as its goal a greater ease of performing the most inferior of the steps in mobilization.

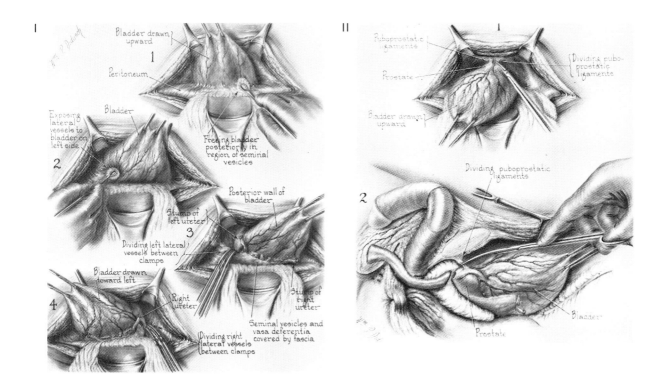

FIG. 178
Total cystectomy without lymphade-nectomy. Abdominal stage after ure-teral diversion, perineal mobiliza-tion of prostate and seminal vesicles, and division of inferior vesical pedi-cles. I. 1, 2. Dissection behind and lateral to bladder. 3, 4. Division of branches from umbilical arteries. II. 1. Division of puboprostatic liga-ments. 2. Same in sagittal view. Note previous perineal mobilization. III. 1. The freed specimen. 2, 3. Drainage and closure. (From Lowsley and Kirwin, 1956.)

In the female with benign disease the vagina and uterus may be left intact. In this case the origin of the uterine artery should be preserved.

Total cystectomy without lymphadenectomy in the female can be performed through the vagina. It was recommended by Marshall and Schnittman (1947), particularly for carcinoma of the urethra, bladder neck, or trigone. An *en bloc* removal is done of the labia minora, the vestibule, the bladder and urethra with the perivesical tissues, and the upper anterior wall of the vagina.

In total cystectomy with lymphadenectomy an *en bloc* removal is performed of the bladder and ureteral stumps, with all the cellular tissue about the bladder—the abdominal vas deferens, the prostate, and seminal vesicles, in the male, the uterus with its adnexa and all, or almost all, of the vagina, in the female; and the lymph nodes and cellular tissue from the iliac vessels to the aortic bifurcation. The dissection of the lymphatics resembles that described in Chapter 5.

The operation may be done entirely from above, ending in the male with division of the membranous urethra. Removal of the entire urethra to the glans penis may be indicated in multicentric urothelial tumors. The urethra is quite easily removed in its entire length from above, by traction and scissor dissection along its wall. In the female all the urethra is removed, but the lower vagina is retained. An additional perineal dissection is desirable in either sex when the tumor is low or when irradiation fibrosis is present. It may be done at the same sitting as the abdominal operation. In the male, the perineal dissection is done first. It resembles that done for a radical prostatovesiculectomy; the membranous urethra is sectioned, and the mobilized prostate and seminal vesicles with their covering fascia are pushed into the pelvis (see Fig. 193). In the female, the perineal stage generally follows the completed mobilization of the organs from above. Additional removal of the rectum completes an exenteration of the pelvis if that is required.

REfERENCES

Begg, R. C.: The urachus: Its anatomy, histology and development. J. Anat. 64:170–183, 1930.

Bennett, A. H.: Exstrophy of bladder treated by ureterosigmoidostomies. Long-term evaluation. Urology 2:165–168, 1973.

Braithwaite, J. L.: The arterial supply of the male urinary bladder. Brit. J. Urol. 24:64–71, 1952.

Campbell, M. F.: Anomalies of the Bladder. Chapter 38 *in* Urology, Campbell, M. F., and Harrison, J. H., Eds., 3rd ed. Vol. 2. Philadelphia, W. B. Saunders, 1970.

Chisholm, T. C.: Exstrophy of the Urinary Bladder. Chapter 73 *in* Pediatric Surgery, Mustard, W. T., Ravitch, M. M., Snyder, W. H., Jr., Welch, K. J., and Benson, C. D., Eds., 2nd ed. Vol. 2. Chicago, Year Book Medical Publishers, 1969.

Darget, R., Ballanger, F., and Odano: La vascularisation de la prostate. Son intérêt chirurgical. J. Urol. (Paris) 63:341–349, 1957.

Didusch, W. P.: A Collection of Urogenital Drawings, New York, American Cystoscope Makers, Inc., 1952.

Farabeuf, L.-H.: Les vaisseaux sanguins des organes génito-urinaires du périnee et du pelvis. Paris, Masson, 1905.

Glenn, J. F., and Boyce, W. H., Eds.: Urologic Surgery. New York, Hoeber Medical Division, Harper & Row, 1969.

Goss, C. M., Ed.: Anatomy of the Human Body, by Henry Gray, 29th American ed. Philadelphia, Lea & Febiger, 1973.

Hendren, W. H.: Ureteral reimplantation in children. J. Pediat. Surg. 3:649–664, 1968.

Hutch, J. A.: A new theory of the anatomy of the internal urinary sphincter and the physiology of micturition. Invest. Urol. 3:36–58, 1965.

Hutch, J. A., and Amar, A. D.: Vesicoureteral Reflux and Pyelonephritis. New York, Appleton-Century-Crofts, 1972.

Kaufman, J. J.: Urethral compression operations for the treatment of post-prostatectomy incontinence. J. Urol. 110:93–96, 1973.

Kelly, H. A., and Burnam, C. F.: Diseases of the Kidneys, Ureters and Bladder, with Special Reference to the Diseases in Women. New York, Appleton, 1914.

Lapides, J., Ajemian, E. P., Stewart, B. H., Breakey, B. A., and Lichtwardt, J. R.: Further observations on the kinetics of the urethrovesical sphincter. J. Urol. 84:86–94, 1960.

Leadbetter, W. F.: Surgery for Malignant Disease of the Bladder. Chapter 8 *in* Glenn and Boyce, *op cit.,* 1969.

Lowsley, O. S., and Kirwin, T. J.: Clinical Urology, 3rd ed. Baltimore, Williams & Wilkins, 1956.

Marshall, V. F., and Schnittman, M.: Vaginal cystectomy. J. Urol. 57:848–857, 1947.

Muellner, S. R., and Fleischner, F. G.: Normal and abnormal micturition: A study of bladder behavior by means of the fluoroscope. J. Urol. 61:233–243, 1949.

Paquin, A. J., Jr.: Surgery of the Ureteropelvic Junction. Chapter 6 *in* Glenn and Boyce, *op cit.,* 1969

Parker, A. E.: The lymph collectors from the urinary bladder and their connections with the main posterior lymph channels of the abdomen. Anat. Rec. 65:443–460, 1936.

Pierce, J. M., Jr.: Exposure of the membranous and posterior urethra by total pubectomy. J. Urol. 88:256–258, 1962.

Scott, R., Jr., and Carlton, C. E., Jr.: Surgery for Benign Disease of the Bladder. Chapter 7 *in* Glenn and Boyce, *op cit.,* 1969.

Smith, M. J. V., and Lattimer, J. K.: The management of bladder exstrophy. Surg. Gynec. Obstet. 123:1015–1018, 1966.

Stephens, F. D., and Smith, E. D.: Ano-Rectal Malformations in Children. Chicago, Year Book Medical Publishers, 1971.

Symington, J.: The Topographical Anatomy of the Child. Edinburgh, Livingstone, 1887.

Talbot, H. S.: Functional disorders of the urinary bladder. New Eng. J. Med. 258:643–648, 1958.

Tanagho, E. A.: Interpretation of the Physiology of Micturition. Chapter 2 *in* Hydrodynamics of Micturition, Hinman, F. A., Jr., Boyarsky, S., Pierce, J. M., Jr., and Zinner, N. R., Eds. Springfield, Charles C Thomas, 1971.

Waterhouse, K., Abrahams, J. I., Gruber, H., Hackett, R. E., Patil, U. B., and Peng, B. K.: The transpubic approach to the lower urinary tract. J. Urol. 109:486–490, 1973.

Woodburne, R. T.: The sphincter mechanism of the urinary bladder and the urethra. Anat. Rec. 141:11–20, 1961.

Woodburne, R. T.: Anatomy of the bladder and bladder outlet. J. Urol. 100:474–487, 1968.

Young, H. H., and Davis, D. M.: Young's Practice of Urology. Philadelphia, W. B. Saunders, 1926.

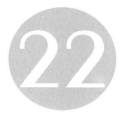

MALE GENITAL ORGANS

THE TESTIS, EPIDIDYMIS, SPERMATIC CORD, AND SCROTUM

From the time of its earliest appearance at the upper lumbar level, the testis projects forward in the primitive peritoneal cavity, the constituents of its pedicle entering the organ from behind. It maintains this relationship throughout its descent. As the testis reaches the iliac fossa it is preceded by the peritoneal diverticulum, known as the processus vaginalis, and guided by the fibrous gubernaculum, which extends from its lower pole through the inguinal canal to the bottom of the scrotal sac (Fig. 179).

The extensions of the body wall about the testis, including the cremaster muscle, constitute the sheaths about the testis and the spermatic cord. After descent the processus is normally obliterated, except for that portion around the testis which remains as the tunica vaginalis (see Chapter 2).

Figure 180 emphasizes some topographical relationships of the testis. Note that the original orientation to its vessels and nerves is maintained, that is, they all enter from behind at the 'mediastinum testis' (Fig. 180 II). The situation is comparable to the attachment of the mesentery, and the mesothelium of the parietal tunica vaginalis continues as a visceral layer on the tunica albuginea, or fibrous capsule. When hydrocele distends the tunica vaginalis, the testis retains its posterior position.

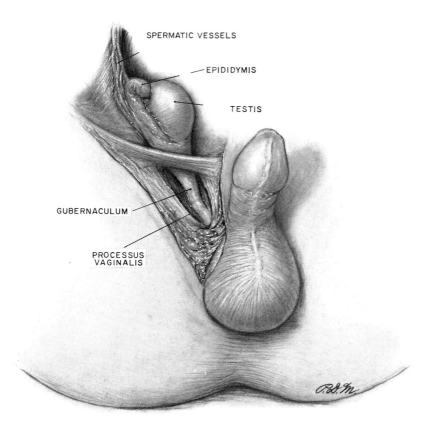

SPERMATIC VESSELS

EPIDIDYMIS

TESTIS

GUBERNACULUM

PROCESSUS
VAGINALIS

FIG. 179
Descent of the testis. Drawn from a fetus approximately 5 months of age.

Undescended testis is the most common developmental anomaly affecting this structure. Ectopia, in which the testis migrates to the superficial fat of the perineum or abdominal wall, is relatively rare, whereas the absence of one or both testes or the presence of a supernumerary testis is extremely rare. Failure of union of the epididymis and testis occurs most often with lack of descent (Gray and Skandalakis, 1972).

Steps in the operation for undescended testis consist of finding the testis, mobilizing it and the cord so that the testis may be brought down into the scrotum without tension, and fixing it within the scrotum to prevent retraction (see Gross, 1953). The testis may be palpable on opening the inguinal canal, but it may lie higher and one may have to explore upward behind the peritoneum. When it lies relatively low a patent processus is frequently present, with a 'congenital' inguinal hernia (see page 38). Wide incision of the transversalis fascia in the posterior wall of the inguinal canal and division of the inferior epigastric vessels allow the mobilized

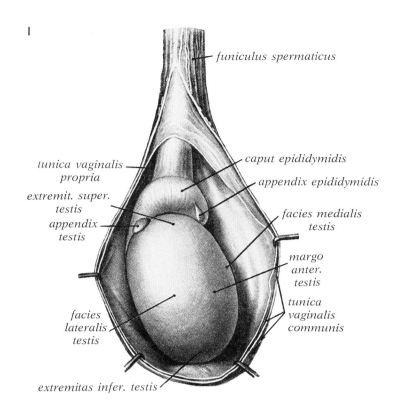

I

funiculus spermaticus

tunica vaginalis
propria

caput epididymidis

appendix epididymidis

extremit. super.
testis

facies medialis
testis

appendix
testis

margo
anter.
testis

tunica
vaginalis
communis

facies
lateralis
testis

extremitas infer. testis

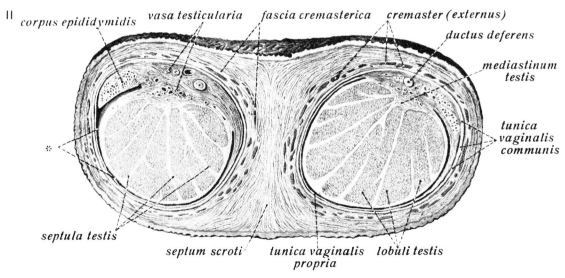

II

corpus epididymidis

vasa testicularia

fascia cremasterica

cremaster (externus)

ductus deferens

mediastinum
testis

tunica
vaginalis
communis

*

septula testis

septum scroti

tunica vaginalis
propria

lobuli testis

FIG. 180

*Topography of the testes. I. Right testis seen from in front. The epididymis lies posterolateral with its head on the upper pole of the testis. II. Cross section of the scrotum and testes. The elements of the cord enter the testis posteriorly, where they lie medial to the epididymis. * (asterisk) = cavity of the tunica vaginalis. (From Sobotta, 1933.)*

spermatic cord to extend downward medially and in a more direct path. The mobilization is done by sectioning the gubernaculum, and then dissecting the connective tissues about the vas deferens into the pelvis and about the neuro-vascular elements of the cord high upward behind the peritoneum. The blood vessels must be preserved. Division of the testicular artery produces an atrophied and useless testis in 85 per cent (Mixter, 1924; Wangensteen, 1927). The scrotum is forcibly dilated with the fingers. The testis is held by a single traction suture through the tunica albuginea at its lower pole, the gubernaculum being too friable. Harrison and Barclay (1948) noted that the branches of the testicular artery are end-arteries. They ramify beneath the tunica albuginea and can be interrupted by deep suturing. The testis is anchored to the septum of the scrotum by the traction suture, or the suture is passed through the scrotum and attached to the thigh.

Within the spermatic cord, the vas is easily identified by palpation as a hard cord 3 or 4 mm. thick. lying posteriorly among the veins. Its artery (Fig. 181) lies alongside the vas and varies from being threadlike to 1 mm. in diameter (Harrison, 1949). Harrison found that the deferential communicates with the testicular artery via the epididymal branch of the latter, at the lower pole of the testis. Only occasionally was the deferential as large as or larger than the testicular, which varied from 0.7 to 1.1 mm. in diameter. The cremasteric artery, a branch of the inferior epigastric, is most variable in size, but always the smallest. While the three arteries communicate with each other, division of the testicular, in the young or old, almost always results in atrophy and occasionally in necrosis of the testis. This has been seen in operations for undescended testis, division of the cord in hernia repair (Chapter 3), or during kidney transplantation (Penn *et al.,* 1972). Hydrocele is also a known complication after surgery involving the cord.

The pampiniform plexus of veins tends to divide into a larger anterior group surrounding the testicular artery and a smaller posterior group (Fig. 181). The invariable left-sidedness of a varicocele, except in situs inversus or consequent to venous obstruction, is thought to be related somehow to the termination of the left testicular vein in the left renal vein. Venous division for varicocele is usually car-

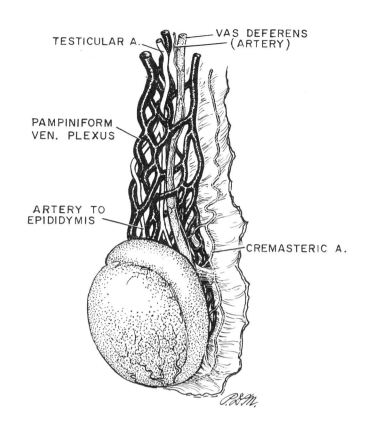

FIG. 181
Arterial supply to the testis.

ried out high in the inguinal canal, where the plexus is reduced to one or two veins. The operation is considered comparable in effect to saphenous division for leg varices. Excision of the varicocele mass is sometimes performed, but the testicular artery should not be divided.

The lymphatics of the testis travel within the spermatic cord and end in the aortic and renal lymph nodes. Resection of the cord and aortic lymphadenectomy often accompany orchiectomy for carcinoma of the testis (see Chapter 5). It is worth noting that the lymphatics of the scrotum and of the penis drain to the inguinal nodes.

Torsion of the testis creates an acute emergency since it involves twisting of the pedicle and may cause hemorrhagic infarction of the testis. It is based on a developmental fault, inadequate fixation, and therefore excessive mobility of the testis within the tunica vaginalis or of the cord and testis together. In the first instance the usual attachment of the posterior border of the testis is more like a free pedicle ('bell-clapper' deformity). In the second, the cord and the coverings of the testis are fixed loosely within the scrotal fascia. Early operative treatment consists of reduction of the torsion and suture fixation to prevent recurrence. Since the fault is bilateral and torsion of the second testis is a frequent occurrence, fixation should be performed on both sides.

THE PENIS AND URETHRA

The components of the penis are shown in Figure 182. Two congenital malformations are known in which the corpus spongiosum is absent or deformed and the enclosure of the urethra is lacking in part or entirely. In the relatively common hypospadias (Fig. 183), the penis is open on its perineal aspect. The penis and scrotum are often additionally malformed. In the rare epispadias (Fig. 184), the penis fails to fuse in its abdominal aspect. The opening may be limited to the urethra alone, or the malformation may be continuous with exstrophy of the bladder (see Chapter 21). Epispadias and hypospadias may affect females in a comparable way.

The arterial supply of the penis through the deep and dorsal arteries stems from the internal pudendal artery. An accessory pudendal artery, often constituting the deep ar-

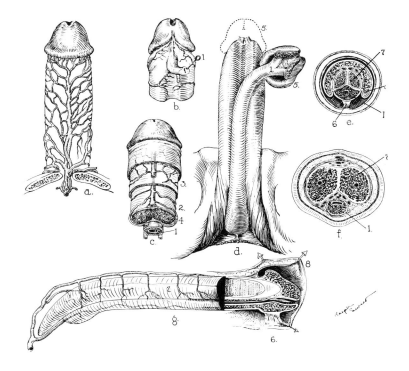

FIG. 182
Elements of the penis. a. The deep dorsal vein, and b, its ventral tributaries: 1, the corpus spongiosum. c. The venous circulation of the penis in cross section: 1, corpus spongiosum and the bulbo-urethral veins; 2, 3, branches of deep dorsal and superficial dorsal veins; 4, branches of veins from the corpus spongiosum. d. Relation of corpus spongiosum (1) and glans (5) to corpora cavernosa. e. Cross section through glans: 1, corpus spongiosum; 5, lateral lip of glans; 6, frenulum of prepuce; 7, corpus cavernosum. f. Cross section through middle of penis: 1, corpus spongiosum; 7, corpus cavernosum. g. Distribution of dorsal and deep arteries: 6, frenulum of prepuce; 8, the prepuce. (From Hinman, 1935.)

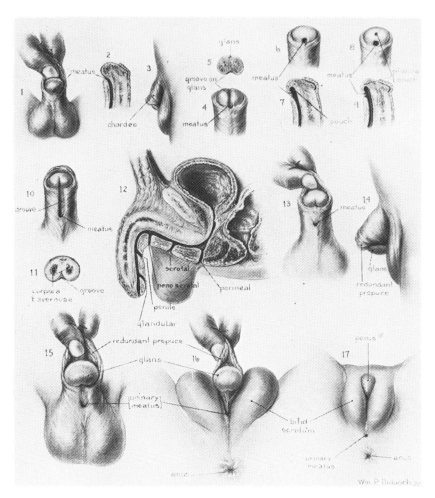

FIG. 183

Hypospadias of various grades in the male, from the simplest, or glandular, type (1, 2, 3), to the perineal type (17). 12. A composite of different grades. (From Lowsley and Kirwin, 1956.)

tery to the penis, may arise independently from the internal iliac or obturator artery and course on the upper surface of the pelvic diaphragm and beneath the pubic arch (see Fig. 175).

The two corpora cavernosa are said to possess good intercommunications through the intervals of the penile septum. In the treatment of priapism, Grayhack and his colleagues (1964) thus used a saphenous vein shunt placed to one of the corpora. They visualized the cavernous spaces by angiography, filling both corpora from a single right-sided injection; the corpus spongiosum did not fill. Schmidt (1971) proposed and used an internal shunt made between the involved corpus cavernosus and the uninvolved corpus spongiosum.

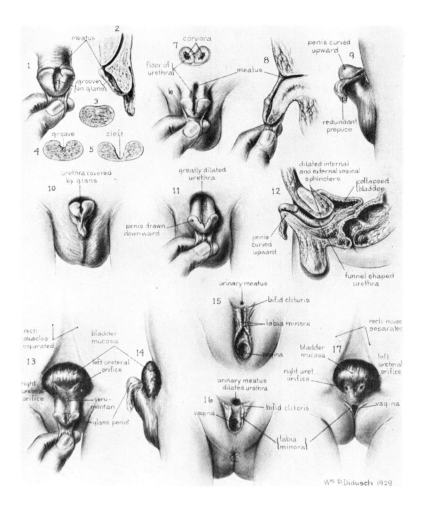

FIG. 184

Epispadias of various grades in the male and female. 1 to 5. Glandular epispadias in the male, the rarest and mildest form. 6 to 12. Penile epispadias: without incontinence (6 to 9); with incontinence (10 to 12). 13, 14. Complete epispadias with exstrophy of the bladder. 15 to 17. Epispadias in the female: without exstrophy of the bladder (15, 16); with exstrophy (17). (From Lowsley and Kirwin, 1956.)

The lymphatics of the penis travel to the superficial and deep inguinal nodes. Carcinoma of the penis may be treated by partial penectomy and radiotherapy, or by *en bloc* resection of the penis and subcutaneous fat and lymph nodes from one inguinal region to the other, including the fat of the suprapubic and suprainguinal areas. As with other groin dissections, the lymphadenectomy may be extended to the iliac region (see Chapter 5).

Rupture of the urethra may occur in any of its divisions. When it occurs close to the apex of the prostate, the resulting hemorrhage and urinary extravasation extend extraperitoneally. Rupture of the membranous urethra generally involves perforation of the inferior layer of the urogenital diaphragm. In this case the extravasation extends beneath the superficial fascia of the perineum, scrotum, and lower abdominal wall. It is initially prevented from extending to the posterior perineum or the thighs by the attachment of the fascia (Colles' fascia) to the posterior edge of the urogenital diaphragm and to the ischiopubic rami (but not to the front of the pubes). The extravasation takes the same pathway after rupture of the penile urethra once the deep fascia of the penis (Buck's fascia) is perforated, initially or by the resulting infection. However, as Tobin and Benjamin (1949) emphasize, infection can spread within the superficial fascia into other regions, no matter where this fascia is attached deeply. Urine and the infection also tend to follow along vessels and nerves into deeper territories of the abdominal wall or into the ischiorectal fossae, or along the spermatic cord.

Exposure of the membranous urethra is usually made through an incision like that for the initial steps of perineal prostatectomy (see below). The membranous urethra and bladder may be simultaneously exposed by section of the pubic bones (p. 325). The penile urethra may be exposed by incision over the perineal surface of the penis through the corpus spongiosum.

THE PROSTATE: RESECTIONS FOR BENIGN HYPERPLASIA AND FOR CARCINOMA

The blood and lymphatic vessels of the prostate and seminal vesicles are intimately connected with those of the bladder, as described in Chapter 21 and shown in Figure 185. The distribution of arteries within the gland is particularly pertinent to transurethral resection. Flocks (1937) and Clegg (1955) demonstrated that the two to five prostatic arteries divide into capsular and urethral groups. The capsular arteries penetrate the prostate to be distributed mainly to the outer zone containing the main prostatic glands (Fig. 186). The urethral group of arteries pass through each side of the bladder neck at about the positions of 7 to 11 o'clock on the left and 1 to 5 o'clock on the right, as the urethra is viewed through the cystoscope. They turn distally beneath the mucosa to supply the mucosal and submucosal glands located in the internal zone of the prostate, and therefore supply the mass constituting

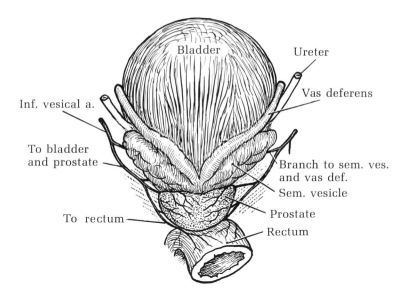

FIG. 185
Posterior view of distribution of inferior vesical arteries in the male. The origin of the deferential artery from the inferior vesical is exceptional. (From Albarran, 1909.)

hyperplasia (Fig. 187) and the mucosa itself short of the colliculus (verumontanum).

The prostate is described as consisting of five lobes: two lateral lobes, the anterior lobe in the ventral midline, the middle lobe in the posterior midline above the passage of

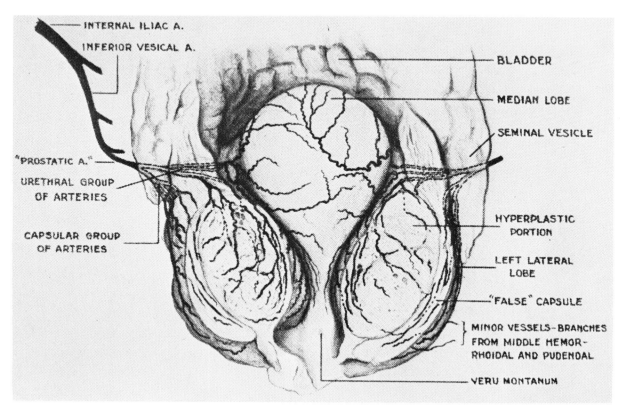

FIG. 186
Distribution of the prostatic arteries. (From Flocks, 1937.)

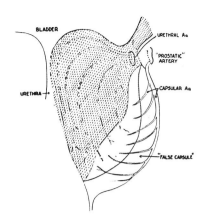

FIG. 187
The arterial supply from the urethral arteries to hyperplastic tissue of the prostate. The hyperplastic tissue is stippled. Note the compression of the outer zone to form the 'false capsule.' (From Flocks, R. H., in Nesbit, R. M.: Transurethral Prostatectomy, 1943. Courtesy of Charles C Thomas, Publisher, Springfield, Illinois.)

the ejaculatory ducts, and the posterior lobe below the ducts. Hyperplasia originates in the inner zone of glands in any of these lobes except the posterior, which is a site of predilection for carcinoma (Young and Davis, 1926). The enlarging mass of hyperplasia compresses the outer zone of the prostate into a 'false capsule.' Transurethral resection is most often performed for benign hyperplasia. Making the initial electrosurgical cuts at the bladder neck interrupts the urethral group of arteries proximal to their longitudinal course, and renders avascular large distal masses of the gland. The dissection seeks to remove enough gland to lay bare the circular muscle of the bladder neck, and the false capsule distally (Flocks, 1937; Nesbit, 1943; Baumrucker, 1968). Moderate bleeding may be seen from the interruption of terminal twigs of the capsular arteries.

Suprapubic prostatectomy (Fig. 188) and the retropubic

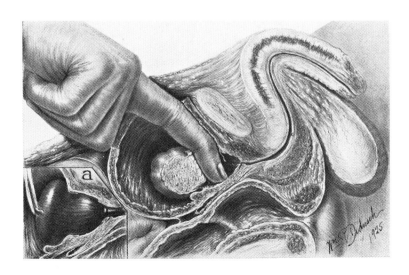

FIG. 188
Suprapubic prostatectomy. (From Young and Davis, 1926.)

operation devised by Millin (1947) (Fig. 189) both enucleate the mass of hyperplastic tissue from the surrounding false capsule. In the suprapubic operation the bladder is entered and the prostate approached from above. In the retropubic procedure, the incision is made directly through the anterior part of the capsule of the prostate itself. In both procedures the mucosa of the prostatic urethra is re-formed mainly through mucosal regeneration.

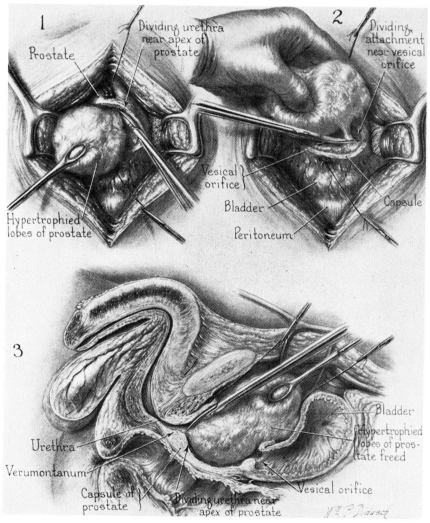

FIG. 189

Retropubic prostatectomy for benign disease. 1. The anterior wall of the prostate has been incised; the distal prostatic urethra is being divided. The hypertrophied part of the gland has been freed by blunt dissection. 2. One adherent part is being divided. 3. The division of the prostatic urethra distally is located. The initial freeing of the prostatic mass has involved breaking through the mucous membrane just distal to the internal meatus (vesical orifice). After removal of the specimen, the mucous membrane will be tacked down, and the anterior incision closed over an in-dwelling catheter. (From Lowsley and Gentile, 1948.)

Carcinoma of the prostate spreads by contiguous growth, notably to the seminal vesicles, and by lymphatic and venous extension. Transurethral or suprapubic prostatectomy can only be palliative when the lesion is malignant. The retropubic approach is, however, adaptable for both benign and malignant lesions, and the same is true of the perineal approach. When used for carcinoma the prostatectomy is termed radical, and is extended to remove the entire prostate as well as the seminal vesicles, with or without their investing fascia—the anterior layer of the rectovesical septum. Partial cystectomy may be included in either operation if the tumor is found growing into the bladder neck. The lymphatic pathway is essentially the same as from growths in the lower bladder, and lymphadenectomy is much the same as for cancer of the bladder or the cervix; that is, by removal of lymph-bearing tissue from the pelvic floor and along the iliac vessels (see Chapters 5, 26). Lymphadenectomy can accompany the retropubic radical prostatectomy, or it can be done separately if the perineal operation is performed.

Retropubic prostatovesiculectomy is shown in Figure 190. It differs in several ways from the procedure for benign hyperplasia. The dorsal vein of the penis and the puboprostatic ligaments are divided, and then the membranous urethra. Further dissection stays anterior to the rectovesical septum. This mobilizes the entire prostate, the seminal vesicles, and the lower bladder. The bladder is sectioned proximally, either just above the base of the prostate or higher, if some of the trigone is involved. In that event a bladder neck is reconstructed prior to anastomosis to the urethra.

The perineal relations of the prostate, its investment by the rectovesical septum (Denonvilliers) (Figs. 191, 192), and the position of the inferior vesical arteries (see Fig. 185) are pertinent to the performance of perineal prostatectomy (Young and Davis, 1926).

The steps in radical perineal prostatectomy and subtotal cystectomy in a case of carcinoma of the trigone are shown in Figure 193. Note that the mobilization of the bladder is adequate to permit transplantation of the ureter in the reconstructed bladder, prior to its anastomosis to the urethra. Perineal prostatectomy for benign disease is begun in the same way, but the prostate, once presented to the incision with the aid of a tractor introduced through the penis, and

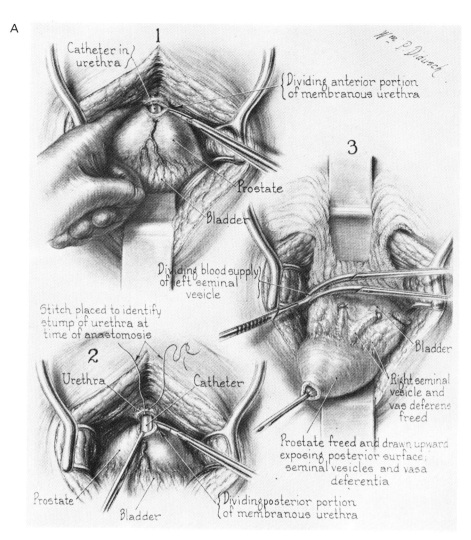

FIG. 190

Radical retropubic prostatovesiculectomy and partial cystectomy for cancer of the prostate.

A. 1. The dorsal vein of the penis and the puboprostatic ligaments have been divided. Division of the membranous urethra. The finger protects the rectum.   2. Completion of division of the urethra.   3. Posterior mobilization.

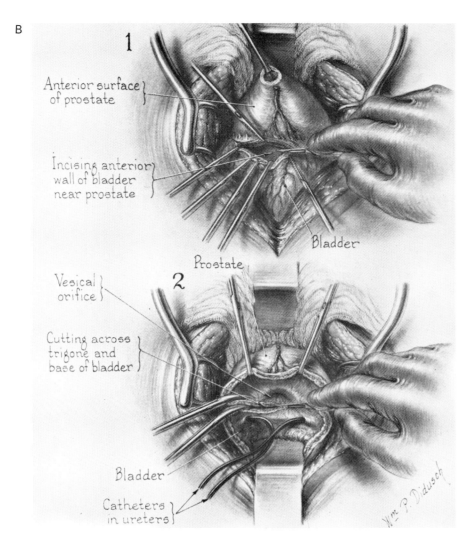

B

1

Anterior surface of prostate

Incising anterior wall of bladder near prostate

Bladder

Prostate

2

Vesical orifice

Cutting across trigone and base of bladder

Bladder

Catheters in ureters

Wm. P. Didusch

FIG. 190
Radical retropubic prostatovesiculectomy and partial cystectomy for cancer of the prostate (continued).
    B. 1. Bladder incised anteriorly.   2. Incision of bladder posteriorly completes freeing of the specimen. Anastomosis will be made between residual bladder and the membranous urethra. (From Memmelaar, 1949.)

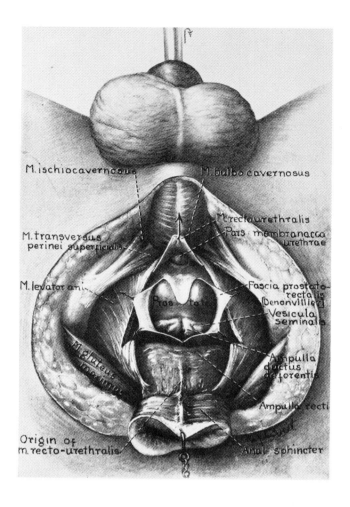

M.ischiocavernosus
M.bulbocavernosus

M.rectourethralis
Pars membranacca urethrae

M.transversus perinei superficialis

Fascia prostato-rectalis (Denonvillier)

M.levator ani

Vesicula seminalis

Prostata

M.gluteus maximus

Ampulla ductus deferentis

Ampulla recti

Origin of m.recto-urethralis

Anal sphincter

FIG. 191

Fascias about the perineal organs. The ischiorectal fat and the superficial fascia of the region have been removed. The central tendon of the perineum and the rectourethralis muscle have been divided, allowing posterior retraction of the rectum, whose thin rectal fascia (posterior layer of rectovesical septum) has been cut from the prostatic apex. The membranous urethra is exposed through the urogenital diaphragm, the inferior layer of which is retracted anteriorly.

The prostate and seminal vesicles are seen through the window in the shiny white anterior layer of the rectovesical septum. These structures are brought into good view by the intraurethral prostatic tractor introduced through the penis. (From Anson and McVay, 1971.)

exposed by a window in the anterior layer of the rectovesical septum, is then simply incised and the hyperplastic masses removed from within the false capsule.

Transsacral removal of the prostate is not widely practiced, but the approach is said to give better access for determining the extent of a carcinoma in the vicinity of the seminal vesicles, and for the urethral reconstruction, than that offered by the standard perineal approach (Parry and Dawson, 1969). The patient is placed prone. The perineal dissection involves removal of the coccyx, and of the sacrum below the sacral hiatus. One levator ani muscle is partially divided to allow lateral retraction of the anorectum, which is usually mobilized by separating the two layers of the rectovesical septum, as in Figure 192.

FIG. 192

The rectovesical septum (Denonvilliers) in sagittal section. Three surgical pathways are indicated. 1. A little-used pathway between the posterior layer and the rectal wall. It carries the danger of perforation of the rectum. 2. The early stage in the Young approach between the heavy anterior and the thinner posterior (rectal) layer of the septum. 3. The subsequent pathway through the anterior layer, used for benign and most often for malignant disease of the prostate. Note the attachment of the anterior layer to the peritoneum above, and the attachment of both layers to the apex of the prostate and urogenital diaphragm below. (From Tobin and Benjamin, 1945. By permission of Surgery, Gynecology & Obstetrics.)

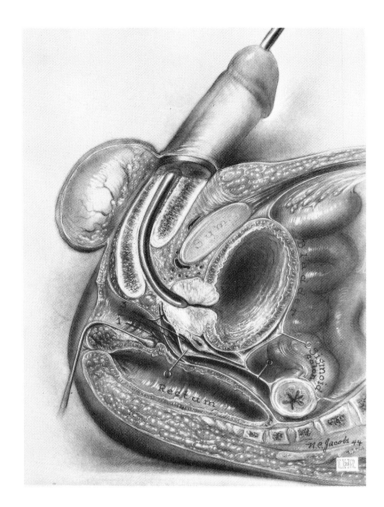

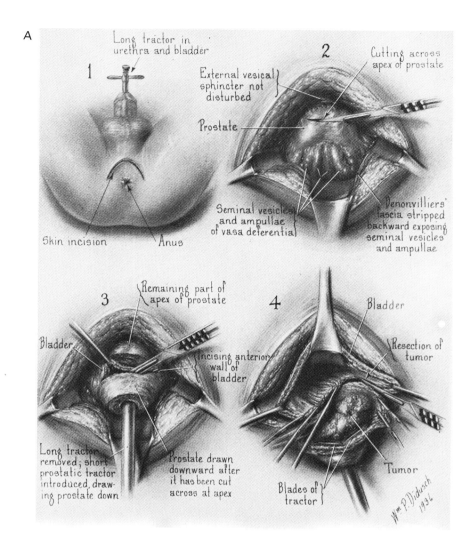

FIG. 193

Steps in radical perineal prostatovesiculectomy and partial cystectomy for carcinoma of the bladder trigone.

A. Excision. 1. Skin incision, long prostatic tractor introduced. 2. The prostate and seminal vesicles exposed; the anterior layer of rectovesical fascia displaced; incision across distal prostate. 3. Traction on prostate allows section through anterior wall of bladder, then, 4, through trigone proximal to tumor, which has involved orifice of left ureter.

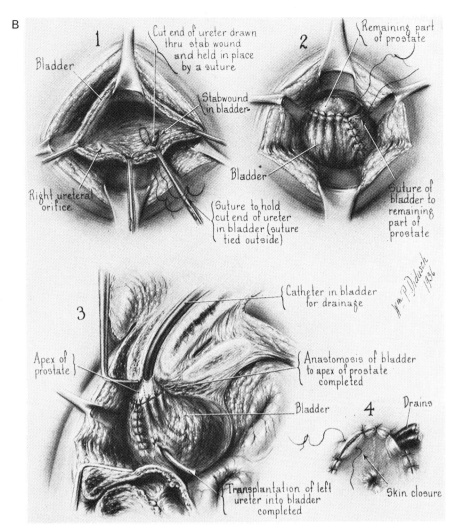

FIG. 193

Steps in radical perineal prostatovesiculectomy and partial cystectomy for carcinoma of the bladder trigone (continued).

B. Reconstruction. 1. Implantation of left ureter. 2,3. Reconstruction of the bladder and its anastomosis to the urethra. 4. Skin closure. (From Shaw, 1937.)

REFERENCES

Albarran, J.: Médicine opérataire des voies urinaires. Paris, Masson, 1909.

Anson, B. J., and McVay, C. B.: Surgical Anatomy, 5th ed. Philadelphia, W. B. Saunders, 1971.

Baumrucker, G. O.: Transurethral Prostatectomy. Technique, Hazards, and Pitfalls. Baltimore, Williams & Wilkins, 1968.

Clegg, E. J.: The arterial supply of the human prostate and seminal vesicles. J. Anat. 89:209–216, 1955.

Flocks, R. H.: The arterial distribution within the prostate gland. Its role in transurethral prostatic resection. J. Urol. 37:524–548, 1937.

Flocks, R. H.: Arterial Distribution within the Prostate Gland: Its Role in Transurethral Prostatic Resection. Chapter 1 in Transurethral Prostatectomy, Nesbit, R. M. Springfield, Charles C Thomas, 1943.

Gray, S. W., and Skandalakis, J. E.: Embryology for Surgeons. The Embryological Basis for the Treatment of Congenital Defects. Philadelphia, W. B. Saunders, 1972.

Grayhack, J. T., McCullough, W., O'Conor, V. J., Jr., and Trippel, O.: Venous bypass to control priapism. Invest. Urol. 1:509–513, 1964.

Gross, R. E.: The Surgery of Infancy and Childhood. Its Principles and Techniques. Philadelphia, W. B. Saunders, 1953.

Gross, R. E.: An Atlas of Children's Surgery. Philadelphia, W. B. Saunders, 1970.

Harrison, R. G.: The distribution of the vasal and cremasteric arteries to the testis and their functional importance. J. Anat. 83:267–282, 1949.

Harrison, R. G., and Barclay, A. E.: The distribution of the testicular artery (internal spermatic artery) to the human testis. Brit. J. Urol. 20:57–66, 1948.

Hinman, F.: The Principles and Practice of Urology. Philadelphia, W. B. Saunders, 1935.

Lowsley, O. S., and Gentile, A.: Retropubic prostatectomy. J. Urol. 59:281–296, 1948.

Lowsley, O. S., and Kirwin, T. J.: Clinical Urology, 3rd ed. Baltimore, Williams & Wilkins, 1956.

Memmelaar, J.: Total prostatovesiculectomy—retropubic approach. J. Urol. 62:340–348, 1949.

Millin, T.: Retropubic Urinary Surgery. Edinburgh, Livinstone, 1947.

Mixter, C. G.: Undescended testicle. Operative treatment and end-results. Surg. Gynec. Obstet. 39:275–282, 1924.

Nesbit, R. M.: Transurethral Prostatectomy. Springfield, Charles C Thomas, 1943.

Parry, W. L., and Dawson, C. B.: Surgery for Malignant Disease of the Prostate. Chapter 10 in Urologic Surgery, Glenn, J. F., and Boyce, W. H., Eds. New York, Hoeber Medical Division, Harper & Row, 1969.

Penn, I., Mackie, G., Halgrimson, C. G., and Starzl, T. E.: Testicular complications following renal transplantation. Ann. Surg. 176:697–699, 1972.

Schmidt, J. D.: Intracorporal shunt procedure for priapism. Arch. Surg. 103:409–410, 1971.

Shaw, E. C.: Perineal and vaginal cystectomy with transplantation of the ureters. J. Urol. 37:850–857, 1937.

Sobotta, J.: Atlas of Human Anatomy. Translated by McMurrich, J. P. Vol. II. The Viscera Including the Heart, 3rd English ed. New York, Stechert, 1933.

Tobin, C. E., and Benjamin, J. A.: Anatomical and surgical restudy of Denonvilliers' fascia. Surg. Gynec. Obstet. 80:373–388, 1945.

Tobin, C. E., and Benjamin, J. A.: Anatomic and clinical re-evaluation of Camper's, Scarpa's, and Colles' fasciae. Surg. Gynec. Obstet. 88:545–559, 1949.

Wangensteen, O. H.: The undescended testis. An experimental and clinical study. Arch. Surg. 14:663–731, 1927.

Young, H. H., and Davis, D. M.: Young's Practice of Urology, Philadelphia, W. B. Saunders, 1926.

SECTION 7
FEMALE PELVIS AND PERINEUM

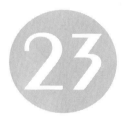

pelvic support;
perineum; displacements

STRUCTURES CREATING PELVIC SUPPORT

The pelvic organs rest on the pelvic and urogenital dia-phragms. Each diaphragm consists of muscle clothed by fascia above and below. The levator ani muscles of the pelvic diaphragm extend across the pelvic outlet from side to side (Fig. 194). The potential gap between the two muscles anteriorly is compensated for by the urogenital diaphragm, whose upper fascia is the same as that of the pelvic dia-phragm, that is, the pelvic fascia (Fig. 195). The muscles and inferior fascia of the urogenital diaphragm are located on a plane inferior to that of the muscles and inferior fascia of the pelvic diaphragm (see Figs. 197, 198).

Superior to the pelvic and urogenital diaphragms lie peritoneal and subperitoneal ligaments which are of addi-tional significance in maintaining pelvic support (Fig. 196). Normal anteversion of the uterus is maintained by the for-ward pull on the fundus of the round ligaments and the backward pull on the cervix of the uterosacral ligaments. The uterus is canted forward on the pelvic floor, preventing its being pushed downward through the vagina, as occurs when the long axes of these two organs are identical (see Fig. 201).

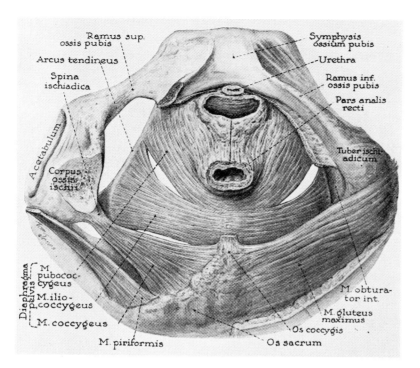

Labels on figure:
Ramus sup. ossis pubis
Arcus tendineus
Spina ischiadica
Acetabulum
Corpus ossis ischii
Diaphragma pelvis
M. pubococcygeus
M. iliococcygeus
M. coccygeus
M. piriformis
Symphysis ossium pubis
Urethra
Ramus inf. ossis pubis
Pars analis recti
Tuber ischiadicum
M. obturator int.
M. gluteus maximus
Os coccygis
Os sacrum

FIG. 194

Levator ani muscles from below. The three constituent portions are seen, the pubococcygeus and coccygeus extending from bony origins, the iliococcygeus from the arcus tendineus. They blend medially with the walls of the urethra, vagina, and rectum, as indicated. The urogenital diaphragm has been removed; a portion remains attached to the left conjoined rami of pubis and ischium. (From Curtis et al., 1942. By permission of Surgery, Gynecology & Obstetrics.)

The positions of the uterine artery and the ureter within the parametrium are shown in Figure 196 II. Wider relationships of the pelvic blood vessels and the ureter are displayed in Figure 39.

CONSTITUENTS OF THE PERINEUM

The superficial fascia of the perineum possesses a deep membranous layer (Colles). On its removal the anal and urogenital triangles are disclosed, divided by the two superficial transverse perineal muscles, meeting at the central point of the perineum (Figs. 197, 198).

The distribution of the internal pudendal artery and of the pudendal nerve to the female perineum are shown in Figure 198. The venous drainage of the perineum is partly through the venae comitantes of the internal pudendal artery, and partly through the deep dorsal vein of the clitoris. This vein passes behind the arcuate ligament of the symphysis pubis and anterior to the urogenital diaphragm to end in

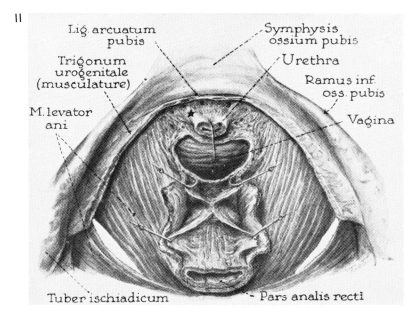

FIG. 195

Pelvic fascia in the female. I. Seen from above, there is continuity of transversalis, iliac, and obturator fascias and the superior fascia of the pelvic diaphragm, all parts of the continuous endoabdominal fascia (see Fig. 2). The fascia of the pelvic diaphragm covers the upper surface of the levator ani muscles, and the urogenital diaphragm. It continues medially as the visceral fascias of the rectum, uterus, vagina, and bladder and urethra. The pelvic fascia is pierced behind the arcuate ligament by the deep dorsal vein of the clitoris. (From Curtis et al., 1939. By permission of Surgery, Gynecology & Obstetrics.) II. Below, the visceral fascia blends with the walls of the tubular organs, but vaginal and anal fascias can be created by sharp dissection. Most of the fascia on the levator ani muscles has been removed. The small portion on the medial edges of the muscles lifted by the anterior hooks is part of the pubocervical or vesicovaginal ligaments, or pillars of the bladder (puboprostatic ligaments in the male). The star indicates special fibers to the urethra from the levator ani muscle, similar to those which extend to the vagina and anal canal. (From Curtis et al., 1942. By permission of Surgery, Gynecology & Obstetrics.)

the venous plexus about the base of the bladder (prostatic plexus in the male) (see Fig. 177).

The sensory supply of the perineum and pelvis is considered in Chapter 24, and the lymphatics of the region are considered in Chapter 26.

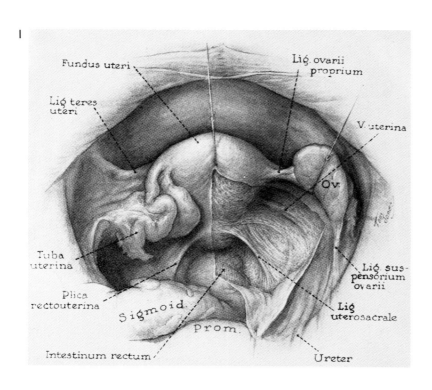

I

Fundus uteri

Lig. ovarii proprium

Lig. teres uteri

V. uterina

Ov.

Tuba uterina

Plica rectouterina

Lig. suspensorium ovarii

Sigmoid.

Lig. uterosacrale

Prom.

Intestinum rectum

Ureter

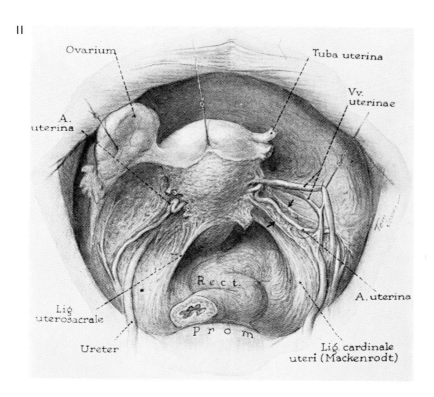

II

Ovarium

Tuba uterina

Vv. uterinae

A. uterina

Lig. uterosacrale

Rect.

Prom.

Ureter

A. uterina

Lig. cardinale uteri (Mackenrodt)

FIG. 196
Peritoneal and subperitoneal ligaments of the female pelvis. In I the peritoneum has been removed from the right parametrial tissues. II shows the structures within the broad ligament. The thickened part beneath the uterine vessels is the cardinal ligament, continuous posteriorly with the uterosacral ligament. (From Curtis et al., 1940. By permission of Surgery, Gynecology & Obstetrics.)

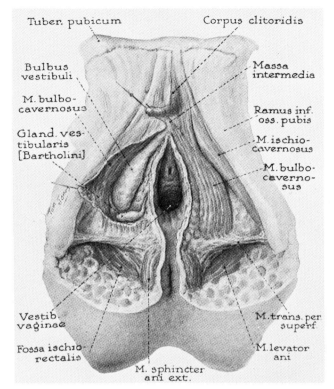

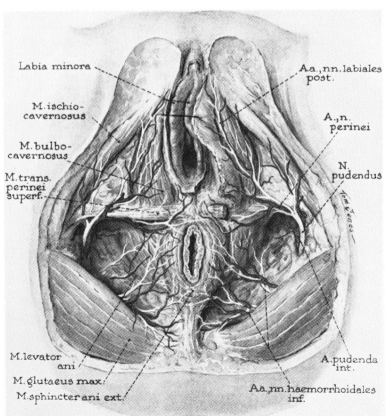

FIG. 197
Perineal structures in the female. On the subject's left side the superficial perineal pouch has been opened by removing the superficial fascia including its deep stratum of Colles' fascia. On the subject's right, the deep perineal compartment has been opened by partial reflection of the bulbocavernosus muscle and the inferior fascia of the urogenital diaphragm. (From Curtis et al., 1942. By permission of Surgery, Gynecology & Obstetrics.)

FIG. 198
Arteries and nerves of the perineum in the female. The dorsal artery and nerve to the clitoris lie in the deep compartment and are not here displayed. (From Curtis and Huffman, 1950.)

EPISIOTOMY; REPAIR OF ANAL SPHINCTER

Episiotomy is done during obstetrical delivery to avoid excessive perineal stretching or laceration. Figure 199 A shows the perineal and levator musculature during delivery. In median episiotomy, the incision is made in the posterior midline of the lower vagina and through the central point of the perineum. It offers a little increase in size of the outlet of the birth canal. Its danger lies in its possible extension by laceration into the sphincter ani muscle. After delivery, there is an ample view into the incision, facilitating repair (Fig. 199 B). The pubococcygeus muscle, covered by its ensheathing fascia, can be felt on each side. The two muscles can be sutured together to offset any perineal attenuation caused by the delivery. If the sphincter ani muscle has been torn, its two retracted ends must be sought and brought together (Fig. 200).

A mediolateral episiotomy creates more room and safeguards the sphincter ani muscle. It passes through the stretched bulbocavernosus and transverse perineal muscles, and some of the levator ani. Repair of the levator ani is aided by its ensheathment of fascia. The divided perineal muscles are not separately identified, these structures and their fascia being sutured as a single layer (Fig. 199 C).

NATURE OF POSTPARTUM DISPLACEMENTS; STRESS INCONTINENCE

Childbirth may give rise to considerable relaxation of pelvic and perineal supports, sometimes augmented by gross laceration of the perineum. The commonest manifestations are cystocele (with or without urethrocele) and rectocele. Each presents as a bulging through the vagina (Fig. 201). Enterocele, a less common lesion, is a herniation of bowel through the rectouterine pouch (of Douglas). An enterocele is usually accompanied by a rectocele, but the higher bulge it causes is separated from the rectocele by a usually discernible groove. It is usually based on the presence of a deep rectouterine pouch.

Stress incontinence is a frequent accompaniment of cystocele. It may be useful to consider this problem before

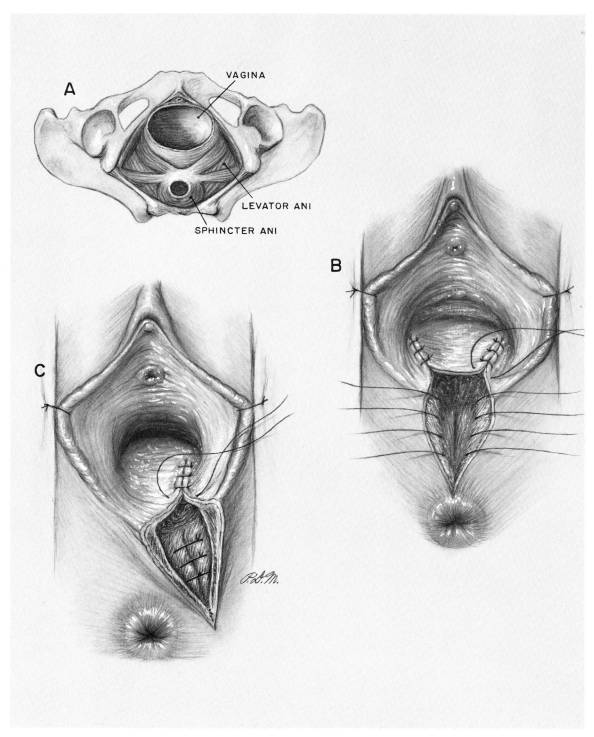

FIG. 199

Parturient perineum: Episiotomy and repair. A. Musculature of the pelvic floor in parturition, distended by the presenting part of the fetus. B. Repair of perineal laceration and of median episiotomy. The pubococcygeus muscles, covered by their fascia, are to be approximated by sutures. C. Repair of mediolateral episiotomy. The divided levator ani muscle has been sutured. The vaginal wall and perineum await repair. (A after Bumm, 1908.)

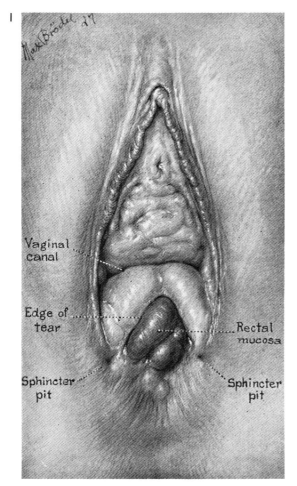

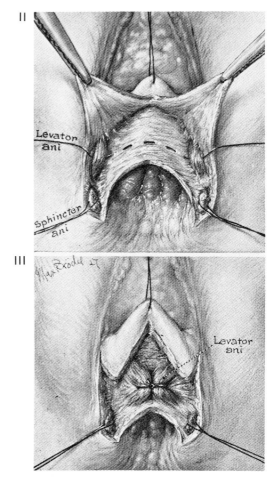

Fig. 200
Late repair of third-degree perineal laceration. I. Preoperative condition. II. Delineation of levator ani muscles and the ends of the torn external anal sphincter. III. Suture of levator ani muscles. The external sphincter awaits approximation. (From Kelly, 1952.)

going on to other aspects of deficiencies of pelvic support. Stress incontinence is based on inadequacy of the pubococcygeus muscles and associated fascias behind the urethrovesical junction (see Chapter 21). The lesion is classified as type I when the widening of the posterior urethrovesical angle is the major change seen in the lateral cystourethrogram (Fig. 202). It is classified as type II when the pelvic relaxation is more severe, and the bladder neck and proximal urethra have fallen away from the pubis, in addition to the loss of the posterior urethrovesical angle.

Operative repair of type I stress incontinence usually consists of restoration of the urethrovesical angle by suturing

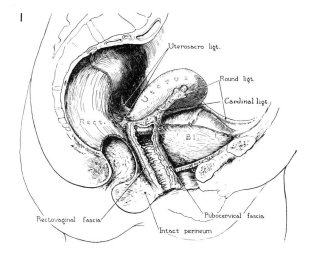

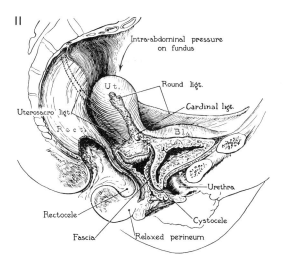

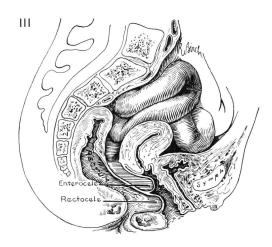

FIG. 201

Topography of cystocele, rectocele, and en-
terocele in sagittal section. I. Normal pel-
vis. II. Cystocele, rectocele, and uterine ret-
roversion and prolapse. III. Relationship of
enterocele to rectocele. (From Te Linde and
Mattingly, 1970.)

the pubocervical fascia and nearby perineal tissues across
the posterior aspect of the angle, in performing cystocele
repair (see Fig. 206). Kelly (1913) first proposed this, calling
it a plication of the urethral sphincter, which is partly true.
He advised an exposure through a short longitudinal incision
in the anterior vaginal wall centered on the bladder neck.
He identified the bladder neck by tugging on a previously
introduced urethral catheter with a 'mushroom tip' (now a
balloon type, as in Fig. 205). The vagina is ''dissected away
for a distance of 2 to 2.5 cm. around the neck of the bladder. . . . The finger should be able to grasp at least one half
or two thirds of the neck of the bladder, including the contiguous urethra.'' Kennedy (1937) advised greater mobilization to free the urethra from distortion by scar, and allow

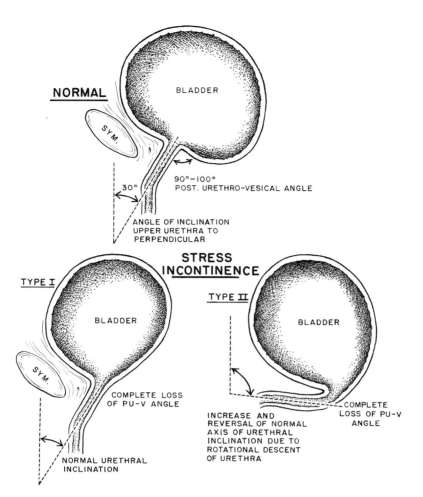

NORMAL

BLADDER

SYM.

90°–100°
POST. URETHRO-VESICAL ANGLE

30°

ANGLE OF INCLINATION
UPPER URETHRA TO
PERPENDICULAR

**STRESS
INCONTINENCE**

TYPE I

BLADDER

SYM.

COMPLETE LOSS
OF PU-V ANGLE

NORMAL URETHRAL
INCLINATION

TYPE II

BLADDER

COMPLETE
LOSS OF PU-V
ANGLE

INCREASE AND
REVERSAL OF NORMAL
AXIS OF URETHRAL
INCLINATION DUE TO
ROTATIONAL DESCENT
OF URETHRA

FIG. 202
*Urethrovesical relationships in stress
incontinence as seen by cystou-
rethrography. (After Green, 1971.)*

better placement of sutures. ''By a blunt dissection, the
urethra is separated from the median posterior margin of the
ramus . . . and the separation carried into the paravesical
space. . . . Sometimes in this separation, one may encoun-
ter a branch of the inferior vesical artery which is usually
on the bladder and should be ligated.'' Furniss (1937) reported injuring a ureter in the deep dissection.

Green (1971) advises that one should try to produce a
posterior urethrovesical angle of 90 degrees. If one pays no
attention to the angle and simply elevates the bladder in the
cystocele repair, the angle may be further widened and incontinence produced or made worse. If prolapse of the
uterus is a prominent feature in the case, vaginal hysterectomy is generally added (see Fig. 217). The operation of
cardinal ligament fixation (Manchester-Fothergill operation)

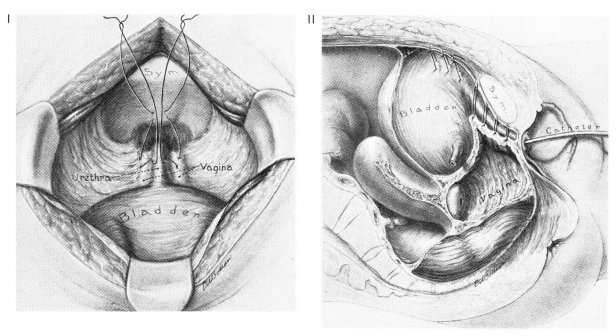

FIG. 203

Suprapubic suspension of bladder neck and urethra. I. Initial sutures. II. Parasagittal view of completed procedure. (*From Te Linde and Mattingly, 1970, after Marshall* et al., *1949.*)

is occasionally done when there is elongation of the cervix and moderate uterine prolapse (see Fig. 208).

In type II stress incontinence suspension of the bladder neck and proximal urethra is often performed from above— the Marshall-Marchetti-Krantz operation, as reported by Marshall and his colleagues (1949) (Fig. 203).

Finally, when previous surgical attempts have failed, a suprapubic suspension of the urethrovesical angle by a sling of fascia lata or other material may be performed (Fig. 204).

OPERATIONS FOR DEFICIENCIES OF PELVIC SUPPORT

Operations done for weakness of the pelvic floor include anterior and posterior colporrhaphy, with correction of cystocele and rectocele (Figs. 205–208). The dissection is first carried immediately beneath the mucous membrane of the vagina, in order to avoid the large veins lying deep to the vaginal fascia.

In performing anterior colporrhaphy, once the mucous

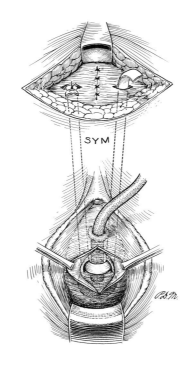

SYM

FIG. 204
Suprapubic sling suspension of ure-
throvesical junction. (From Copen-
haver, 1960.)

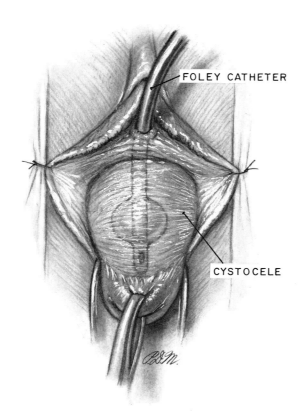

FOLEY CATHETER

CYSTOCELE

FIG. 205
Relationship of cystocele to cervix
and vagina. The balloon-tipped cath-
eter within the bladder indicates the
limits of this organ.

membrane has been dissected to each side, the bladder is separated from the uterovaginal fascia by blunt and some sharp dissection to a level which will allow the cystocele to be elevated, and the urethrovesical junction to be identified (Figs. 205, 206). Pulling the uterus backward tenses the pubocervical fascia on each side—the so-called bladder pillars. This fascia is the deepest layer available for reposi-

I

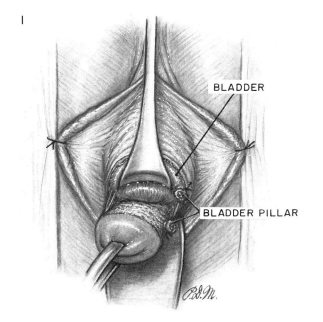

II

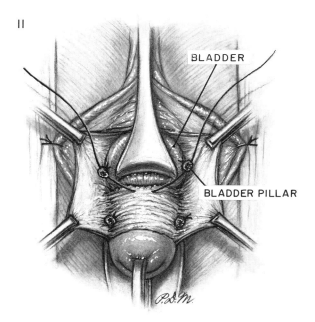

III

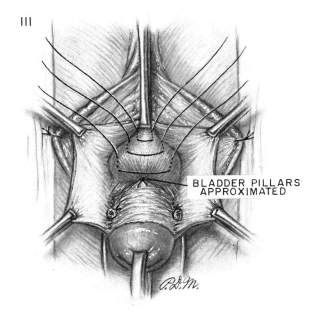

FIG. 206
Repair of cystocele, or anterior colporrhaphy. I. The limits of the cystocele have been defined. II. The urethrovesical angle is restored by suture approximation of the divided bladder pillars. III. Further plication sutures elevate the bladder. Excess vaginal wall will be excised before final closure of that layer.

tioning the posterior urethrovesical angle and reducing the cystocele (see Stress Incontinence, above). If the fascia is attenuated, wide bites of the needle may still produce a strong suture line but the operator must be aware of the proximity of the ureters. More superficially the musculofascial perineal tissues are also sutured.

The dissection in posterior colporrhaphy (Fig. 207) discloses the medial borders of the levator ani muscles, covered by their fascia. They are sutured together in the midline to constitute the strongest part of the rectocele repair. This is augmented anteriorly and somewhat superficially by suturing the relaxed perineal tissues anteriorly, and the fascia about the anal canal posteriorly.

If an enterocele is present, the sac is entered after the initial exposure—the contents are reduced and the neck is sutured. The uterosacral ligaments are identified, as in performing vaginal hysterectomy (see Fig. 217). The ligaments are brought together in the midline before proceeding with the suture of the levator ani muscles. An enterocele may also be corrected from above, by closure of the rectouterine pouch, placing the sutures through the peritoneum and the uterosacral ligaments. This is the same procedure as in the Moschowitz correction of prolapse of the rectum (see Chapter 17). If the sphincter ani muscle has been torn in a peri-

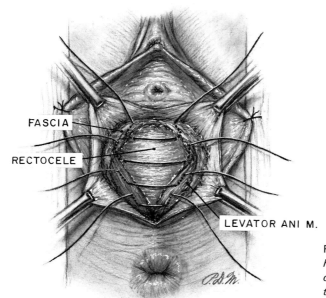

FASCIA

RECTOCELE

LEVATOR ANI M.

FIG. 207
Repair of rectocele, or posterior colporrhaphy. Elevation of the rectal bulge will be maintained by approximating the levator ani muscles deeply, aided by suture of the perineal fascias.

neal laceration, its ends are sought and sutured together (see Fig. 200).

The choice of procedures available for prolapse of the uterus is discussed by Colcock (1949). A slight degree of prolapse is correctable by colporrhaphy alone, but this operation is inadequate in the presence of more severe uterine descent. Cardinal ligament fixation (Manchester-Fothergill) and amputation of the cervix is occasionally chosen if the cervix is elongated and prolapse is moderate (Fig. 208). Vaginal hysterectomy is often done for severe prolapse, with careful attention to suture of the divided ligaments in the repair. In the uterine interposition (Watkins-Wertheim) operation, the cervix is amputated, the vesicouterine peritoneum opened, and the uterine fundus is anteflexed and fixed between the bladder and anterior vaginal wall (Fig. 209). In an elderly patient, a partial (LeFort) or total colpocleisis, or obliteration of the vaginal lumen, gives good support of the uterus with low operative risk. Abdominal suspension of the uterus can be accomplished by shortening the round liga-

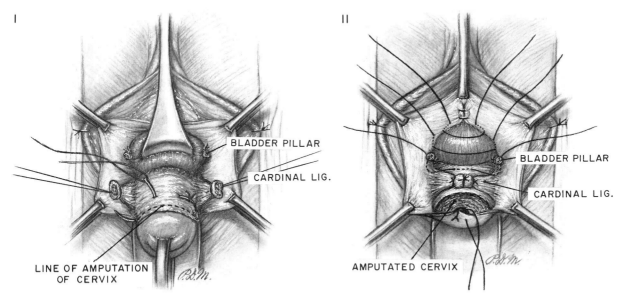

FIG. 208
Cervical amputation and cardinal ligament fixation for uterine prolapse (Manchester-Fothergill operation). I. Initial dissection. The bladder pillars have been divided and the cystocele dissected free and retracted. The cardinal ligaments have been freed from their lateral attachment on the cervix. Suture ligation of blood vessels to the cervix anticipates amputation of that structure. II. The cardinal ligaments are united anterior to the shortened cervix and the vaginal mucosa is sutured over the surface. Elevation of the cystocele is proceeding as in anterior colporrhaphy.

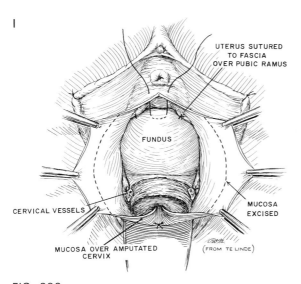

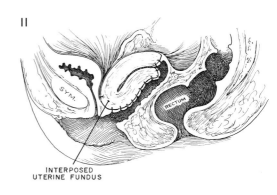

FIG. 209

Uterine interposition (Watkins-Wertheim) operation. I. The bladder has been freed from the anterior vaginal wall and pushed upward. The peritoneum has been entered and the uterus anteflexed so as to place the fundus behind the bladder. The cornua of the uterus have been sutured to the fascia over the pubic rami; suture fixation of vagina to uterus has begun. The cervix has been amputated, as it often is if badly lacerated. II. Position of organs at conclusion of the procedure. (From Colcock, 1949.)

ments in front, and the uterosacral ligaments behind. Ventral fixation of the fundus to the anterior abdominal wall gives somewhat more certain support.

References

Bumm, E.: Grundriss zum Studium der Geburtshilfe, 5th ed. Wiesbaden, J. F. Bergmann, 1908.

Colcock, B. P.: Treatment of prolapse of the uterus. Surg. Clin. N. Amer. 29:847–860, 1949.

Copenhaver, E. H.: Recurrent stress incontinence of urine following unsuccessful surgery. Surg. Clin. N. Amer. 40:751–760, 1960.

Curtis, A. H., Anson, B. J., and Ashley, F. L.: Further studies in gynecological anatomy and related clinical problems. Surg. Gynec. Obstet. 74:709–727, 1942.

Curtis, A. H., Anson, B. J., and Beaton, L. E.: The anatomy of the subperitoneal tissues and ligamentous structures in relation to surgery of the female pelvic viscera. Surg. Gynec. Obstet. 70:643–656, 1940.

Curtis, A. H., Anson, B. J., and McVay, C. B.: The anatomy of the pelvic and urogenital diaphragms, in relation to urethrocele and cystocele. Surg. Gynec. Obstet. 68:161–166, 1939.

Curtis, A. H., and Huffman, J. W.: A Textbook of Gynecology, 6th ed. Philadelphia, W. B. Saunders, 1950.

Furniss, H. D.: Discussion on Kennedy, W. T.: *op cit.,* 1937.

Green, T. H., Jr.: Gynecology. Essentials of Clinical Practice, 2nd ed. Boston, Little, Brown, 1971.

Kelly, H. A.: Incontinence of urine in women. Urol. Cutan. Rev. 17:291–293, 1913.

Kelly, H. A.: Complete Tear of the Perineum. Rectovaginal Fistula. Chapter 5 *in* Lewis' Practice of Surgery, Vol 10. Hagerstown, W. T. Prior, 1952.

Kennedy, W. T.: Incontinence of urine in the female, the urethral sphincter mechanism, damage of function, and restoration of control. Amer. J. Obstet. Gynec. 34:576–589, 1937.

Marshall, V. F., Marchetti, A. A., and Krantz, K. E.: The correction of stress incontinence by simple vesicourethral suspension. Surg. Gynec. Obstet. 88:509–518, 1949.

Te Linde, R. W., and Mattingly, R. F.: Operative Gynecology, 4th ed. Philadelphia, J. B. Lippincott, 1970.

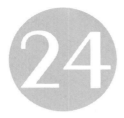

sensory innervation
of the female genitalia;
denervation procedures

SENSORY PATHWAYS

A knowledge of the pathways for sensation from the female genitalia is important in the planning of procedures to denervate painful lesions, particularly those of malignant disease.

For the viscera, as for somatic structures, the cell bodies of the sensory neurons lie in ganglia outside of the central nervous system. For the abdomen and pelvis these ganglia are the posterior root ganglia of spinal nerves. Viscerosensory fibers are peculiar in that they tend to traverse autonomic pathways on their way from viscera. It must be expected therefore that at least some of the sensory nerves from the genitalia will be included with the autonomic fibers of the ovarian and the superior and inferior hypogastric plexuses and their subsidiaries (Fig. 210; see also Chapter 6).

The external genitalia are supplied by the pudendal and adjacent somatic nerves, consistent with the somatic origin of these parts. The connective tissues and lymph nodes

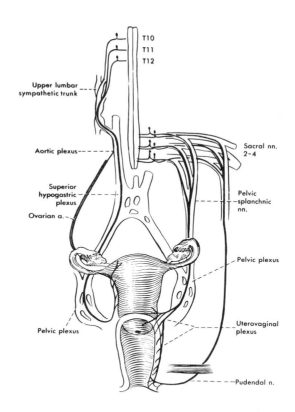

FIG. 210
Afferent nervous pathways from the female genitalia. (From Hollinshead, 1971.)

about the pelvic viscera, of special significance as the site of extension of cancer, are innervated by the sacral spinal nerves, partly through the inferior hypogastric plexus, partly by direct fine branches embedded in the fascia of the pelvic diaphragm. These sacral branches also innervate the cervix, and the vagina above the introitus; they travel as a plexus about the uterine artery and can be anesthetized by a paracervical block.

DENERVATION PROCEDURES

Two procedures—presacral neurectomy and pudendal neurectomy—are done to partially denervate the genitalia. Presacral neurectomy has proved useful in primary dysmenorrhea, and pudendal neurectomy in treating the pain of vaginismus and of vulval carcinoma or pruritus. Neither of these procedures is effective in the pain of uterine carcinoma, as Meigs (1940) and White and Sweet (1969) have emphasized. The pain in this condition is due to invasion beyond the uterus, often including the sacral nerve trunks.

Cordotomy with bilateral section of the spinothalamic tracts may be used at this stage (White and Sweet).

Presacral Neurectomy

Presacral neurectomy, formerly performed in both men and women in attempts to relieve pelvic pain, or to modify the motor function of pelvic organs, has in late years come to be done only for primary dysmenorrhea.

The presacral nerves are more or less plexiform, as the synonym 'superior hypogastric plexus' implies (Fig. 211). The nerves are the inferior continuation of the pre-aortic plexus, merging as they descend with the paired inferior hypogastric plexus. The adjacent inferior mesenteric plexus sends a variable contribution to the superior hypogastric plexus; some branches also come from the fourth lumbar

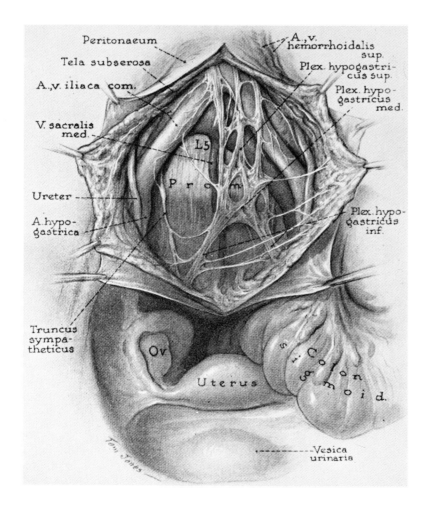

Fig. 211

The presacral plexus—the interconnected strands, here three in number, are labeled superior and middle hypogastric plexuses. They continue over the sacral promontory in the paired inferior hypogastric plexuses. On the left the presacral plexus is in continuity with the inferior mesenteric plexus along the superior rectal (hemorrhoidal) vessels. The left common iliac and the median sacral vein are significant related structures. The sympathetic trunks are usually not seen at operation, being overlain by the iliac veins. (From Curtis et al., 1942. By permission of Surgery, Gynecology & Obstetrics.)

sympathetic ganglia, traveling posterior or occasionally anterior to the common iliac vessels. These relationships are further shown in Figures 50, 51 (Chapter 6), which also show the subsidiary plexuses which reach the pelvic viscera in the various ligaments, partly around the visceral arteries.

Surgical exposure of the presacral nerves is through the peritoneum over the aortic bifurcation and between the iliac vessels. The exposure does not extend as low or as wide as the dissection in Figure 211. Elaut (1932) emphasized that the nerves often lie to the left of the midline. Further, the pelvic mesocolon may lie directly over them so that the inferior mesenteric vessels or their branches must be displaced to the left. The ureters are usually seen in the field adherent to the overlying peritoneum. Injury to the left common and internal iliac and middle sacral vessels must be avoided. The plexus is removed within the interiliac trigone from the aortic bifurcation to just below the sacral promontory. White and Sweet say that the operation may fail if one does not divide the contributions from the inferior mesenteric plexus and from the fourth lumbar sympathetic ganglia. Some small lymph trunks and nodes may be removed with the presacral nerves.

The pain of primary dysmenorrhea is usually relieved, without interfering with menstruation, pregnancy, or parturition. The denervation usually does away with the pain of the first stage of labor so that delivery may be precipitate. There is no certain effect on function of the rectum or bladder, or on pain originating in these organs or in the cervix or in other genital organs of either sex. Exceptionally, presacral neurectomy has resulted in atony of the bladder. It is probable that this is due to too low a dissection, with interruption of the sacral branches to the inferior hypogastric plexus. In the male dog, presacral neurectomy prevents ejaculation, but there is no firm evidence that it does so in man (Van Duzen *et al.,* 1947; see also Chapter 6).

Pudendal Neurectomy

Most of the perineum can be denervated by dividing the branches of the pudendal nerves and the pudendal branches of the posterior cutaneous nerves of the thigh. Both nerves arise from the 'sacral plexus'—that portion of the lumbosacral plexus below the origin of the sciatic nerve (see Fig. 50).

The course of the pudendal nerve parallels that of the internal pudendal artery which it accompanies. Originating in the pelvis from the 2nd, 3rd, and 4th sacral nerves, it leaves through the sciatic foramen below the sciatic nerve. It turns around the external surface of the ischial spine, to enter the perineum through the lesser sciatic foramen in company with the internal pudendal artery and vein (Fig. 212).

In the perineum it runs in the pudendal canal ('Alcock's canal') in the fascia covering the obturator internus muscle. The branching of the pudendal nerve into the perineal nerve and the dorsal nerve of the clitoris (or penis) may take place before or during its course in the canal. The first branch of

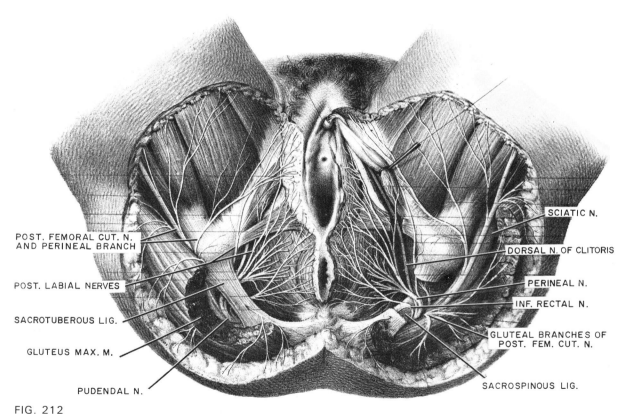

FIG. 212

Perineal branches of pudendal and posterior femoral cutaneous nerves. On the subject's left, the sacrotuberous ligament has been sectioned to show the pudendal nerve, already divided into its three primary branches, entering the perineum by turning around the sacrospinous ligament. The obturator fascia has been removed, displaying the course of the perineal nerve and the dorsal nerve of the clitoris. An unusual number of twigs to the levator ani muscle are shown. (From Hirschfeld and Leveillé, 1853.)

the pudendal, the inferior rectal (hemorrhoidal), is supplemented in its motor supply to the external anal sphincter by the anal branch of the perineal, which arches backward to meet the sphincter. Two or more superficial branches of the perineal—the posterior labial (or, in the male, scrotal) branches—run forward, crossing or penetrating the transverse perineal muscle in their course. The lateral posterior labial anastomoses quite regularly with an anterior branch of the perineal branch of the posterior cutaneous nerve of the thigh. Deep perineal branches are both motor and sensory, supplying the muscles of the perineum and the bulb of the vestibule.

The posterior cutaneous nerve of the thigh—entirely sensory—originates from the 1st, 2nd, and 3rd sacral nerves. It leaves the pelvis through the greater sciatic foramen and is distributed to the skin of the posterior thigh and popliteal space. One early division, the perineal branch, runs medially and beneath the superficial fascia about 2 cm. lateral to the ramus of the ischium to supply a small posterior and larger anterior branch to the lateral part of the perineum. The anterior branch communicates with a lateral posterior labial nerve. An inconstant cutaneous branch of the pudendal nerve perforates the sacrotuberous ligament. It may communicate with the perineal branch of the posterior cutaneous nerve of the thigh, or replace it (Roberts et al., 1964).

The fields of the perineum innervated by the pudendal and adjacent nerves are shown in Figure 213. There is considerable overlap in this innervation.

Denervation of the perineum has been accomplished mainly by division of the pudendal nerve and the perineal branch of the posterior cutaneous nerve of the thigh. An incision is made on each side medial to the conjoined rami of ischium and pubis, starting between the ischial tuberosity and anus, and extending forward. Tavel (1902) uncovered the obturator internus fascia in the anterior part of the ischiorectal fossa, locating the pudendal canal by palpating the internal pudendal artery. The canal is opened, and the nerve trunk, or its branches, is identified. Learmonth and his associates (1933) first identified the posterior labial nerves on the transverse perineal muscle, then traced them back to the pudendal trunk. The anal branch of the perineal is saved, but the rest of the perineal nerve and the dorsal nerve of

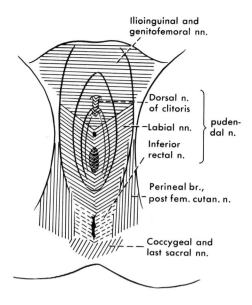

Ilioinguinal and
genitofemoral nn.

Dorsal n.
of clitoris

Labial nn.

Inferior
rectal n.

puden-
dal n.

Perineal br.,
post fem. cutan. n.

Coccygeal and
last sacral nn.

FIG. 213
*Cutaneous territories of nerves to the
female perineum. (From Hollinshead,
1971.)*

the clitoris are divided or excised. The perineal branch of
the posterior cutaneous nerve of the thigh is likewise divided, after having been identified through its communication with the lateral of the posterior labial nerves, or by
seeking it just lateral to the conjoined rami. The two communicating nerves run in the cleft deep to the membranous
layer (Colles) of the superficial fascia (Roberts *et al.*).

REFERENCES

Curtis, A. H., Anson, B. J., and Ashley, F. L.: Further studies in
gynecological anatomy and related clinical problems. Surg.
Gynec. Obstet. 74:309–727, 1942.

Elaut, L.: The surgical anatomy of the so called presacral nerve.
Surg. Gynec. Obstet. 55:581–589, 1932.

Hirschfeld, L., and Leveillé, J. B.: Névrolgie ou description et
iconographie du système nerveux et des organes des sens de
l'homme avec leur mode de préparation. Paris, Baillière, 1853.

Hollinshead, W. H.: Anatomy for Surgeons, 2nd ed. Vol. 2. The
Thorax, Abdomen, and Pelvis, New York, Harper & Row,
1971.

Learmonth, J. R., Montgomery, H., and Counseller, V. S.: Resection of sensory nerves of perineum in certain irritative conditions of the external genitalia. Arch. Surg. 26:50–63, 1933.

Meigs, J. V.: Pelvic pain and its relief. New Eng. J. Med.
222:187–190, 1940.

Roberts, W. H., Habenicht, J., and Krishingner, G.: The pelvic and perineal fasciae and their neural and vascular relationships. Anat. Rec. 149:707–720, 1964.

Tavel, E.: La résection du nerf honteux interne dans le vaginisme et le prurit de la vulve. Rev. Chir. 25:145–163, 1902.

Van Duzen, R. E., Slaughter, D., and White, B.: The effect of presacral neurectomy on fertility of man and animals. J. Urol. 57:1206–1209, 1947.

White, J. C., and Sweet, W. H.: Pain and the Neurosurgeon. A Forty-Year Experience. Springfield, Charles C Thomas, 1969.

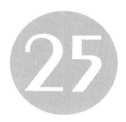

Hysterectomy for benign disease

BLOOD SUPPLY OF THE UTERUS AND VAGINA

The distribution of the uterine and ovarian arteries to the uterus is shown in Figure 214. The uterine artery arises most commonly from high on the anterior division of the internal iliac artery, near the umbilical artery or in common with it (see Fig. 39). It may come off the proximal internal pudendal or inferior vesical artery (Roberts and Krishingner, 1967). The vaginal artery may be as large as the uterine. Roberts and Krishingner noted that the vaginal arises somewhat oftener from the internal pudendal within the pelvis than from the uterine. Vaginal branches may arise from adjacent vessels (Fig. 215). As the uterine artery approaches the uterus it crosses above the ureter about 1.5 cm. lateral to the lower cervix. Here it gives off its cervical and vaginal branches. Large uterine veins are found both above and below the ureter.

Ligation of the internal iliac artery, usually bilateral, is a maneuver sometimes employed to overcome bleeding from the uterus or vagina. Ischemic complications are rare (see Chapter 4).

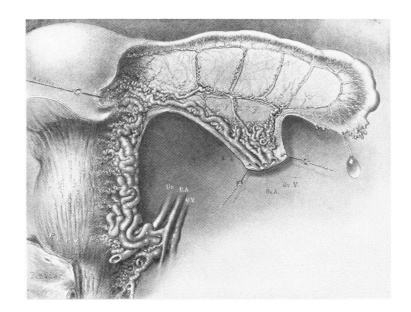

FIG. 214
Communication of uterine and ovarian blood vessels. The specimen is viewed from in front. The round ligament has been removed; its stump is being retracted. The uterine artery crosses above the ureter, but substantial cervical and vaginal branches and veins lie beneath the ureter as well. A pedunculated hydatid of the uterine tube is present. (From Kelly, 1901.)

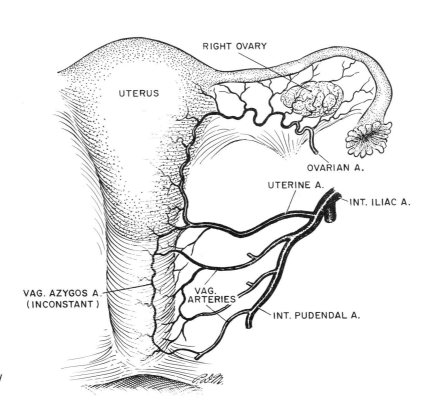

FIG. 215
Arterial supply to the vagina, viewed from behind.

ABDOMINAL HYSTERECTOMY
FOR BENIGN DISEASE

Division of the broad ligament, along with the uterine tube, round ligament, and the ovarian artery, gives access to the uterine vessels and the ureter lateral to the cervix on the lateral cervical or cardinal ligament (Fig. 216). The ureter is usually identified only by palpating its hard consistency in operations for benign diseases. Many prefer to divide the vesicouterine peritoneum initially to displace the bladder from the cervix and upper vagina, to give a safer approach to the uterine artery and the ureter.

The posterior aspect of the cervix and vagina come into view after division of the uterosacral ligaments and the overlying peritoneum. Placing this division close to the midline avoids the area of the ureters and blood vessels. Excision of the uterus with the attached upper vagina can now be done. The pelvic floor is made firm by including the ends of the divided ligaments in the vaginal and peritoneal closure.

The ureter is subject to injury near the uterus when the uterine artery is ligated during hysterectomy. More remotely, the ovarian vessels cross superolateral to the ureter at the pelvic brim, over the iliac bifurcation. Here the ureter may also be injured during ovariectomy. Again it is vulnerable on the side wall and floor of the pelvis when operation is carried here because of pelvic adhesions or during radical hysterectomy for carcinoma of the cervix (see Chapter 26).

Some fascial relationships may be emphasized. The vesical fascia in front and the heavier uterovaginal fascia behind join in a vesicovaginal fascia, or septum, which is opened to allow for a safer mobilization of the bladder prior to its anterior displacement from the vagina. A bit of the uterovaginal fascia is opened when the uterine vessels are cut close to the cervix. This division may be carried around the front of the lower cervix to make the uterus more mobile. An extensive venous plexus lies deep to the fascia, and its division also allows ligation of these veins before the vagina is opened. Posteriorly, endometriosis may fix the rectum to the lower uterus, and posterior incision of the fascia on the cervix allows one to push back the rectovaginal septum to protect the rectum. In performing hysterectomy for cancer

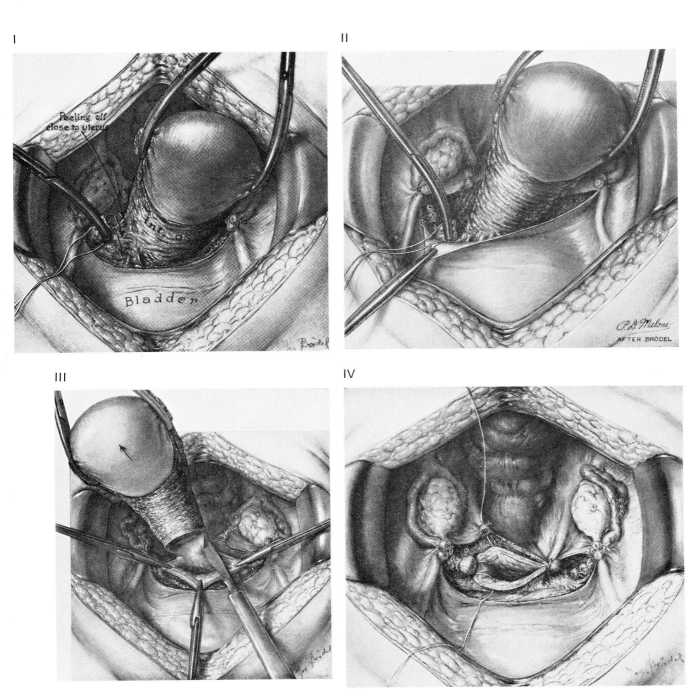

FIG. 216

Abdominal hysterectomy for benign disease. I. The vesicouterine peritoneum has been incised. The round ligament, uterine tube, and utero-ovarian ligament with its contained ovarian vessels have been clamped and divided on each side. The broad ligament is cut to its base, allowing division of the uterine vessels close to the uterus at the level of the internal os. The arrows indicate the direction of dissection to displace these vessels and the ureter farther laterally. II. The last maneuver of I now allows clamping and division of the cardinal ligament and the blood vessels lying inferior to the ureter. III. The vagina, exposed by division of the posterior peritoneum and the uterosacral ligaments, is being sectioned and the uterus removed. IV. The pelvic floor is closed by suturing the divided structures. The suture being placed passes through the vagina and the cardinal and uterosacral ligaments. (From Richardson, 1929. By permission of Surgery, Gynecology & Obstetrics.)

I

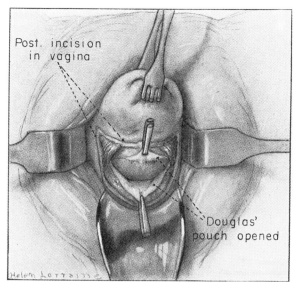

II

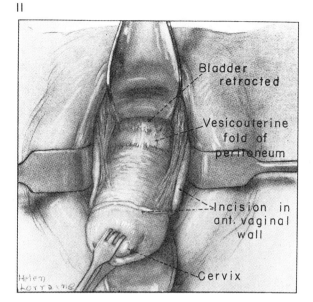

III

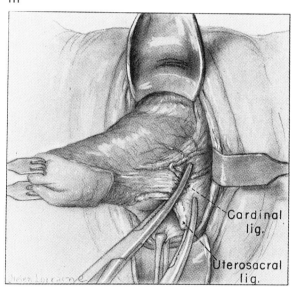

IV

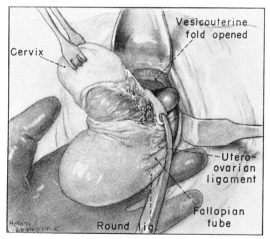

FIG. 217

*Vaginal hysterectomy for benign disease. I. Opening the rectouterine peritoneum between the uterosacral liga-
ments. II. Delineation of the vesicouterine peritoneum between the bladder pillars. III. Division of the uterosacral
and cardinal ligaments and the uterine artery. The clamp on the artery lies close to the ureter. It is safest to place
it snug against the cervix. IV. Downward displacement of the fundus and division of the uterine tube and ligaments
on the fundus. (From Burch, J. C., and Lavely, H. T.: Hysterectomy, 1954. Courtesy of Charles C Thomas, Publisher,
Springfield, Illinois.)*

of either the fundus or the cervix, it is desirable to remove the uterovaginal fascia along with the uterus and upper vagina.

VAGINAL HYSTERECTOMY
FOR BENIGN DISEASE

A posterior incision of the vaginal mucous membrane close to the cervix discloses the uterosacral ligaments, between which the peritoneum is opened (Fig. 217). Further mobility of the uterus is gained by incising the anterior vagina, again close to the cervix, and separating the bladder. This involves a delineation of the 'bladder pillars,' the medial edges of the pubocervical fascia, passing from the sides of the cervix to the sides of the bladder. The vesicouterine peritoneum is opened. This step may precede the posterior entry into the peritoneal cavity.

Downward and lateral traction of the uterus brings into view the uterine artery at the side of the cervix. The uterosacral and then the cardinal ligaments are divided. The ureter is not visualized in ordinary vaginal hysterectomy, its injury being avoided by ligating the artery close to the uterus.

Pushing the fundus out through the posterior peritoneal opening brings the broad, round, and uterovarian ligaments and the uterine tube into view for their sectioning. As in hysterectomy from above, the stumps of the ligaments, the peritoneum, and the vaginal walls are available for closure of the defect in the pelvic floor.

REFERENCES

Burch, J. C., and Lavely, H. T.: Hysterectomy. Springfield, Charles C Thomas, 1954.

Kelly, H. A.: Operative Gynecology. New York. Appleton. 1901.

Richardson, E. H.: A simplified technique for abdominal panhysterectomy. Surg. Gynec. Obstet. 48:248–256, 1929.

Roberts, W. H., and Krishingner, G. L.: Comparative study of human internal iliac artery based on Adachi classification. Anat. Rec. 158:191–196, 1967.

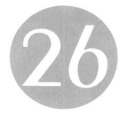

OPERATIONS FOR
MALIGNANT DISEASE

LYMPHATICS OF THE FEMALE GENITALIA

The lymphatics of the female genitalia are shown in Figure 218. The major groups of nodes are the superficial and deep inguinal, external, internal, and common iliac, aortic, and caval. The pathways terminate in the cisterna chyli at the upper renal level (see Chapter 5).

The vulvar and vaginal lymphatics course to the superficial inguinal then to the deep inguinal nodes and upward. The deep inguinal node medial to the femoral vein, shown on the right receiving lymph from the round ligament, is the node of the femoral canal (Cloquet).

Lymph from the uterus follows two pathways, one along the uterine, the other along the ovarian, blood vessels. The first is particularly significant for the cervix. The lymph passes through the parametrial nodes, the most medial of which is named the paracervical, or 'ureteral,' from its proximity to the ureter. The parametrial nodes connect to the internal iliac. The obturator are the most inferior of the internal iliac nodes. An alternate path from the cervix is to the sacral (pararectal) nodes.

The fundus of the uterus is drained by lymphatics along the ovarian blood vessels, joining those from the uterine tube

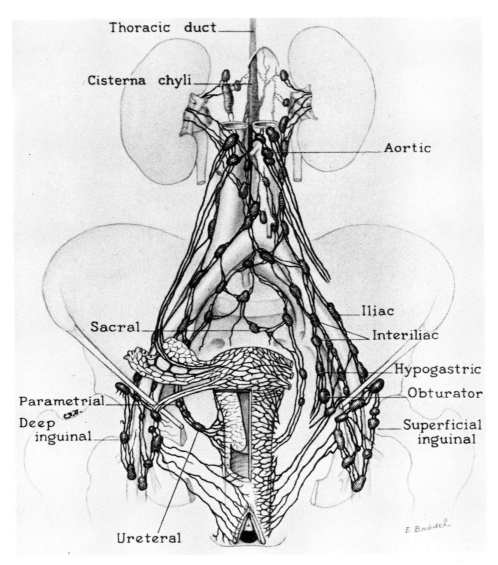

FIG. 218

Lymphatics of the female genitalia. (From Javert, in Surgical Treatment of Cancer of the Cervix, J. V. Meigs, Ed. New York, Grune & Stratton, 1954. By permission of the publisher.)

and the ovary to terminate in the aortic nodes at the renal level.

VULVECTOMY

The extent of vulvar excision as usually practiced is shown in Figure 219. The central incision spares the urethra, but extends into the vagina above the meatal level.

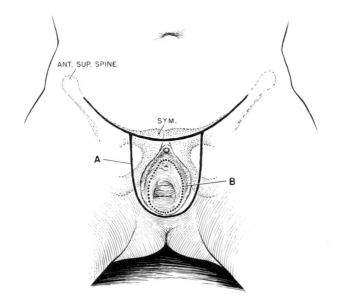

FIG. 219
Incisions for vulvectomy and inguinal lymphadenectomy. Structures between lines A and B are removed. The extensions of the incision are used for the lymphadenectomy.

When the location of the lesion requires it, some of the urethra may be removed. However, if more than the distal half is sacrificed, urinary incontinence may result, and the prognosis for cure is poor in these cases. The vulvar excision includes the clitoris; it is carried down to the fascia which covers the pubes and the conjoined rami, and exposes the bulbocavernosus muscles. Closure is effected by suturing the vaginal mucous membrane to the lateral skin edge. The perineum may be buttressed by bringing together first the levator ani muscles, as in rectocele repair (see Fig. 207, Chapter 23), and then the bulbocavernosus muscles.

Lymphadenectomy of a varied extent is usually added to the vulvectomy. Figure 219 shows the incision extended above the pubes for this procedure. The primary pathway is to the superficial inguinal nodes and along the round ligament (Taussig, 1938). At its least, therefore, the adenectomy consists of removal of the superficial inguinal nodes and the node of the femoral canal, usually with additional opening of the inguinal canal to remove the round ligament to the deep inguinal ring, plus the fat and the occasional nodes of the canal. The lymphadenectomy may be extended to the deep inguinal and the external iliac and common iliac nodes, with a varying portion of the internal iliac nodes (see Chapter 5).

OPERATION FOR CANCER OF THE FUNDUS

Figure 218 shows that the primary lymphatic flow from the fundus is upward to join the ovarian stream. Such flow is evidenced by the frequent spread of carcinoma from the fundus to the tube and ovary. Downward spread along the paracervical route generally occurs only when the tumor has invaded the cervix. The operation for cancer of the fundus is usually a hysterectomy as for benign disease, but with removal of the uterovaginal fascia, and with bilateral salpingo-oophorectomy. Some do perform a radical, or Wertheim, hysterectomy, as for carcinoma of the cervix.

OPERATIONS FOR CANCER OF THE CERVIX

Operations for carcinoma of the cervix take into account the lymphatic spread to paracervical tissue along and inferior to the uterine artery, thence to the iliac nodes. The posterior channels draining into sacral and aortic nodes are less frequent paths of dissemination (Plentl and Friedman, 1971). Upward spread along the ovarian path is uncommon; indeed Meigs (1962) often did not remove the ovary in young patients.

Operation for microinvasive carcinoma of the cervix can consist of a hysterectomy such as is used for benign disease, or it may be enlarged in scope to include some of the features of radical hysterectomy.

Radical hysterectomy for carcinoma of the cervix—the procedure described by Wertheim (1911)—consists of a hysterectomy and salpingo-oophorectomy, with excision of much of the vagina and parametrial tissue. Removal of the parametrium is facilitated by division of the uterine vessels lateral to the well-visualized ureter. Wertheim added lymphadenectomy to the hysterectomy only when the nodes were enlarged.

Meigs and his colleagues were, to a large extent, responsible for the development of a radical hysterectomy combined with pelvic lymphadenectomy (Meigs, 1954, and in Pack and Ariel, 1962; Parsons and Ulfelder, 1968). Two major complications are peculiar to this operation. The first, and commonest, is ureteral fistula, which Meigs (1954)

I

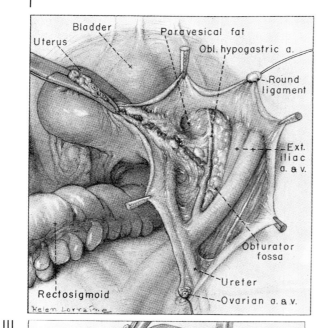

Bladder
Uterus
Paravesical fat
Obl. hypogastric a.
Round ligament
Ext. iliac a. & v.
Obturator fossa
Ureter
Rectosigmoid
Ovarian a. & v.

Helen Lorraine

II

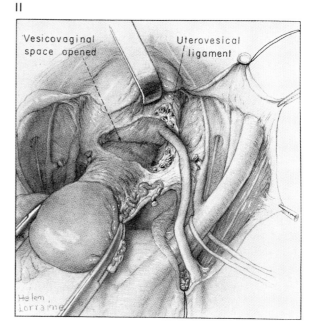

Vesicovaginal space opened
Uterovesical ligament

Helen Lorraine

III

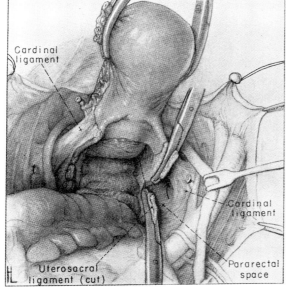

Cardinal ligament
Cardinal ligament
Uterosacral ligament (cut)
Pararectal space

FIG. 220

Radical hysterectomy and pelvic lymphadenectomy. (From Burch, J. C., and Lavely, H. T.: Hysterectomy, 1954. Courtesy of Charles C Thomas, Publisher, Springfield, Illinois.) I. Initial subperitoneal exposure. The ovary, uterine tube, and part of the round ligament are shown excised. The uterine artery extends from its common origin with the obliterated hypogastric artery. II. Lymph node–bearing tissue has been removed from about the iliac vessels. The genitofemoral nerve on the psoas muscle is the lateral limit of this removal. The obturator nerve is exposed passing into the obturator canal. The obturator artery is encountered here, coming either from the internal iliac or the external iliac artery. The accompanying vein may be very large (see Fig. 30). The bladder has been separated extensively from the vagina, leaving the vaginal fascia in place. The plane of dissection is free of large vessels in the midline. The uterine artery has been divided lateral to the ureter, whose pelvic course is now fully exposed. Its termination is visualized by division of the 'uterovesical' (vesicouterine) ligament (superior part of 'pillars of the bladder'). III. Dividing the uterosacral ligament gives access to the cardinal ligament. Blunt dissection beneath it (arrow) allows passage into the paravesical space and isolates the ligament for section (clamp), as in IV.

IV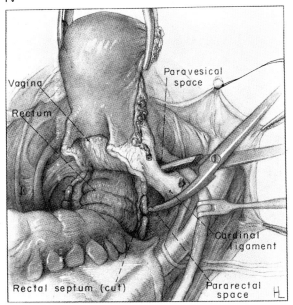

V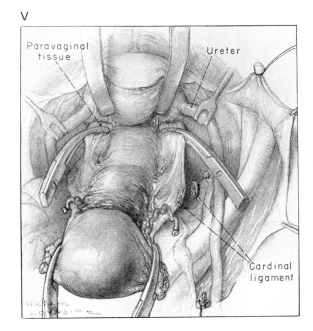

FIG. 220

Radical hysterectomy and pelvic lymphadenectomy (continued).

IV. Posteriorly the pararectal space is cleared of lymphatic tissue. This entails division of the 'rectal septum' (lateral ligament of the rectum), containing the middle rectal artery. V. Paravaginal tissue, continuous with both the cardinal ligament and the vesicouterine ligament, is now being divided, anticipating removal of a large segment of the vagina and final freeing of the specimen.

related to ischemia incident to division of supply to the ureter from the uterine, vaginal, and internal iliac arteries (see Fig. 164). The second is the rare postoperative rupture of a major pelvic vessel, usually an artery, attributed to infection adjacent to vessels denuded by the dissection (Brunschwig and Brockunier, 1960).

The procedure shown in Figure 220 is taken from Burch and Lavely (1954). We will mention points about the operation that Meigs thought noteworthy. Meigs paid little attention to the node of the femoral canal, removing it only when it was apparent. He found that the first branch of the internal iliac artery usually coursed medially to the ureter. He saved this vessel and left the sheath of the ureter ('adventitia') intact to preserve the longitudinal anastomoses that extend from this artery to the ureteral branches of the uterine and vaginal arteries, whose parent vessels had been sacrificed (see Fig. 164). For similar reasons he retained that part of the pararectal peritoneum adherent to the upper pelvic portions of the ureter.

In the posterior dissection Meigs removed most of the

peritoneum of the cul de sac, retaining the upper part to which he left the ureters attached. He advised removing the presacral area of fat and nodes "just as is done in a presacral neurectomy, but the nerves are not deliberately removed." He did not dissect between the sacrum and rectum. Dividing the cardinal ligament (Meigs' 'web') exposes the levator ani. Meigs saved the inferior hypogastric plexus seen on the muscle.

Radical vaginal hysterectomy for carcinoma of the cervix was first performed by Schuchardt (1893), who initially made use of resection of the sacrum as in the Kraske operation (see Chapter 1), then developed his 'paravaginal' incision for this perineal approach. This procedure, now generally termed the Schauta-Amreich, offers an alternative to the Wertheim operation. The exposure is adequate to visualize the ureter, and allows the removal of considerable parametrial and paravaginal tissue, although it is probably somewhat less than that obtainable from above. Moreover lymphadenectomy, if desired, must be separately performed by transperitoneal or extraperitoneal exposure. Good descriptions of the operation are given by Schauta (1908) and by Bastianse, Mitra, and Navratil (all in 1954).

RADICAL HYSTERECTOMY EXTENDED TO OTHER PELVIC ORGANS

Extension of carcinoma of the cervix to the rectum or bladder may be managed by total exenteration of the pelvis, that is, by removal of the bladder, uterus and vagina, and the rectum, along with lymphadenectomy. Anterior or posterior exenteration is the term applied, respectively, to resection of the bladder or rectum added to the radical hysterectomy. Details of the procedures are given in Meigs (1954), by Parsons (1962), Parsons and Ulfelder (1968), and Bricker (1970).

Total exenteration requires diversion of the urinary stream, as by implanting the ureters into a pedicled segment of ileum leading to a cutaneous stoma, and diversion of the bowel by a separate colostomy. The usual procedures for cystectomy (see Chapter 21) and for sigmoid resection (see Chapter 18) are added to those of radical hysterectomy, except that the maneuvers for separating the bladder and rectum from the uterus and vagina are omitted. The upper pelvic portions of the ureters are mobilized early, leaving them attached to some peritoneum, for implantation into the chosen bowel segment. Likewise the colon is divided, anticipating colostomy. The view of the lateral wall of the pelvis, exposed by displacing the pelvic organs medially, will resemble that seen in Figure 39 II.

Total exenteration may be done entirely from above, dividing the pelvic and urogenital diaphragms around the urethra, vagina, and rectum, cutting through the entire thickness of perineum. In anterior or posterior exenteration, the most distal parts of the tubular organs may be allowed to remain if tumor has not extended to the perineum. If the perineal parts are to be removed, separate perineal dissection is performed.

The lymphadenectomy of the pelvis in total exenteration is rendered more complete by removal of the internal iliac artery and vein, and by the dissection proceeding as a clean sweep across the floor of the pelvis. The internal iliac trunks are left intact in anterior or posterior exenteration, to prevent ischemic damage to the organs remaining.

REFERENCES

Bastianse, M. A. van B.: Radical Vaginal Hysterectomy. Chapter 6, essay 1, *in* Meigs, J. V., Ed., *op. cit.,* 1954.

Bricker, E. M.: Pelvic exenteration. Advances Surg. 4:13–72, 1970.

Brunschwig, A., and Brockunier, A.: Postoperative rupture of major vessels after radical pelvic operation. Amer. J. Obstet. Gynec. 80:485–489, 1960.

Burch, J. C., and Lavely, H. T.: Hysterectomy. Springfield, Charles C Thomas. 1954.

Javert, C. T.: The Lymph Nodes and Lymph Channels of the Pelvis. Chapter 2, essay 2, *in* Meigs, J. V., Ed., *op. cit.,* 1954.

Meigs, J. V.: Radical Hysterectomy with Bilateral Dissection of the Pelvic Lymph Nodes. Chapter 5, essay 2, *in* Meigs, J. V., Ed., *op. cit.,* 1954.

Meigs, J. V.: Surgical Treatment of Cancer of the Uterine Cervix. Chapter 10 *in* Pack, G. T., and Ariel, I. M., Eds., *op. cit.,* 1962.

Meigs, J. V., Ed.: Surgical Treatment of Cancer of the Cervix. New York, Grune & Stratton, 1954.

Mitra, S.: Radical Vaginal Hysterectomy. Chapter 6, essay 2, *in* Meigs, J. V., Ed., *op. cit.,* 1954.

Navratil, E.: Radical Vaginal Hysterectomy. Chapter 6, essay 3, *in* Meigs, J. V., Ed., *op. cit.,* 1954.

Pack, G. T., and Ariel, I. M., Eds.: Treatment of Cancer and Allied Diseases, 2nd ed. Vol. VI. Tumors of the Female Genitalia. New York, Harper & Row, 1962.

Parsons, L.: Exenteration of the Pelvic Organs for Extensive Cancer of the Female Genital Tract. Chapter 18 *in* Pack, G. T., and Ariel, I. M., Eds., *op. cit.,* 1962.

Parsons, L., and Ulfelder, H.: An Atlas of Pelvic Operations, 2nd ed. Philadelphia. W. B. Saunders. 1968.

Plentl, A. A., and Friedman, E. A.: Lymphatic System of the Female Genitalia. The Morphologic Basis of Oncologic Diagnosis and Therapy. Philadelphia, W. B. Saunders, 1971.

Schauta, F.: Die erweiterte vaginale Totalexstirpation des Uterus bei Kollumkarzinom. Wien, Šafář, 1908.

Schuchardt, K.: Eine neue Methode der Gebärmutterexstirpation. Centralb. Chir. 20:1121–1126, 1893.

Taussig, F. J.: A study of the lymph glands in cancer of the cervix and cancer of the vulva. Amer. J. Obstet. Gynec. 36:819–832, 1938.

Wertheim, E.: Die erweiterte abdominale Operation bei Carcinoma colli uteri. Auf Grund von 500 Fällen. Berlin. 1911. (Note: The text minus the case reports is also given in English translation by Grad, H., in Amer. J. Obstet. 66:169–232, 1912.)

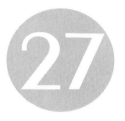

CESAREAN SECTION

SEGMENTS OF THE UTERUS AT TERM; CLASSICAL CESAREAN SECTION

The several methods of cesarean section will be better understood if we define the so-called uterine segments. The uterus at term is divisible into a heavier upper and a thinner lower segment, demarcated externally by a transverse furrow located near the vesicouterine fold of peritoneum (Fig. 221). Internally, the boundary is shown by the transverse physiological contraction ring. The ring is made of heavy uterine muscle, and a prominent vein lies within. Prior to effacement of the cervix in labor, the lower segment consists only of the isthmus, the part of the corpus adjacent to the cervix. As labor commences the cervix dilates and elongates, so that by the second stage the lower uterine segment includes the cervix. The contraction ring is now located at a higher level. Abnormally, the ring may constrict and prevent the passage of the fetus ('pathologic contraction ring,' or Bandl's ring). The upper uterine segment, the major source of expulsive force, is heavier in musculature and more vascular than the lower.

In the classical cesarean section the uterus is exposed by a vertical transperitoneal incision, then opened by a vertical cut in the upper segment, this part being intraperitoneal. The pregnant uterus will usually be found canted somewhat

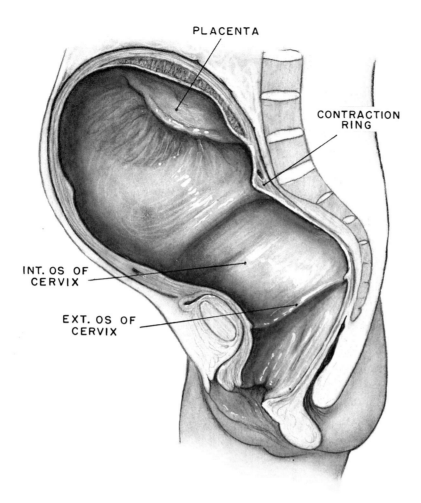

PLACENTA

CONTRACTION
RING

INT. OS OF
CERVIX

EXT. OS OF
CERVIX

FIG. 221
Segments of the parturient uterus
seen from within, in frozen section
of a woman dying in the second
stage of labor. (After Braune, 1872.)

to the right. The incision, in the midline of the uterus, passes
through the least vascular zone, where branches from the
paired uterine vessels intercommunicate.

LOWER SEGMENT CESAREAN SECTIONS

Advantages claimed for lower segment cesarean sections
include less damage to the uterine musculature (thus less
danger of rupture with future pregnancies) and a better
chance of limiting potential infection since the bladder and
peritoneum fall back over the uterine incision at the conclusion of the procedure.

Lower segment sections can be either transperitoneal or
retroperitoneal. In the transperitoneal procedure, once the
abdomen is opened, the peritoneum on the anterior uterine

surface is incised proximal to the vesicouterine reflection, to allow downward displacement of the bladder, thus uncovering the lower uterine segment, covered by its gray and glistening uterine fascia (Fig. 222). Pregnancy causes a loosening of the peritoneal attachment to the uterus, facilitating its mobilization. The incision in the lower segment is usually transverse, taking advantage of the direction of the blood vessels and the transverse orientation of the muscle bundles in this segment. Extension too far laterally into the extraperitoneal fatty tissue endangers the uterine artery and veins and the ureters. Greater length of incision is often gained by making it crescentic or V shaped.

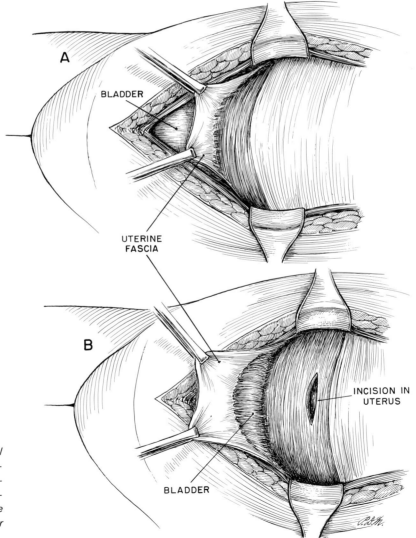

FIG. 222
Lower segment transperitoneal cesarean section. A. A flap of peritoneum and uterine fascia is reflected from the lower uterine segment. B. The incision is being made through the uterine wall. (After Willson, 1969.)

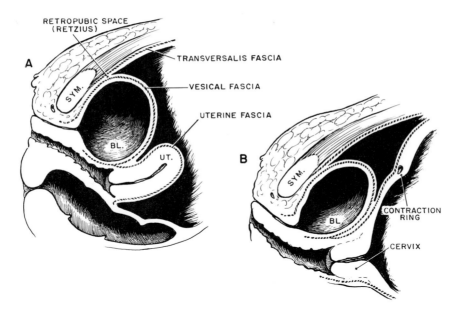

FIG. 223
Fascias of the vesicouterine region. A. In a non-gravid subject, with distended bladder. B. At term, with non-effaced cervix. (After Ricci and Marr, 1942.)

The goal of preventing peritonitis in cases of potential infection, as after premature rupture of the membranes, prolonged labor, or repeated vaginal examination, has led to the development of several techniques for extraperitoneal lower segment cesarean section. Reference to Figure 223, which depicts the fascias diagrammatically, will aid in understanding these procedures, one of which, the Waters supravesical extraperitoneal section (Waters, 1940), is shown in Figure 224. An extraperitoneal incision is made; the vesical fascia is opened anteriorly. With the bladder retracted this fascia is then incised posteriorly. The bladder is displaced downward, and the lower uterine segment is exposed. Note that the mobilization of the bladder entails division of the urachus, which is hypertrophied during pregnancy.

Other extraperitoneal cesarean operations, such as the Latzko, in which the bladder is pushed to one side, are described by Ricci and Marr (1942).

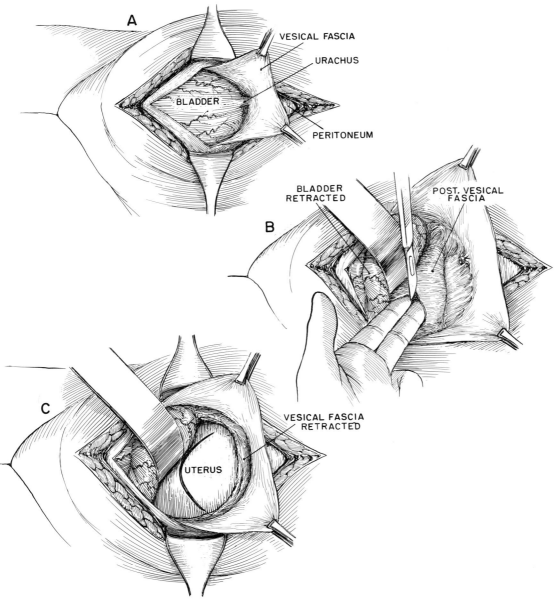

FIG. 224

Extraperitoneal cesarean section. A. The exposure is extraperitoneal. The vesical fascia is opened over the distended bladder. The urachus is a prominent structure. B. The bladder has been emptied and lifted away from the posterior part of the vesical fascia, which is now incised below the uterovesical peritoneal fold. C. The freed peritoneum and vesical fascia retreat upward. The bladder is retracted downward. The lower uterine segment encased in the uterine fascia is now exposed. The line of incision in the uterus is indicated. (After Waters, 1940, and Willson, 1969.)

REFERENCES

Braune, W.: Die Lage des Uterus und Foetus am Ende der Schwangerschaft. Suppl. to Topographisch-Anatomischen Atlas. Leipzig, Von Veit, 1872.

Ricci, J. V., and Marr, J. P.: Principles of Extraperitoneal Caesarean Section. Philadelphia, Blakiston, 1942.

Waters, E. G.: Supravesical extraperitoneal cesarean section. Presentation of a new technique. Amer. J. Obstet. Gynec. 39:423–434, 1940

Willson, J. R.: Atlas of Obstetric Technic, 2nd ed. St. Louis, C. V. Mosby, 1969.

iNdEx

Page numbers in **boldface** indicate illustrations.
Page numbers followed by "t" indicate tables.

Appendix, vermiform, anterior extraperitoneal abscess
      and, 7
   colonoscopy of, **230–231**
   duplications of, 223
   intraperitoneal abscess and, 30, 32t
   in neonate, 28
   teniae and, 228
Appendix fibrosa hepatica, aberrant biliary ducts and, 156
Arc of Riolan, 235
Arcuate veins of kidney, 299, **299**
Arteria radicularis magna, 62–63
Arteriomesenteric duodenal obstruction, 131–132
Artery(ies). See *Aorta; specific arteries.*
Asplenia, 29, 145
Atresia, anorectal, 248t, **249**, 314
Autonomic nervous system, 86–97. See also *specific
      nerves.*
   abdominal components of, 86–89, **87–89**
Azygos continuation anomaly, 158
Azygos vein, aortic exposure and, 61
   as collateral, 75–76
   portasystemic communications and, 203
   vertebral venous system and, **74,** 75

BARE AREAS OF MESENTERY, 215
Bassini operation, 43
"Bell-clapper" deformity, 335
Bile duct. See also *Cystic duct; Hepatic duct.*
   anatomy of, 188–191
   anomalies of, 186–187, **188–189**
   atresia of, 193, **193**
   distal subtotal pancreatectomy and, 134, **135–136**
   exposure of, 194–195
      hazards of, 195
   in gastrectomy, 115, **116,** 117
   lymph nodes of, 190–191, **190**
   length of, 190
   pancreatoduodenectomy and, 137, **141**
   portal vein branching and, 153
   stenosis of, 194
   supraduodenal, 188–191
   terminal, 191–193, **192**
Biliary apparatus, embryologic development of, 101, **102,**
      103
   intraperitoneal abscess and, 31, 31t
Billroth operations, 115, **116**
Bladder, abdominal hysterectomy and, 382, **383**
   agenesis of, 315
   anterior colporrhaphy and, **366,** 367–368, **367**
   arteries of, 321–323, **322–323**
      prostate and, 339, **340**
   "base plate" of, 321
   in children, **27,** 28, 316, **316**
   collecting vein of, 323
   congenital abnormalities of, 314–316
   diverticulum of, 315
      surgical approaches for, 325–326
   duplication of, 294, 315
   exstrophy of, 314–315, 336, **338**
   fascia of, 3, **6**
      in female, **357**
   functional mechanism of, 319–320, **320**
   fundus of, topography of, 316–317
   herniation of, 39–40, **41**
   hypoplasia of, 315
   innervation of, 324–325
      abdominoperineal resection and, 272
      congenital aganglionic megacolon and, 250

ischemic necrosis of, 61–62, 68
   ligament of, 322–323
      total cystectomy and, 326
   lower segment cesarean section and, 397–398,
      397–399
   lymphatics of, 324
   neck of, exposure of, 325
      stress incontinence and, 362–365, **364–365**
   pelvic exenteration and, 392–393
   pillars of, 316, **357**
      in anterior colporrhaphy, 367–368, **367**
      in Manchester-Fothergill operation, **369**
      in radical hysterectomy, **390**
      in vaginal hysterectomy, **384,** 385
   presacral neurectomy and, 375
   in radical hysterectomy, **390**
   resection of. See *Cystectomy.*
   in suprapubic prostatectomy, **341,** 342
   topography of, 316–317, **318**
   septum of, 315
   surgical approaches to, 17, 325–326. See also
      Cystectomy.
      plastic repair of, 325–326
   trigone of, 317, **318**
      carcinoma of, perineal prostatectomy and, 343,
         348–349
         total cystectomy for, 328
      lymphatics of, 324
      urachal cysts and, 315–316
      ureteral reflux and, 317, 319
      in vaginal hysterectomy, **384,** 385
   veins of, 323–324, **324**
Blood vessels. See *specific arteries and veins.*
Brandl's ring, 395
Broad ligament, anorectal carcinoma and, 271
   hysterectomy and, abdominal, 382, **383**
      vaginal, 385
   parametrial abscess and, 8–9, **8**
   structures within, **358**
Brödel's "white line," 302, **302**
Bronchial veins, portasystemic communications and, 203
Buck's fascia, urethral rupture and, 339
Bulbocavernosus muscle, **359**
   episiotomy and, 360
   vulvectomy and, 388
Bulbo-urethral veins, **336**
Bypass graft, for superior mesenteric artery embolism, 64,
   64

CALCULI, renal, 301, 303
   ureteral, 305
Calices, renal, 300–301, **300**
   nephrotomy incision and, 303
Calot's triangle, 187
Cancer. See *specific organs.*
Cantlie's interlobar line, 149, **150**
Capsular arteries, prostatic, 339, **340**
Carcinoma. See also *specific organs.*
   iliac lymphadenectomy and, 82
Cardia, 113, **114,** 119. See also *Stomach.*
Cardinal ligament, **358**
   hysterectomy and, abdominal, **383**
      radical, **390–391,** 392
      vaginal, **384,** 385
   uterine prolapse and, 364–365, 369, **369**
Caudate lobe, definition of, 150, **151,** 152, 152t
Cecum, colonoscopy of, 229, **230–231**
   intestinal graft and, 240

Extraperitoneal space of Retzius, 316
Exstrophy of bladder, 314–315, 336, **338**

Falciform ligament, liver lobulation and, 149–150
  umbilical venous catheterization and, 207–208
Fallopian tube. See *Uterine tube.*
Falx inguinalis, anatomy of, 37, **38**
  inguinal hernia repair and, 43, **49,** 51
Fascia. See also *specific names and organs.*
  abdominal wall, surgical approaches to, 3–7, **4–6**
  urethral rupture and, 338–339
Fascia of Gerota. See *Renal fascia.*
Fascia propria, in rectal resection, 271, **275**
Fat, retroperitoneal, 3, **6,** 7
Fecal continence. See *Continence.*
Femoral artery, in inguinal lymphadenectomy, **81,** 82
Femoral canal node, 386
  in inguinal lymphadenectomy, 82
  in radical hysterectomy, 391
  vulvectomy and, 388
Femoral circumflex arteries, as collaterals, 68
Femoral cutaneous nerve, course of, 375, **376,** 377
  in inguinal lymphadenectomy, 81–82, **81**
  pudendal neurectomy and, 375–378, **376, 378**
Femoral hernia. See *Hernia.*
Femoral nerve, inguinal ligament repair and, 43
  lumbar sympathectomy and, 93
Femoral ring, anatomy of, 37, **38**
Finney pyloroplasty, 118
Fissure(s), anal, 246
  of liver, **150,** 152–153
Fistula, anal, 252–254, **253–254**
Fold of Kohlrausch, 245
Foregut, definition of, 214
Fundus, gastric, 113, **114**
Fusion fascia, of mesentery, 215–216

Gallbladder, arteries of, 186, **188**
  cholecystectomy, 187–188, **188–189.** See also
    Cholecystectomy.
  congenital anomalies of, 186, **188–189**
  ducts of, 186
    anomalies of, 186, **188–189**
  hepatic ducts and, aberrant, 155
  lymphatics of, 186
  nerves of, 186
  in pancreatoduodenectomy, 137, 139, **140**
  right hepatic artery and, 155
  subcostal incision for, 10
  valves of Heister, 187–188
  veins of, 186
Ganglia, celiac. See *Celiac ganglia.*
  of lumbar sympathetic trunks, 92
Gastrectomy, for benign disease, 114–117, **115–118**
  complications of, 115, 117, **117–118**
  indications for, 114–115
  procedure for, 115, **116**
  for cancer, 119–122, **120–121**
    approaches to, 119
    extent of, 119–122, **120–121**
    lymphadenectomy with, 119–121
    reconstruction following, 119
  hepatic artery ligation and, 168
  middle colic artery injury and, 235
Gastric artery(ies), in bile duct exposure, 195
  in gastrectomy, for benign disease, 115, **116,** 117
    for cancer, 120

hepatic artery and, aberrant, 120
  left, gastropancreatic fold and, 166
    hepatic artery and, variations in, **167,** 168
    splenic artery and, 139
  in splenectomy, 143
  supramesocolic viscera and, vascular relationships,
    103–105, **104**
  vagotomy and, 108, **111**
Gastric nodes, liver and, 169
Gastric veins, course of, 200–201, **201**
  in distal splenorenal shunt, 206, **206**
Gastrocolic ligament, in distal subtotal pancreatectomy,
  135, 137
  in gastrectomy, **116**
  pancreas and, approaches to, 133
  splenic exposure and, 143
Gastroduodenal artery, in bile duct exposure, 195
  duodenal ulcer and, 115
  gastrectomy and, for cancer, 120, **121,** 122
  hepatic artery and, 166
  pancreas and, 125, **126, 128–130**
Gastroduodenal node, **190,** 191
Gastroduodenal rotation, 102–103
Gastroduodenostomy, for benign disease, 115
  pyloroplasty and, 118
Gastroepiploic artery(ies), in gastrectomy, 115, **116**
  pancreas and, 125, **126, 128, 130,** 133
  in splenectomy, 143
  supramesocolic viscera and, vascular relationships,
    103–105, **104**
Gastroepiploic veins, course of, 201–202, **201**
  in distal splenorenal shunt, 206, **206**
Gastroesophageal varices, coronary vein and, 201
  distal splenorenal shunt for, 206, **206**
Gastrohepatic ligament, 132–133
  in pancreatoduodenectomy, 139
Gastrojejunostomy, for benign disease, 115, **116**
  Roux loop formation, 239
Gastropancreatic folds, 166
Gastroschisis, 221
Gastrosplenic ligament, 143
Genital system. See also *specific organs and topics.*
  accessory suprarenal glands and, 283
  female, cancer of, operations for, 387–393, **388,**
    390–391
    cesarean section, 395–399, **396–399.** See also
      Cesarean section.
    episiotomy repair, 360, **361–362**
    hysterectomy, for benign disease, 380–385, **381,**
      383–384. See also *Hysterectomy.*
    lymphatics of, 386–387, **387**
    pelvic support, operations for deficiencies of, 365,
      367–370, **366–370.** See also *Cystocele;*
      Enterocele; Rectocele.
    structures creating, 355–356, **356–359**
    perineum, constituents of, 356–357, **359**
    postpartum displacements, 360, 362–365, **363.** See
      also *Cystocele; Enterocele; Rectocele.*
    sensory pathways of, 372–373, **373**
      denervation procedures, 373–378, **374, 376, 378**
    stress incontinence, 360, 362–365, **364–366**
  male, arteries to, **322,** 323
    lymphatic trunks, **79**
    organs of, 331–351. See also *specific organs.*
    veins of, 323, **324**
Genitofemoral nerve, in lumbar sympathectomy, 94
  in radical hysterectomy, **390**
Glans penis, **336**
Glisson's capsule, 174, **176**

Peritonitis, cesarean section and, 398
  intraperitoneal abscess and, 30–31
Peri-ureteral nodes, 324
Permeation, cancer spread and, 264
Peyer's patches, 228
Pfannensteil incision, 11
Phrenic artery(ies), splenic artery and, 139
  suprarenal arteries and, 283, **284**
  suprarenal gland exposure and, 286, **287**
  vertebral level of origin, 55, 56t
Phrenic nerves, liver and, 164, 169
Phrenic vein, hepatic vein and, 158
  suprarenal vein and, 285
Phrenicocolic ligament, 143
Pleura, anterior abdominal incisions and, 13–14
  retroperitoneal approaches and, 18–19, **18–19**
Plexus pelvicus, **90**
Plexus pudendus, **89**
Plicae transversales, 244
Polar artery, **141**
Polyps, rectal, 276
Polysplenia, 29, 145
Portacaval shunt, 203–204
Portal pedicle. See also *specific structures.*
  lymph nodes of, 190–191, **190**
  nerves of, 190
Portal sheath, 174, **176**
Portal vein. See also *Portal venous system.*
  bile duct and, 190
  branches of, intrahepatic, 150, 151, 153–154,
    153
  as collateral, 75
  in distal subtotal pancreatectomy, **135,** 137
  gallbladder and, 186
  in gastrectomy, **121,** 122
  hemorrhage of, 164
  hepatic artery and, 128, **130,** 166–168, **167**
  hilar relationships of, 177, **182**
  ligation of, 169
  lymph nodes of, 190–191
  pancreas and, 127, **127–128,** 130
  in portacaval shunt, 203–204
  in portal sheath, 174, 176, **176**
  umbilical venous catheterization and, 206–208,
    207
  variations of, 199–202, **200–201**
Portal venous system, 199–210. See also *Portal vein.*
  course and tributaries of, 199–202, **200–201**
  portasystemic communications and, 202–203
  portasystemic shunts, 203–205, **204–205**
  splenorenal shunt, distal, 206, **206**
  umbilical-portal catheterization, 206–208
  valves of, 202–203
Portasaphenous shunt, 208
Portasystemic communications, 202–203, **202**
  mesentery fixation and, 215
Posterior retroperitoneal abscess, 7–8
Postrenal cava, 72t
Pouch of Douglas, rectal prolapse and, 254, 256
Pre-aortic nervous plexus, presacral nerves and, 374
Prepuce, **336**
Prerenal cava, 72t
Presacral abscess, 251–252
Presacral nerves, 324, 374–375, **374**
  aortic exposure and, 60
Prevertebral fascia. See *Psoas fascia.*
Prevesical abscess, 7–8
Priapism, treatment of, 337
Primary retroperitoneal incision, 17

Processus vaginalis, inguinal hernia and, 38–39
  in neonate, 26
  testicular descent and, 331–332, **332**
Proctosigmoidectomy, perineal, 256, **256–257**
Prostate, arterial supply to, 339–340, **340**
  bladder relationship to, 317
  carcinoma of, bladder neck and, 326
    resections for, 343, **344–345,** 346, **346–349.** See
      also *Prostatectomy.*
    site of, 341
  collecting vein of, 323, **324**
  "false capsule" of, **340–341,** 341
  hyperplasia of, arterial supply and, 339–340, **340–341**
    resection for. See *Prostatectomy.*
    site of, **340–341,** 341
  lobulation of, 340–341
  lymphatics of, 324
  rectovesical abscess and, 8
  resection of, 339–349, **340–342, 344–349.** See also
    Prostatectomy.
  retroperitoneal approach, 17
  total cystectomy and, with lymphadenectomy,
    328
    without lymphadenectomy, 326, **327**
  veins of, 323, **324**
Prostatectomy. See also *Prostatovesiculectomy.*
  perineal, for benign disease, 343–344
    for malignancy, 343, **348–349**
  radical, 343, **344–345**
  retropubic, for benign disease, 341–342, **342**
    for malignancy, 343, **344–345**
  stress incontinence and, 321
  suprapubic, for benign disease, 341–342, **341**
    cystotomy and, 325
    for malignancy, 343
  transsacral, 346
  transurethral, for benign disease, 341
    for malignancy, 343
Prostatic artery, origin of, 65
Prostatitis, **318**
Prostatovesical venous plexus, 323
Prostatovesiculectomy, radical, 328, **348–349**
  retropubic, 343, **344–345**
Psoas abscess, 7–8
Psoas fascia, abdominal wall and, surgical approaches to, 3,
  6,
  in lumbar sympathectomy, 94
  psoas abscess and, 7–8
Psoas muscles, intraperitoneal spaces and, 29
  lumbar sympathetic trunks and, 92, 94
Pubic bones, bladder exposure and, 325, 339
  bladder exstrophy and, 314
Pubocervical fascia, in anterior colporrhaphy, 367–368,
  367
  stress incontinence and, of, 363
  in vaginal hysterectomy, 385
Pubocervical ligaments, 316, **357**
Pubococcygeus muscle, female, **356**
  episiotomy and, 360, **361–362**
  stress incontinence and, 320–321, 362
Puboprostatic ligaments, in prostatovesiculectomy, 343,
  344
  total cystectomy and, 326, **327**
Puborectalis sling, 243
  in congenital aganglionic megacolon, 251
  fecal continence and, 245, 247–248, 273
  in imperforate anus, 249–250, **249–250**
  rectal prolapse and, 255–256, **255**
Pubovesical ligaments, 316

Pudendal artery, accessory, 65, 336–337
  internal, bladder and, **322**, 323, **323**, 325
    intestinal blood supply and, **233**, 235
    origin of, 65, **67**
    perineum and, 356, **359**
    pudendal neurectomy and, 376–377
    uterine and vaginal blood supply, 380, 381
Pudendal canal, pudendal neurectomy and, 376–377
Pudendal nerve, **89**, 356, **359**
  anal sphincter innervation and, 246
  course of, 375–376, **376**
  female genitalia innervation and, 372
  perineal approach and, 21
  resection of, indications for, 373
    procedure for, 375–378, **376–378**
  urethra and, 325
Pudendal nodes, anorectal drainage and, 261, 264
Pudendal veins, bladder and, 323, **324**
Puestow procedure, 129
Pull-through technique, of rectal resection, 273–274, **274**
Pulmonary veins, portasystemic communications and, 203
Pyelotomy, 301
Pyloric canal, 113
Pyloric lymph nodes, 120
Pyloric vein, 113, **114**, 115, 201
Pyloroplasty, 118–119
Pylorus, 113, **114**
Pyramidalis muscle, **4**
Pyramids, renal, 300

Quadrate lobe, definition of, 150, 152, 152t
Quadratus lumborum muscle, 3, **6**
  psoas abscess and, 8

Rami communicantes, 86, 92
Rectal artery(ies), anterior anorectal resection and, 269–270
  collateral arteries and, 57, **57**, 238
  intestinal blood supply and, **233**, 234–236
  in radical hysterectomy, **391**
  in rectal prolapse repair, **255**
  origin of, 65, **67**
  sigmoid colon resection and, 268–269
Rectal crypt, abscess of, 252
Rectal fascia, in anterior perineal resection, 274, **275**
  in transsacral resection, **276**, 277
Rectal folds, 244–245, **252**
  anorectal lymphatic territories and, 261
  in anterior resection, 269–270, **270**
Rectal lymphatics, 78, **79**, 261
Rectal nerve, pudendal nerve and, **376**, 377
Rectal septum, in radical hysterectomy, **391**
Rectocele, 360, **363**
  colporrhaphy for, 365, 368, **368**
Rectosigmoid colon, colonoscopy of, **230–231**
  in imperforate anus, 250
  resection of, collaterals for, 238–239
    pull-through technique, 273–274
    transsacral, **276**
Rectourethral fistula, 248, 249, **249–250**
Rectourethralis muscle, 271
Rectouterine pouch, enterocele and, 360, 368
  rectal prolapse and, 254
Rectovaginal fistula, 248, 249, **249**
Rectovaginal septum, abdominal hysterectomy and, 382
  lymphatic drainage of, 264
Rectovesical abscess, 7–8, 31, **33**

Rectovesical pouch, abscess of, 7–8, 31, **33**
  level of, 245
  rectal prolapse and, 254, **255–256**, 256
  in transsacral resection, **276**
Rectovesical septum, in abdominoperineal resection, 271
  lymphatic drainage of, 264
  prostatectomy and, 343, 346, **346–347**
  rectal resection and, 274
Rectum. See also *Anorectum.*
  carcinoma of, extension of, **262–263**
    resection of. See *Rectum, resection.*
  colonoscopy of, **230–231**
  endometriosis of, 382
  fascia of, in female, **357**
  levator ani muscles and, in female, **356**
  lymphatic drainage of, 261, 263, 264
  posterior relationships of, **275–276**
  presacral neurectomy and, 375
  prolapse of, 254–257, **255–257**
    complete, definition of, 254
      treatment of, 255–257, **255–257**
    etiologic factors, 254–255
    incomplete, definition of, 254
      treatment of, 255
    pull-through technique for, 273
  resection of, for carcinoma, pull-through technique, 273–274, **274**
    sphincter-saving, 273–277, **274–276**
      anterior perineal approach, 273, 274, **275**, 276
      transsacral, 273, 276–277, **276**
      types of, 273
    urinary incontinence and, 321
  pelvic exenteration and, 392–393
  for prolapse, 256–257, **256–257**
  total cystectomy and, 328
  sphincter of. See *Sphincter.*
  topography of, 228
Rectus abdominus muscles, **4–5**
  anterolateral incision and, 9–11, **10–11**, 17
  bladder exposure and, 325
  in bladder exstrophy, 314
  hernia repair and, 43, **49**, 51
  subcostal incision and, **15**
  in suprarenal gland exposure, 285
Renal. See also *Kidney.*
Renal artery(ies), accessory, 56, 298
  collateral arteries for, 58, 298
  divisions of, extrarenal branches, **304–305**, 305
    variations in, 297–298
    interlobar branches, 297, **297**
    renal segmentation and, 295–298, **295–297**
  dual, 298
  exposure of, 60, 63
  multiple, 298
  pancreas and, relationship to, 128
  supernumerary, 298
  suprarenal arteries and, 283
  vertebral level of origin, 56t
Renal collar, 60, 72t, 299
Renal fascia, 3, **6**, 7
Renal pelvis. See *Kidney.*
Renal plexus, 86
Renal sinus, 301
Renal vein, 298–300, **299**
  aortic exposure and, 60
  as collateral, 75
  occlusion of, 299–300
  pancreas and, relationship to, 128, **129**
  portasystemic communications and, 203